W9-BOO-651

STUDY GUIDE

to accompany

EGAN'S
FUNDAMENTALS
OF
RESPIRATORY CARE

EGAN'S
FUNDAMENTALS
OF
RESPIRATORY CARE
EIGHTH EDITION

Stephen F. Wehrman, RRT, RPFT

Professor/Program Director

Respiratory Care Program

Kapi'olani Community College

University of Hawaii

Honolulu, Hawaii

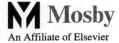 Mosby

An Affiliate of Elsevier

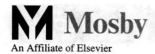

Mosby

An Affiliate of Elsevier

11830 Westline Industrial Drive
St. Louis, Missouri 63146

Study Guide to accompany Egan's Fundamentals of Respiratory Care   ISBN 0-323-02209-X
Copyright © 2003, Mosby, Inc. All rights reserved.

No part of this publication may be reproduced or transmitted in any form or by any means, electronic or mechanical, including photocopying, recording, or any information storage and retrieval system, without permission in writing from the publisher. Permissions may be sought directly from Elsevier's Health Sciences Rights Department in Philadelphia, PA, USA: phone: (+1) 215 238 7869, fax: (+1) 215 238 2239, e-mail: healthpermissions@elsevier.com. You may also complete your request on-live via the Elsevier Science homepage
(http://www.elsevier.com), by selecting 'Customer Support' and then 'Obtaining Permissions'.

Although for mechanical reasons all pages of this publication are perforated, only those pages imprinted with a Mosby, Inc. copyright notice are intended for removal.

Notice

Respiratory Care is an ever-changing field. Standard safety precautions must be followed, but as new research and clinical experience broaden our knowledge, changes in treatment and drug therapy may become necessary or appropriate. Readers are advised to check the most current product information provided by the manufacturer of each drug to be administered to verify the recommended dose, the method and duration of administration, and contraindications. It is the responsibility of the licensed prescriber, relying on experience and knowledge of the patient, to determine dosages and the best treatment for each individual patient. Neither the publisher nor the editor assumes any liability for any injury and/or damage to persons or property arising from this publication.

Previous edition copyrighted 1999

Acquisitions Editor: Mindy Copeland
Developmental Editor: Shelly Dixon
Publishing Services Manager: Pat Joiner
Project Manager: Karen M. Rehwinkel
Cover Design: Mark A. Oberkrom

Printed in the United States

Last digit is the print number: 9   8   7   6   5   4   3   2

This book is dedicated to my dad, Robert Wehrman,
who taught me how to think,
and my mom, Susan Wehrman,
who taught me that it is what you do with your mind that matters.

Eager for Egan!

> "The one real object of education is to get you in the condition of continually asking questions."
> **Bishop M. Creighton**

Dear Student:

The year was 1977. I had just started school to become a respiratory technician. My first textbook was *Egan's Fundamentals of Respiratory Therapy*. I have to confess, that I had to read everything three times to understand it. Egan really bent my brain out of shape! I was really glad to graduate and be done with the difficult task of understanding that book. When I began teaching, there was Egan waiting for me! A new edition and a new challenge. Twenty years, and four editions later, I finally began to apply myself to the problem! I knew that this was a good book, full of almost all the information my students would need to know as they prepared for this exciting career. But how was I going to get them to read it, use it, and make sense of the information?

My students gave me the answer! They said: "You know how to make it easy to understand. You know what to emphasize. Why don't you write us a guide...?" The rest is history. The problem for all students of health care is information overload. This is just as true for teachers as it is for anyone else. It is just as true for you as it was for me 25 years ago. This workbook will help you

learn and help you sort out some of the important information you will need to succeed in practice and to pass your board exams. If you want to get the most out of this book and the textbook, here's what you should do. First, read the assigned chapter in Egan. Read lightly, using a highlighter pen to mark important points that jump out at you. Next, open the workbook and Egan together. Complete the workbook as you review the material in Egan. I suggest you note the page numbers where you found the answers. I've been careful to look up those answers in the text, and have provided your instructors with a key. Sometimes you will come to problems where you have to really think or answer on your own. There are also experiments you can do at home or in the lab to help you understand.

At the end of each chapter you will find questions written in the same style the NBRC uses on the Entry-Level and Written Registry Examinations. You'll also find something new—internet tools. I use the internet all the time as I teach and you will find lots of great websites and references to help you in this endeavor. When you graduate and are preparing for your boards, you'll find *Egan's Fundamentals* and this workbook waiting to help you prepare.

Learning how to be a Respiratory Care Practitioner is a challenging, fun, difficult, and sometimes painful experience. Don't ever give up along the way. Your instructors, textbooks, and clinical faculty are all there to help you succeed. You've chosen a dynamic and exciting field that will always keep you on your toes!

Aloha,

Steve

P.S. I'd like to acknowledge some of the wonderful people who made this book possible. My wife Cathy, son James, and daughter Jessica who supported; colleagues Ken and Aaron who suggested; editors Mindy Copeland, Shelly Dixon, and Karen Rehwinkel; who encouraged; and most important of all, my students, who are always the best inspiration.

P.P.S. Want to talk? Your feedback, questions, or comments are welcome at **wehrman@hawaii.edu**

CONTENTS

CHAPTER 1

Quality and Evidence-Based Respiratory Care

> "Quality is never an accident.
> It is always the result
> of intelligent effort."
>
> **John Ruskin**

Everyone expects quality, from the goods we buy to the services we receive. Healthcare is no different. You want to work for a quality-oriented organization. You try to deliver quality care to your patients. Patients expect to be treated by qualified providers and to get the best care at all times. In Chapter 1 we look at what quality means in the healthcare setting and at specific ways we can monitor and achieve quality in the respiratory care profession. We'll also look at the trend toward using evidence-based methods for determining best practices in our profession.

► WORD WIZARD

Before you can understand quality care, you need to know the specific terms used to describe quality. Once you've read the first chapter of *Egan's*, try your hand at completing this crossword puzzle.

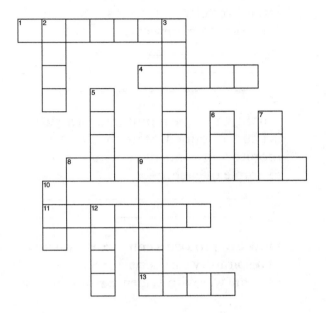

ACROSS

1. _____ director. The physician who helps manage your department
4. Body that reviews health care companies such as hospitals
8. Recognition
11. Characteristic reflecting excellence
13. Credentializing organization for respiratory care

DOWN

2. Original author of your textbook
3. Permission to practice
5. Someone like you...
6. Informal training in the workplace
7. Agency that regulates drugs
9. Therapist _____ protocols
10. Improvement that is ongoing in nature
12. College of chest doctors

Copyright © 2003, 1999 Mosby, Inc. All rights reserved.

► MEET THE OBJECTIVES

Chapter 1 presents five main objectives for learning. How well do you understand these important ideas about delivering the best care?

1. Providing quality care to the patient involves many dimensions. Name at least three elements that are part of quality respiratory care.
   A. _____
   B. _____
   C. _____

2. Quality must be monitored to assure it is being obtained. State the two basic monitoring strategies and give one example of each.
   A. _____
   B. _____

3. How can protocols enhance the quality of respiratory care services? Support your answer with evidence from the text.

4. What are the four essential components of a disease management program?
   A. _____
   B. _____
   C. _____
   D. _____

5. Evidence-based medicine specifies precise methods for analyzing data and making decisions. Give a brief explanation of the three main components of this process.
   A. _____
   B. _____
   C. _____

► CHAPTER HIGHLIGHTS

Fill in the blanks to identify eight key points from Chapter 1.

6. The _____ director is professionally responsible for the clinical function of the respiratory care department.

7. Ordering too many respiratory care services is called _____ and hinders delivery of quality care.

8. Specific guidelines for delivering appropriate respiratory care services are called _____ .

9. The _____ Respiratory Therapist is the highest credential in the profession.

10. Respiratory care credentialing examinations are administered by the _____ .

11. Personnel _____-_____ is the method most frequently cited as the optimal strategy for decreasing redundancy of patient care activities.

12. An ongoing form of quality assurance that puts emphasis on quality and cost-effectiveness is called _____ Quality _____ .

13. The two major forms of credentialing in health fields are state _____ and voluntary _____ .

► CASE STUDIES

Case 1

Mary Young, a 25-year-old woman, has returned to a medical/surgical nursing unit

Copyright © 2003, 1999 Mosby, Inc. All rights reserved.

after an appendectomy. She has no history of lung disease and is wearing a nasal cannula at 3 L/min. Ms. Young is alert and oriented with a respiratory rate of 18 breaths/min and a heart rate of 82 beats/min. Her SpO_2 (pulse oximeter reading) is 99% on the nasal cannula. Her physician orders "Respiratory Therapy Protocol," and you are asked to assess this patient.

▶ *Use the protocol on p. 10 in Egan's (Figure 1-2) to help you answer the following questions.*

14. What are the clinical signs of hypoxia and hypoxemia? Name at least three.
    A. _____
    B. _____
    C. _____

15. Using the oxygen therapy protocol, determine whether the oxygen therapy is appropriate for this patient. Support your answer with information from the textbook.

16. What action would you recommend at this time?

Case 2

Mr. Parker Day, a 54-year-old man with a history of asthma and cigarette smoking, was admitted to the hospital for a hernia repair. After the procedure, his chest radi-ograph shows elevated diaphragms with bilateral atelectasis. The pulse oximetry reading is 95% on room air. The heart rate is 84 beats/min; blood pressure, 110/78 mm Hg; respiratory rate, 20 breaths/min; and temperature, 36.8° C. Breath sounds are decreased bilaterally with apical wheezes. Mr. Day has a weak, nonproductive cough. He is alert and oriented.

17. Develop a specific respiratory care plan for this patient. Write your plan in the space below.

Respiratory care practitioners (RCPs) routinely plan, deliver, and assess the effects of care.

▶ **BOARD EXAM BUSINESS**

The National Board for Respiratory Care (NBRC) expects you to be able to participate in the development of care plans. You might expect to see five questions in this area on the Entry Level examination. The following questions are similar in style to the ones on the boards. If you're a beginner, you will need to look up the therapeutic interventions and disease management options in other parts of your text.

18. A patient with chronic obstructive pulmonary disease complains of difficulty breathing when he is walking. His SpO_2 is 88% at rest. Which of the following would you recommend?
    A. Oxygen therapy
    B. PEEP therapy
    C. Antibiotic therapy
    D. Aerosolized bronchodilator therapy

Copyright © 2003, 1999 Mosby, Inc. All rights reserved.

19. An alert 18-year-old patient is admitted with difficulty breathing. A diagnosis of asthma is determined, and you are asked to instruct the patient in the use of an MDI. An MDI is a device used for
    A. Oxygen therapy
    B. PEEP therapy
    C. Antibiotic therapy
    D. Aerosolized bronchodilator therapy

20. A patient with pneumonia is receiving oxygen via nasal cannula at 2 L/min. The SpO_2 is 89%. The heart rate is 110 beats/min, and the respiratory rate is 24 breaths/min. Which of the following would you recommend?
    A. Increase the liter flow to the cannula
    B. Intubate and begin mechanical ventilation
    C. Initiate aerosolized bronchodilator therapy
    D. Initiate postural drainage

21. Incentive breathing devices are primarily used in the treatment of
    A. Patients with emphysema
    B. Postoperative patients
    C. Patients with adult respiratory distress syndrome
    D. Patients with pulmonary fibrosis

▶ FOOD FOR THOUGHT

22. Protocol-based therapy and quality assurance efforts don't always work (seems amazing, I know). Discuss some of the reasons you think these two strategies might fail.

23. Respiratory care practitioners don't just work in acute care hospitals. They work in pulmonary labs, sleep labs, home care, skilled nursing facilities, and physician offices. What do you think might be different about delivery and assessment of quality care in these settings? What would be similar to acute care?

▶ INFORMATION AGE

Computers have become invaluable tools in the practice of respiratory care. The World Wide Web is a good place to search for current information. Keep in mind the rules for evaluating information found on the Web (see Chapter 6), because approximately 80% of this information is neither scientific nor educational in nature.

The Centre for Evidence-Based Medicine in Oxford, England, has a good website for this topic:
www.cebm.net

The best site for respiratory care protocols and clinical practice guidelines is the American Association for Respiratory Care (AARC).
www.aarc.org

You can link from this site to the national guideline clearinghouse:
www.guideline.gov/index.asp

Copyright © 2003, 1999 Mosby, Inc. All rights reserved.

Safety, Communication, and Recordkeeping

"Good communication is just as stimulating as black coffee, and just as hard to sleep after."
Anne Morrow Lindbergh

Safety first. How many times have we heard that one?

Say the right thing at the right time. How do you do that?

Nobody loves paperwork. The hospital environment is swimming in it.

Chapter 2 combines a huge amount of information that can be difficult to swallow all at once. I hope you don't choke! I'm going to break the material into bite-sized pieces, and you see if you can digest it. It's important.

▶ WORD POWER

Read Chapter 2 in your textbook to see if you can fill in the missing words.

You'll Get a Charge Out of This

The medical center is filled with electrical equipment. Everything has a three-pronged plug. The third prong is the neutral wire, or _____ , which helps prevent electrocution. For this reason, no outside electrical devices are allowed in the hospital unless they are checked out by the biomedical staff. Electrocution can occur in the form of a _____ shock. This might happen if you were standing on a wet floor, and a power cord fell onto the floor. Many power cords are detachable, so this is a potential hazard. Always clean up spills. A small shock, or _____ shock, is a hazard to patients who have pacemakers, ECG leads, and indwelling heart catheters.

A shock can result in ventricular _____ and death! This can happen if the ground wire breaks, so don't ever roll beds or other equipment over electrical power cords. Report frayed cords and take suspect equipment out of use.

Burn, Baby, Burn

Because high oxygen concentrations are used in respiratory care, fire is a real hazard.

Even though oxygen is _____ and does not burn, it greatly speeds up an existing fire. In fact, oxygen is necessary for fires to exist. For a fire to start, you also need _____ material and heat. Remove any of these three, and the fire will go out. You must make sure that ignition sources such as _____ are not allowed when oxygen is in use. Most hospitals will call a "Code Red" if a fire exists, and you must respond. One of the RCP's responsibilities in a fire is to shut off the zone valve to the affected area if the fire is near a patient using oxygen (see Chapter 34).

Copyright © 2003, 1999 Mosby, Inc. All rights reserved.

▶ KEEP IT MOVING!

Anyone who stays immobile in a bed for too long will suffer consequences. No couch potatoes allowed in the hospital! We need to ambulate patients as soon as their condition is stable.

Here are some guidelines for safe ambulation. Number them 1 through 7 in the correct order.

_____ Dangle the patient.
_____ Sit the patient up.
_____ Assist the patient to a standing position.
_____ Encourage slow, easy breathing.
_____ Lower the bed and lock the wheels.
_____ Move the IV pole close to the patient.
_____ Provide support while walking.

▶ I CAN'T HEAR YOU

Communication plays a big part in your ability to gain patient cooperation, evaluate progress, and make recommendations for care. What you do (nonverbal) is just as important as what you say (verbal). Communication also plays a role in your satisfaction on the job. Exchanging information and working out problems with other members of the healthcare team are an everyday part of hospital life.

▶ MEET THE OBJECTIVES

Chapter 2 presents 14 objectives for learning. We've already covered some of them. How well do you understand safety and communication?

1. Name at least three risks that are common among patients receiving respiratory care.
   A. _____
   B. _____
   C. _____

2. Describe one way to minimize risk for each of the three common hazard areas named in question 1.
   A. _____
   B. _____
   C. _____

3. What is the main reason you should use good body mechanics?

4. State at least two factors you should monitor during patient ambulation. (There are five total.)
   A. _____
   B. _____

5. Name at least four of the many factors that influence the communication process.
   A. _____
   B. _____
   C. _____
   D. _____

Copyright © 2003, 1999 Mosby, Inc. All rights reserved.

6. The text lists five ways to improve your effectiveness as a sender of messages. Describe two of these that apply to you. Give examples of situations in which you communicated well (or not).

7. Name four sources of conflict in healthcare organizations. Give an example of each.
   A. _____
   B. _____
   C. _____
   D. _____

8. What is a medical record? Who owns the record? Who is allowed to read it?

9. State one legal and one practical essential of recordkeeping.
   A. _____
   B. _____

10. One of the most common formats that RCPs (and others) use in charting is the SOAP format. What does SOAP mean (besides something you use in the shower)? Give examples of information you would chart for each category.

▶ **CHAPTER HIGHLIGHTS**

Fill in the blanks to identify eight key points from Chapter 2.

11. You should begin _____ as soon as a patient's condition is stable.

12. A _____ is a small current that enters the body through external catheters and can cause ventricular fibrillation.

13. Avoid electrical shocks by always _____ your equipment.

14. You can minimize fire hazards by removing flammable materials and ignition sources from areas where _____ is in use.

15. _____ skills play a key role in your ability to achieve desired patient outcome.

16. Accommodating, avoiding, collaborating, competing, and compromising are basic strategies for handling _____ .

Copyright © 2003, 1999 Mosby, Inc. All rights reserved.

17. A medical record is a _____ document.

18. You must _____ each treatment you provide.

► CASE STUDIES

Case 1

The physician orders ambulation for Mr. C. Lunger, who is wearing oxygen. The nurse asks you to assist. Mr. Lunger is wearing a nasal cannula running at 2 L/min. After 5 minutes of walking, you notice that the patient is breathing at a rate of 24 breaths/min and using his accessory muscles of ventilation. His skin appears sweaty, and he is exhaling through pursed lips.

19. What equipment will you need *before* you try to walk with this patient?

20. What observations are important to note in this situation? What action would you take?

Case 2

You are caring for a patient who is on a mechanical ventilator. You need to transport the patient to Radiology for a CT scan. The nurse unplugs the IV pump and pulse oximeter from the *back* of each unit. The pumps and the pulse oximeter are now run-

ning on their battery systems. As you prepare to leave, you notice the power cords are still plugged into the wall outlets. The doctor and the nurse are anxious to get the transport underway.

21. Describe the actions you would take if you were to encounter this situation.

22. What potential conflict and communication problems exist? How will you deal with them?

► BOARD EXAM BLUES

By now you should be asking the question, "Does any of this apply to my board examinations?" The answer is yes! The *CRT Content Outline*, distributed to exam candidates by the NBRC, states in the examination matrix: "In any patient care setting, the respiratory therapist communicates relevant information to members of the healthcare team." More specifically, you should be able to:

1. *Explain* therapy to patients in terms they can understand
2. *Document* a treatment correctly
3. *Note responses* to therapy, including vital signs, adverse reactions, and interpretation of subjective and attitudinal responses to therapy
4. *Verify computations* and correct errors

Copyright © 2003, 1999 Mosby, Inc. All rights reserved.

5. *Communicate clinical information* to other healthcare practitioners
6. *Communicate to avoid conflicts* and to maintain scheduling and sequencing of treatments
7. *Communicate results of therapy* and alter therapy according to protocols

Wow! The Board must really care about this stuff! You will probably see two or three questions on this specific material (more on this subject in Chapter 14). Try the following problems, in board exam style.

23. A respiratory care practitioner has completed SOAP charting in the progress notes after a bronchodilator treatment. While signing the chart form, she notices that the wrong amount for the medication has been entered. Which of the following actions should be taken?
    I. Draw one line through the error
    II. Notify the physician of the error
    III. Write "Error" and initial
    IV. Recopy the progress notes
    A. I only
    B. I and II only
    C. I and III only
    D. IV only

24. An asthmatic patient has orders for albuterol by medication nebulizer every 2 hours. During the shift the patient's condition improves, and the order is changed to every 4 hours. In regard to the new frequency, what action should you take?
    I. Note the new order in your charting
    II. Inform the nurse of the order
    III. Notify the respiratory care supervisor
    A. I only
    B. I and II only
    C. I and III only
    D. I, II, III

► FOOD FOR THOUGHT

The two cases are real. Every year people die in work-related fires and electrocutions. The hospital can be a busy, stressful environment, and it is easy to skip some of the steps in the safety process. That's one reason the Occupational Safety and Health Administration (OSHA) requires healthcare institutions to train workers in fire, electrical, blood-borne pathogen, back health, and other safety areas *every year*. We all know friends, patients, and coworkers who have been injured on the job. I hope you're not going to be one of them.

25. What do you think is the most common type of injury in healthcare?

26. On what shift do most injuries, accidents, and patient incidents occur?

► INFORMATION AGE

The World Wide Web contains a wealth of information on safety and legal issues in healthcare.

It might surprise you to know that the US Food and Drug Administration (FDA) has lots of information about safety as it relates to devices:
www.fda.gov

Copyright © 2003, 1999 Mosby, Inc. All rights reserved.

or more specifically you can look at MedWatch, which is the FDA safety information and adverse event reporting site:
www.fda.gov/medwatch/new.htm

The Howard Hughes Medical Institute offers free online safety courses on all kinds of topics:
www.practicingsafescience.org

Use any of the major search engines and you'll get hundreds more like these—anything from needle safety to healthy back practices. The Internet really sheds some light on the subject of medical safety!

Copyright © 2003, 1999 Mosby, Inc. All rights reserved.

Principles of Infection Control

**"The doctor is to be feared
more than the disease."**

Latin Proverb

No one comes to the hospital to get sick! But let's face it, 5% to 10% of all patients who enter a hospital contract an infection while they are there. To make matters worse, as many as 40% of these infections involve the respiratory system. It costs billions of dollars to manage hospital-acquired illness, and even more to pay for lost work time. Patients aren't the only ones who get sick. Each year, thousands of healthcare practitioners are exposed to diseases such as hepatitis, HIV, and tuberculosis, and some of them become infected. (Wow, I'm scaring myself!) Fortunately, there are plenty of simple, easy ways you can protect yourself and your patients. (Personally, I think the freeway is more dangerous than the hospital.)

▶ SLAM THE DOOR ON INFECTIONS

Chapter 3 introduces terms you should know if you want to be able to beat bacteria and viruses. After you read about this timely topic you will be able to solve this puzzle.

Copyright © 2003, 1999 Mosby, Inc. All rights reserved.

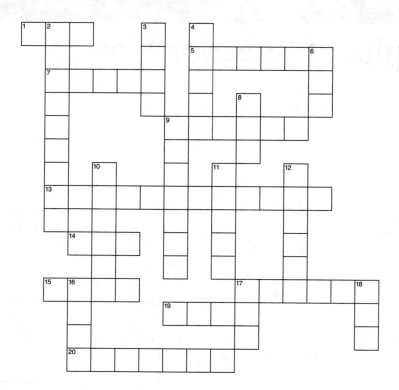

ACROSS

1. Drug resistant, abbrev.
5. Type of acid found in vinegar
7. Watch out or you'll get punctured by this
9. Mosquito, for example
13. Presence of microorganisms in a host
14. Type of plastic
15. Wear this around TB patients
17. Sodium hypochlorite
19. Safety agency
20. Most important and frequent route of transmission

DOWN

2. Clean
3. Type of filter
4. These nebulizers are culprits
6. Center that studies disease
8. Sterilizing gas
9. Water or food are examples of this route of transmission
10. Wear these around body fluids
11. Wash them like your mother told you!
12. Dirty surfaces or equipment
16. Respiratory professional group
17. Put dirty equipment in this before transporting
18. Humidifier that does not use water

► MEET THE OBJECTIVES

Chapter 3 presents 10 objectives for learning. We'll cover some of these later in this chapter. Because your board exams address this topic, let's find out how well you understand the principles of equipment disinfection and sterilization.

1. What is the first step in selecting a method for processing reusable equipment?

Copyright © 2003, 1999 Mosby, Inc. All rights reserved.

2. Describe the pasteurization process and give one limitation of this method of cleaning equipment.

3. Give an example of a high-level chemical disinfectant used in respiratory care. Describe a situation in which you would use this chemical.

4. State the six methods of sterilization. For each method, give an example of applicable equipment to be sterilized.

   Method   *Equipment*
   A. _____   _____
   B. _____   _____
   C. _____   _____
   D. _____   _____
   E. _____   _____
   F. _____   _____

5. State the two types of processing indicators used with sterilization. Give an example of each.

   Indicator   *Example*
   A. _____   _____
   B. _____   _____

6. List the three general barrier methods used to prevent exposure to organisms. Which one is considered the single best way to prevent the spread of infection?
   A. _____
   B. _____
   C. _____

► CHAPTER HIGHLIGHTS

Fill in the blanks to identify 10 key points from Chapter 3.

7. Between _____ and _____ of all nosocomial infections affect the respiratory system.

8. Intermediate-level disinfectants are best used on _____ .

9. _____ is the best choice for high-level disinfection of semicritical respiratory care equipment.

10. Among respiratory care equipment, _____ have the greatest potential to spread infection.

11. Always use _____ fluids for tracheal suctioning and to fill nebulizers and humidifiers.

12. Thoroughly _____ your _____ after any patient contact, even when gloves are used.

13. Use standard (universal) precautions in caring for _____ patients, regardless of their diagnosis or infection status.

14. Wear _____ and _____ during any procedure that can generate splashes or sprays of body fluids.

Copyright © 2003, 1999 Mosby, Inc. All rights reserved.

15. _____ items should be bagged before removal from a patient's room.

16. Exercise extreme caution when handling or disposing of all " _____ ."

► CASE STUDIES

Case 1

You work in the surgical ICU of a large urban hospital. Over the last 2 days, a number of patients in the unit have contracted serious *Staphylococcus aureus* infections.

17. Why are postoperative patients at increased risk of infection?

18. What is the most common source of *Staphylococcus aureus* organisms?

19. Identify three ways to disrupt the route of transmission in this situation.
    A. _____
    B. _____
    C. _____

Case 2

During your third day of clinical, you are assigned to accompany a therapist who has an extremely heavy workload on a medical floor of the hospital. The therapist puts on gloves for each patient contact and asks you to do so also. When you go to wash your hands after the first treatment, the therapist tells you, "We don't have time for that, and besides the gloves will keep our hands clean."

20. Explain the role of gloves in protecting practitioners and preventing the spread of infection.

21. What other concerns does this situation raise?

Case 3

A serious tuberculosis outbreak occurs in a local prison. You are called to the emergency department while four of the sickest patients are being admitted to your hospital for treatment.

22. By what route does tuberculosis spread?

Copyright © 2003, 1999 Mosby, Inc. All rights reserved.

23. When transporting these patients out of the emergency department, what action should you take?

24. What kind of precautions should be taken to prevent the spread of infection once these patients are admitted?

25. What special guidelines exist in regard to cough-inducing and aerosol-generating procedures for patients with active tuberculosis?

26. What other concerns do you have in working with these patients?

▶ WHAT DOES THE NBRC SAY?

You'd be right if you thought your board exams would place an emphasis on infection control. The *CRT Content Outline* for the Entry Level examination has this to say:

"In any patient care setting, the respiratory care practitioner . . . assures cleanliness of all equipment used in providing respiratory care." More specifically, you should:

1. Choose the correct method or agent for disinfection and sterilization
2. Perform disinfection and sterilization procedures
3. Monitor sterilization effectiveness
4. Protect the patient from nosocomial infection
5. Follow infection control policies and procedures

Here are some questions like the ones you might see on the board exam. I have put them in the form of a single case, but they will normally be spread throughout the exam. You can expect at least three questions on infection control on your Entry Level boards.

Questions 1 through 3 refer to the following situation:

Mrs. Ima Marsa is a 72-year-old patient with chronic obstructive pulmonary disease who has a tracheostomy tube after prolonged intubation and mechanical ventilation. She is currently in the medical intensive care unit. After you take her off the ventilator, you need to set up a heated aerosol system with an FIO_2 of 40%.

27. What type of water should be placed in the nebulizer?
    A. Distilled water
    B. Tap water
    C. Normal saline solution
    D. Sterile distilled water

Copyright © 2003, 1999 Mosby, Inc. All rights reserved.

28. To help lower the risk of a nosocomial infection when using heated aerosol systems, the RCP should do which of the following?
    I. Label the equipment with the date and time it is started
    II. Avoid draining condensate into the nebulizer
    III. Remove the capillary tube to reduce the volume of water particles
    IV. Use aseptic technique during the initial setup
    A. I and II only
    B. I, II, and III only
    C. I, III, and IV only
    D. I, II, III, and IV

29. The best way to prevent the spread of infection in the ICU is to:
    A. Ensure that sterilized equipment is used
    B. Wash your hands after every patient contact
    C. Wear gloves when you come in contact with body fluids
    D. Isolate infected patients

30. One of your fellow students comes to clinical with a cold. He asks you not to tell your clinical instructor, because missed clinical days are difficult to make up. What is your reaction to this situation? What are the potential problems with this scenario?

31. The college recommends that you be immunized against hepatitis B before attending clinical. The consent form lists a number of possible side effects of the vaccine, and the vaccination is expensive. What are the pros and cons of vaccines?

What will you choose?

▶ FOOD FOR THOUGHT

Because many hospitalized patients acquire respiratory infections, the RCP is really under a microscope at work. We have to maintain the highest standards of behavior to protect ourselves, our patients, and our loved ones.

▶ INFORMATION AGE

One truly great website can meet many of your needs in the infection control arena: **www.cdc.gov**

This is the site of the Centers for Disease Control and Prevention (CDC). It contains the most current guidelines for infection control in hospitals. You may be surprised to find that handwashing with soap and water is no longer considered the best method. The CDC recommends use of alcohol-based germicides. You will save time (as much as an hour per shift) and decrease the risk of spreading germs by

Copyright © 2003, 1999 Mosby, Inc. All rights reserved.

using these products. The CDC still recommends handwashing when you are grossly contaminated by blood or any other body fluids. You can find the new guidelines at: **www.cdc.gov/handhygiene**

NOTE: The current board exams still emphasize handwashing. We'll see if there are any changes when the NBRC releases the new exams.

Copyright © 2003, 1999 Mosby, Inc. All rights reserved.

Ethical and Legal Implications of Practice

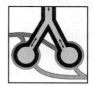

"Ignorance of the law excuses no one from practicing it."

A. Mizner

Malpractice. A word that strikes fear into the hearts of physicians. A word that could strike fear into your heart! Let's face it, we live in a society in which lawsuits are commonplace. You hear about them every day. Do RCPs ever get sued? You bet they do. To make matters worse, the etnical issues that are always present in healthcare are crossing into the legal arena more and more. Should we terminate life support? How can health services be rationed? What if the patient cannot afford the care? Your two safeguards are knowledge and good defensive record-keeping. Chapter 4 provides the tools you need to provide care with confidence.

▶ WORD POWER

Law, like medicine, has a language of its own that most people do not understand. (Shakespeare wrote, "It was Greek to me.") You will need clear comprehension of some basic legal terminology to avoid ending up in court.

The two basic types of law in the United States are public and civil. Public law is further divided into administrative law and _____ law. Healthcare facilities operate under a mountain of regulations set by government agencies. Private, or _____, law protects citizens who feel they have been harmed. The individual who brings a complaint is called the _____, and those accused of wrongdoing are known as _____. A _____ is a civil wrong. These cases can easily involve a healthcare practitioner. There are three types. _____ is failure to perform your duties competently. Cases in which the patient falls, is given the wrong medication, or is harmed by equipment revolve around a provider's duty to anticipate harm and prevent it from happening.

Expert testimony, professional guidelines, and even circumstantial evidence can determine what a reasonable and prudent RCP would do in a given situation. The Latin term _____ _____ _____ (the thing speaks for itself) is sometimes invoked to show that harm occurred because of inappropriate care. When a professional fails to act skillfully, breaches ethics, or falls below a reasonable standard, _____ has occurred. Wrongdoing may be considered intentional or unintentional. Intentional acts include _____, or placing another person in fear of bodily harm, _____, or physical contact without consent. Other common intentional harm occurs through _____, which is verbal defamation of character, and _____, which is written defamation of character. Finally, information

Copyright © 2003, 1999 Mosby, Inc. All rights reserved.

about patients is considered private, or _____, and cannot be shared with anyone who is not involved in their care.

There are two good defenses against all of these problems. The first is to show that actions were not intentional. For example, fainting during a procedure is not a voluntary act. The second defense is to obtain consent from the patient. Consent, whether oral or written, should be obtained from the patient for most procedures. Of course you have to explain the risks and the procedure in clear language the patient can understand.

► CASE STUDIES

Case 1

You get a chance to meet with your fellow students for lunch in the hospital cafeteria during a busy clinical day. One of your classmates is bursting with excitement as you sit down to eat. "You won't believe what I got to do today! I was taking care of Mr. Scanler in the ICU, and he started to go bad and we had to intubate. Then he coded, and I got to do CPR! It was so cool!"

1. What's the problem? What violation has your classmate committed?

2. What are the possible consequences of this scenario?

3. What action should you take?

Case 2

You receive an order to administer a bronchodilator to Daniel Rush, a 27-year-old asthmatic patient. Mr. Rush refuses the therapy, stating, "I just can't take any more of this today!" He appears alert and oriented.

4. Does the patient have a legal right to refuse in this case? Cite evidence from the text to justify your answer.

5. How would you respond to this situation?

6. What other action should you take at this time?

Copyright © 2003, 1999 Mosby, Inc. All rights reserved.

Case 3

After finishing with Mr. Rush, you receive a stat call to the orthopedic floor. The nurse informs you they are having problems with Marie Harme, a 76-year-old woman who recently underwent surgical repair of a broken hip. As you enter the room, you notice that Ms. Harme has removed her oxygen. She is breathing rapidly, and her color is not good. The pulse oximeter shows a saturation of 84%. When you try to get the patient to wear the oxygen, she screams at you to get out of the room.

7. Does the patient have a legal right to refuse in this case? Cite evidence from the text to justify your answer.

8. How would you respond to this situation?

9. Would physical restraints be an option or a possible case of battery?

▶ WHAT ABOUT ETHICS?

No, I haven't forgotten about ethics (Although this subject *is* less clear-cut than the legal implications.) The law sets minimum standards, which we all must try to follow. Ethics, on the other hand, is a set of guidelines for doing your job in a way that is morally defensible. The problem is not that there are a lot of people working in healthcare who are immoral but that there are ethical dilemmas that no one can avoid.

Start at the Beginning

The most famous ethical code in medicine is the Hippocratic oath. We RCPs have our own code of ethics that was developed by the AARC. You can find it on p. 72 in *Egan's*.

I am not going to discuss this subject much longer. It's not that ethical codes are bad. They seek to set general guidelines for behavior within a given professional group. What the codes don't do, however, is help with the really difficult decisions.

Do No Harm versus Save Lives

When two or more "right" choices are in direct conflict, an ethical dilemma exists. A hot topic in medicine and government right now involves how we end our lives, or "assisted suicide." On one hand, we don't want people to suffer needlessly. Watching a terminally ill patient suffer is a sad and demoralizing experience for RCPs. On the other hand, taking someone's life is an equally difficult decision with far-ranging consequences (some of which could be legal). Reducing these issues to simple rules and formulas is not easy, perhaps not even possible. Every ethical principle involves two parts: professional duty and patient rights.

Copyright © 2003, 1999 Mosby, Inc. All rights reserved.

► CASE STUDIES

Case 1

Oscar Mild, a 17-year-old boy, is admitted because of pneumonia. This young man is depressed and has expressed thoughts of ending his life if "my worst fears are true about this illness." Laboratory studies reveal that Mr. Mild is HIV positive. His physician expresses concern to the other caregivers about revealing Mr. Mild's diagnosis to him.

10. Under what circumstances can you lie (or not tell the truth) to patients?

11. What are your feelings about telling the truth to patients?

12. What would you do if Mr. Mild asked you if he has AIDS?

13. What is the problem or issue in this case?

14. Who are the individuals involved?

15. What ethical principles apply here?

16. Who should make the decision to tell Mr. Mild?

17. What is your role as an RCP who is giving this patient treatments?

Ethical Decision-Making Model

Let's apply the model to Case 1 in *Egan's* (p. 78, Box 4-2).

Copyright © 2003, 1999 Mosby, Inc. All rights reserved.

18. Are there short-term consequences to either decision? Long-term consequences?

19. Decide! (What would you do?)

20. How do you proceed after you make your choice?

22. Patients are allowed to refuse even life-sustaining treatment for religious reasons. What about professional caregivers?

23. What would you do if you were the supervisor?

> "I would rather be the man who bought the Brooklyn Bridge than the man who sold it."
>
> **Will Rogers**

Case 2

Johnny M, an RCP, is a deeply religious person who has strong feelings about homosexuality. When he is assigned to provide therapy to Oscar Mild, Johnny objects to the supervisor, saying, "I do not want to take care of him. It is against my religious principles. Assign someone else."

21. What are some of the possible problems for the Respiratory Department that could arise out of this situation?

► CHAPTER HIGHLIGHTS

Fill in the blanks to identify seven key points from Chapter 4.

24. Ethical _____ occur when there are two equally desirable or undesirable outcomes.

25. Professional codes of ethics are general guidelines to identify _____ behavior.

26. The two basic ethical theories are _____ and _____.

27. _____ law deals with the relationships between private parties and the government.

Copyright © 2003, 1999 Mosby, Inc. All rights reserved.

28. Professional _____ is negligence in which a professional has failed to provide the _____ expected, resulting in _____ to someone.

29. Practitioners must carry out their duties with an eye toward _____ themselves in the case of _____ action.

30. A _____ act defines who can perform specified duties in healthcare. The purpose of _____ is to provide for the public's safety.

▶ WHAT ABOUT THOSE BOARD EXAMS?

Sorry, but ethics and legal issues aren't really a part of your examinations to obtain a license to practice respiratory care. Considering the case of an RCP in California accused of so-called mercy killings, perhaps these areas should be on the test!

▶ FOOD FOR THOUGHT

When I go home from work, I usually feel pretty good about what I do for a living. Sometimes I have issues I need to work out.

31. When you have been involved in an ethical dilemma in which you felt the wrong choice was made, how do you resolve the way you feel afterward?

▶ INFORMATION AGE

The Karolinska Institute in Stockholm maintains a dynamite site: **www.mic.ki.se/ Diseases/k1.316.html**

This site is a storehouse of links to hundreds of others on almost every topic in medical ethics from biomedicine to malpractice. Probably the only site you'll need to find up-to-date information on ethics.

Copyright © 2003, 1999 Mosby, Inc. All rights reserved.

Fun with Physics!

> "I find that a great part of the information I have was acquired by looking up something and finding something else along the way."
>
> Franklin P. Adams

Physics is a subject that everyone (everyone normal, that is!) struggles to understand. The purpose of this chapter is to help you figure out what's important and how to apply the information. You don't have to be a rocket scientist to understand physical principles of respiratory care.

▶ UNLOCK YOUR BRAIN

Words are the keys that open your mind so you can start to learn a difficult subject. After you read *Egan's*, you will be able to put the right words into the blanks.

Yes, but It's a Dry Heat . . .

Without humidity, our airways become irritated, and mucus becomes thick and nasty. The actual amount, or weight, of water vapor in a gas is called _____ humidity. As RCPs, we compare the weight of water vapor with the amount it could hold if the gas were fully saturated. This ratio of content to capacity is known as _____ humidity. You hear about this on the weather report every day. I'm more interested in how much vapor gas can hold inside the airways. This amount is called percentage _____ humidity. When inspired gas has less than 100% of its capacity, a humidity _____ exists. Humidifiers are used to make up the difference. When you get a can of icy soda on a hot day, water droplets begin to form on the outside of the can. That's because the air around the can is cooling (cold air does not hold as much water vapor as warm air). When air cools, and gaseous water returns to a liquid form, we say that _____ has occurred. The opposite effect occurs when the drink sits out. Water molecules escape from the liquid into the air. This process is called _____ and adds to the humidity in the air.

Some Like It Hot . . .

Heat moves in mysterious ways—four of them, to be precise. Newborn infants are especially sensitive to heat loss. Keeping a preemie warm can make the difference between life and death. When babies are born, we dry them off to prevent loss through _____.

Then the little one is wrapped in cloth to prevent _____, or loss that occurs when you are touching a cooler object. Finally, we put the infant in an incubator. The incubator provides warmth in two ways. First, a special light _____ heat toward the baby. Second, warm air blows into the incubator. Transfer of heat

Copyright © 2003, 1999 Mosby, Inc. All rights reserved.

through movement of fluids (or gas) is called _____.

▶ *Now that you know some of the important terms, you need to...*

▶ OBEY THE LAWS

Remember the bumper sticker: "Gravity, it's not just a good idea, it's the law!"? Gases have to follow the laws of physics, too. Because RCPs work with different gases, such as oxygen, nitrogen, carbon dioxide, and helium, it's important that you know the laws and how gases behave. In this section, I'll give you examples of gas laws in action, and you tell me which law is being demonstrated.

Example 1

A registered pulmonary function technologist (RPFT) is performing lung testing on a patient. The patient inhales 1.5 L from the spirometer.

1. What will happen to the volume of gas inside the patient's lungs?

2. Gas law?_____

Example 2

A home care therapist places an oxygen cylinder in the van so that she can take it to a client's house. The sun is shining through the window on the cylinder.

3. What will happen to the pressure inside the cylinder as it becomes warmer?

4. Gas law?_____

Example 3

When you start to inhale, your diaphragm drops, and your chest expands. In other words, you increase the size, or volume, of your chest.

5. What happens to the pressure inside your chest?

6. Gas law?_____

▶ TRY IT, YOU'LL LIKE IT!

Here are some safe, easy experiments you can perform in the lab at school or at home.

Experiment 1

Place a dry, empty *glass* soda bottle in the freezer for at least 15 minutes. Take the bottle out, and *immediately* cover the mouth of the bottle with a balloon. Wait a few minutes and watch!

Copyright © 2003, 1999 Mosby, Inc. All rights reserved.

7. What happened to the balloon?

8. Which gas law is responsible for the result?

Experiment 2

Cut a 1-inch strip of notebook paper. Hold one end of the paper to your chin, just below your lip. Blow steadily across the top of the paper.

9. What happened to the paper?

10. What principle is responsible?

Another experiment that shows this same principle can be accomplished with balloons. Blow up two round balloons and tie them off. Attach approximately 1 foot of string to each balloon. Tape the string to a stick (such as a ruler or yardstick) so that the balloons are 6 to 8 inches apart. Blow between the balloons.

11. What happened to the balloons?

Experiment 3

Get a coffee stirrer, an ordinary straw, and a large straw (the kind you use for a milkshake). Now get a couple of cups. Put some water in one cup. Put some honey in the other. (I put a chocolate shake in a third cup!) Suck the water up through each straw. Now try the honey (and/or the shake). To make this more interesting, use a 6-foot length of oxygen-connection tubing. Try the two fluids again.

12. Which tube is easier to suck through?

13. Which fluids are easier to suck up?

14. Which hard to pronounce, French sounding law explains all this?

Copyright © 2003, 1999 Mosby, Inc. All rights reserved.

Because both gases and liquids are fluids, the same rules apply to the inhalation!

► CASE STUDIES

Case 1

A respiratory therapist decides to attend the AARC International Respiratory Congress. To get there, the therapist must travel by air. Before the plane takes off, the flight attendant explains about the oxygen system. The therapist pays attention (unlike everyone else) when he sees the partial rebreathing mask. He also knows that something interesting happens to oxygenation at 30,000 feet.

15. What are the barometric pressure (P_B) and the inspired partial pressure of oxygen (PIO_2) at this altitude?

    P_B _____

    PIO_2 _____

16. A properly fitting oxygen mask can deliver about 70% oxygen to passengers. What would be the PIO_2 with the mask?

17. What gas law did you use to make these conclusions?

Case 2

Respiratory care practitioners frequently draw arterial blood samples to measure the partial pressures of oxygen and carbon dioxide in the blood. Many patients have elevated or decreased body temperatures.

18. What effect does a fever have on these partial pressure readings?

19. A normal arterial carbon dioxide pressure ($PaCO_2$) is 40 torr (mm Hg) at a body temperature of 37° C. Estimate the new $PaCO_2$ for a body temperature of 40° C.

20. Why is temperature correction of arterial blood gas readings controversial?

► MATHEMAGIC

You must be able to perform calculations in the clinical setting and on board examinations. Chapter 5 gives several examples of problems found in both settings. Write the formula, then solve the following problems *without using a calculator*. (Because board examinations do not allow use of electronic

Copyright © 2003, 1999 Mosby, Inc. All rights reserved.

calculators, use a calculator only to check your work.) I always write the formula out first, then plug in the numbers to avoid mistakes, but then I am mathematically challenged. If you're good at it, just skip this step.

21. Convert 30° C to degrees Kelvin.
    Formula _____
    Solution _____
    Answer _____

22. Convert 68° F to degrees Celsius.
    Formula _____
    Solution _____
    Answer _____

23. Convert 40° C to degrees Fahrenheit.
    Formula _____
    Solution _____
    Answer _____

24. At body temperature, gas has a saturated capacity of approximately 44 mg of water vapor per liter. If a gas has an absolute humidity of 22 mg/L, what is the relative humidity?
    Formula _____
    Solution _____
    Answer _____

25. What is the humidity deficit in question 24?
    Formula _____
    Solution _____
    Answer _____

26. Convert a pressure reading of 10 mm Hg to cm H_2O.
    Formula _____
    Solution _____
    Answer _____

27. Convert a pressure reading of 10 cm H_2O) to kilopascals (kPa). *Hint:* It's all right to round the numbers.
    Formula _____
    Solution _____
    Answer _____

28. Air is normally approximately 21% oxygen. Calculate the partial pressure of oxygen in air (PIO_2) when the barometric pressure is 760 mm Hg.
    Formula _____
    Solution _____
    Answer _____

29. Now calculate the PIO_2 that would result with a barometric pressure of 500 mm Hg.
    Formula _____
    Solution _____
    Answer _____

▶ *Math may be difficult for some of us (like me). Getting good at it can make the difference between success and failure on the board exams.*

▶ INFORMATION AGE

Physical principles can be hard to grasp, because you can't always see them in action. Dozens of websites have been posted by science teachers to help students better understand gas laws and physics. Here's a good place to start: **dbhs.wvusd.k12.ca.us/ChemTeamIndex. html**

ChemTeam is a site for helping students learn chemistry and physics. Clicking on "Kinetic Molecular Theory & Gas Laws" will take you to a number of problems and examples.

Copyright © 2003, 1999 Mosby, Inc. All rights reserved.

Or you might try:
jersey.uoregon.edu/vlab/Piston

This one has a cool chamber in which you control the variables to perform gas law experiments. *Vlab* stands for *virtual laboratory*, and there are very clear instructions on how to work the experiments. Pretty good fun!

Copyright © 2003, 1999 Mosby, Inc. All rights reserved.

CHAPTER 6

The Computer is Your Friend

> "The real danger is not that computers will begin to think like humans, but that humans will begin to think like computers."
>
> **Sydney Harris**

Let's face it; we are living in the "Information Age." Microprocessor technology is part of everyday life, and healthcare practitioners use computers every day (I used a computer to write this workbook). If you can learn to use these tools effectively, you will be a more effective RCP. Will this give you more free time? Probably more free time to use the computer!

▶ KEYS TO THE HIGHWAY

Most of the words that describe computers aren't even in the dictionary yet. If you want to travel the information highway, you will need to be able to talk the talk. Let's get started with a few key terms.

▶ COMPUTERESE

The most common computers in use today are personal computers (PCs). Larger computers, called mainframes, are used (by big businesses such as colleges, medical centers, and the IRS) for large applications. Every computer needs _____ ware, such as the central processor, printer, keyboard, and mouse. You also need _____ ware, or programs that are sets of instructions that tell the computer what to do. Information from a computer can be stored on floppy _____, magnetic drives, tapes, or optical memory systems such as _____ -ROMs.

Talk to Me!

Computers can talk to each other through a local network inside the hospital, or they can go outside the institution. The global network of computer networks is called the _____. Your PC can talk to other computers via an analog to digital converter (what a mouthful!) designed to work with acoustic signals. This device can dial the phone and is called a _____.

▶ COMPUTERS IN HEALTHCARE

Clinicians use computers to help interpret data, reach a diagnosis, and automate certain aspects of patient care. Now you need to open your textbook and look up some information about this subject.

Copyright © 2003, 1999 Mosby, Inc. All rights reserved.

1. Give five examples of how a modern hospital information system (HIS) is used by the institution and health care providers.

   A. _____

   B. _____

   C. _____

   D. _____

   E. _____

2. State one example of how computers are used to aid in cardiopulmonary monitoring, and give one example for diagnostic testing.

   A. _____

   B. _____

3. Discuss the difference between open and closed-loop control systems.

4. List four examples of clinical areas in which an RCP might use computer-assisted data interpretation or diagnosis.

   A. _____
   _____

   B. _____
   _____

   C. _____
   _____

   D. _____
   _____

5. Identify the four main nontechnical issues related to the use of computers in healthcare. Explain why these issues are concerns.

   A. _____
   _____

   B. _____
   _____

   C. _____
   _____

   D. _____
   _____

► CASE STUDIES

Case 1

Mark D. Sade, a technical director for a respiratory department in a large urban medical center, knows that asthma mortality is on the rise. He wants to find information about patients admitted to the emergency department with asthma and what happened to them. Mark wants to develop a report on the subject to present to administration. He plans to develop an asthma education program that will require a budget for equipment, personal, and training materials.

6. What type of software program is most useful for gathering specific information on patient populations?

Copyright © 2003, 1999 Mosby, Inc. All rights reserved.

7. What program will Mark use to help prepare the budget for his project?

8. What kind of software will he use to prepare the written report for administration?

9. Students have to write reports, too. What specific program do you use for this task? What do you like about it? What are the limitations?

Case 2

A respiratory care student is asked by her instructor to locate the URL for the AARC so she can access information on clinical practice guidelines (CPGs).

10. What does the term URL mean?

11. What are the three major components of a URL?
    A. _____
    B. _____
    C. _____

12. Identify the three components of the URL for AARC.
    A. _____
    B. _____
    C. _____

13. What action can you take to avoid having to write down or remember the URL for sites you wish to revisit?

▶ PRACTICE MAKES PERFECT!

It isn't good enough to talk the talk. Now you have to walk the walk!

You will need a computer with access to the World Wide Web to practice some of the skills discussed in the text. Most colleges provide a free e-mail account for students and have computers with web access. If yours does not, you can try your local Internet cafe—a coffee shop with computers. Or go to the public library! (As a last resort, you might try a friend who has a computer.)

Activity 1: Information Search

14. Access an index. Yahoo is a popular Internet index (**www.yahoo.com**).

You will need a computer that has a Web browser such as Netscape Navigator or Microsoft Explorer to get started. After you open the browser, enter the Yahoo URL.

Copyright © 2003, 1999 Mosby, Inc. All rights reserved.

Select the heading "Health." Pick one of the topics that relates to Respiratory Care, and spend some time browsing.

15. Conduct a search. Start your browser and open "Net Search," or go directly to the AltaVista search engine (**www.altavista.digital.com**). Now you can enter a keyword or phrase to look for information on a specific topic. Initially, it is alright to use natural language such as "asthma causes," or "what causes asthma" as a keyword. You may find too much information and need to narrow your search. Table 6-2 on p. 130 in your text contains examples of Boolean operators, or special words used in searches. For example, try "asthma AND causes." When you find a site or article that looks worthwhile, bookmark the URL for future reference.

I use Google (**www.google.com**), now considered the top search engine, or Teoma (**www.teoma.com**), Google's main competitor. But watch out. Internet-savvy librarians estimate that 80% to 90% of all information on the Web is nonscientific and not educational!

Activity 2: Evaluate!

Not all the information on the Internet is reliable. You will have to sort through a lot of "junk science," amateur material, and sales and marketing to obtain worthwhile information. Once you have found a website that contains the information you want, you can test it!

▶ *Find a website now, and answer these simple questions:*

Site: _____

16. Is it clear who is sponsoring the page? Look at the URL. Does the address end in "edu" or "gov"? These sites tend to be more reliable than "com" URLs. In any case, it should be very clear who is sponsoring the page.

17. Can you verify the legitimacy of the sponsor? Look for a telephone number or address for more information, not just an e-mail address.

18. Is it clear who wrote the material? And are the author's qualifications evident?

19. Is the information free of spelling, grammar, and typographical errors?

Copyright © 2003, 1999 Mosby, Inc. All rights reserved.

20. Is the information free of advertising?

21. Are there dates on the page to indicate when the material was written or revised?

22. Is it clearly stated when data or statistical information was collected?

The more "Yes" answers you get, the more reliable the information! Refer to Box 6-1 on p. 131 for more information on evaluating websites.

Activity 3: Respiratory Care

23. In this exercise, you will locate a specific document from the AARC website. Open the AARC home page (**www.aarc.org**). Click on "Resources," and find the section titled "Clinical Practice Guidelines." Open the guideline on pulse oximetry. Print this guideline and use it as a study reference. Why? One reason is the reliability of this material. Another good reason is that the NBRC says in its newsletter: "CPGs are a valuable tool for preparing for board examinations." I believe

the AARC website is the single most useful World Wide Web resource for students and practitioners.

▶ FOOD FOR THOUGHT

It is easy to learn how to use the computer for more than just games. Besides those listed earlier, you may want to try these activities:

24. Locate the home page for your college.

25. If your program has a website, locate it and print the home page or find specific information from the page. If you don't have a page, find one from another program. These sites are easily accessed from the AARC website. (You can find my program at **www.kcc. hawaii.edu.** Click on "Programs" and then "Respiratory Care Practitioner.")

26. If you don't have a program website, design one as a class project. Ask your media or learning center to provide skills and access to the campus server. With the new software available, *anyone* can learn to make a website.

27. If your college offers e-mail accounts for students, get the entire class to sign-up. Create an address list for the class, and send messages via e-mail. Ask your instructors to e-mail assignments, the class syllabus, and so on. (Save the trees!)

28. Search any of the websites in Table 6-1 on p. 129 in the textbook. Find a specific article, protocol, practice guideline, or other information that can be linked to a class activity or a personal need. For example, the NBRC site contains information related to the board exams. The AARC site has journals,

Copyright © 2003, 1999 Mosby, Inc. All rights reserved.

protocols, and much more! You can use this site to help write a report or complete a journal assignment.

▶ A FINAL THOUGHT

Personal digital assistants (PDAs) are great tools for students and therapists alike. I have an inexpensive PDA (less than $100) that has the usual calendars, games, and phone book. I have added several *very useful* medical applications. All of them were free downloads! For example, I have a program that allows me to look up almost any drug and check doses, costs, and side effects. I have a blood gas calculator, Henderson-Hasselbach calculator, peak flow and pulmonary function test (PFT) norms, you name it. Most of my students buy PDAs because there is no better digital tool you can get. Fits in your lab coat pocket.

Copyright © 2003, 1999 Mosby, Inc. All rights reserved.

CHAPTER 7

The Respiratory System

> "Anatomy is destiny."
>> **Sigmund Freud**

Remember anatomy? It was one of those required courses, the one where you memorized a lot of body parts. It turns out that structure and function have a lot to do with each other. Anatomy even has clinical applications. In this chapter, we'll be trying to bring anatomy back to life (sounds like Dr. Frankenstein). Before we go there, I just want to check and see if you still remember some important terms that relate to the anatomy of the respiratory system.

Copyright © 2003, 1999 Mosby, Inc. All rights reserved.

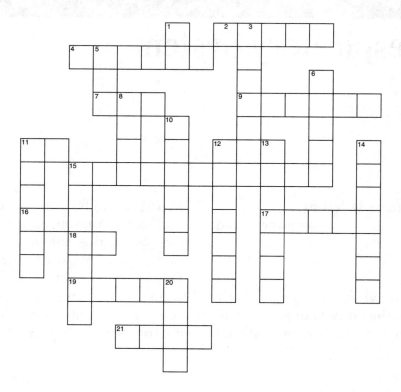

ACROSS

2. Pectoralis _____
4. Cells that produce mucus
7. Type of cells that make up the structure of the alveoli
9. Lining of the airways
11. Chemical name for carbon monoxide
15. Small airways without cartilage
16. Alveolar cells that make surfactant
17. Lobes in the right lung
18. Chemical name for nitric oxide
19. Point where airways and vessels enter the lung
21. Warms, filters, humidifies

DOWN

1. Chemical name for helium
3. _____ apple
5. Pertaining to the mouth
6. Primary anatomical divisions of the lungs
8. Pertaining to the nose
10. _____ abdominus
11. Pertaining to the ribs
12. At the end of the breastbone
13. Opening to the lower airway
14. Nerves to the diaphragm
15. Large airways
20. Cells that store histamine

► FETAL FACTS

Respiratory therapists take care of a wide range of patients from the tiniest preemie to elderly adults. That means you need to know about the ways in which lungs grow and develop.

1. During what stage and week of development is alveolar capillary surface area considered sufficient to support extrauterine life?
   A. Stage _____
   B. Week _____

Copyright © 2003, 1999 Mosby, Inc. All rights reserved.

2. What is the primary organ of gas exchange for the fetus?

3. Describe the umbilical cord blood vessels.

4. The fetus lives in a relatively hypoxic environment. What is considered a major factor that enables the fetus to survive under these conditions?

5. About half of the blood entering the right atrium is shunted to the left atrium through what structure?

6. Why is fetal pulmonary vascular resistance so high?

7. What percentage of blood entering the pulmonary artery actually flows through the lungs? Where does the rest of the blood go?

8. Describe the events that occur in the first few breaths after birth in terms of transpulmonary pressure, blood gases, and circulatory changes.

9. Compare the development of lung structures in newborns, children, and adults.

	New-born	Child	Adult
A. No. of alveoli	_____	_____	_____
B. Surface area	_____	_____	_____
C. Total lung capacity	_____	_____	_____

Copyright © 2003, 1999 Mosby, Inc. All rights reserved.

► THEY AREN'T JUST LITTLE ADULTS . . .

10. Let's compare the head and upper air-ways of adults and babies.

Anatomy	Baby	Adult
A. Head	_____	_____
B. Tongue	_____	_____
C. Nasal passages	_____	_____
D. Larynx	_____	_____
E. Narrow point	_____	_____
F. Dead space	_____	_____
G. Airways	_____	_____

11. Describe the breathing pattern of preterm infants.

12. Compare the metabolism of a healthy infant with that of an adult.

13. What are considered a normal tidal volume and respiratory rate for a newborn?

14. Why do infants experience severe hypoxemia more readily than adults do?

► A PICTURE IS WORTH A THOUSAND . . .

Rather than talk about adult anatomy, there's something else I want you to do. Identify the structures I've labeled in these figures.

Copyright © 2003, 1999 Mosby, Inc. All rights reserved.

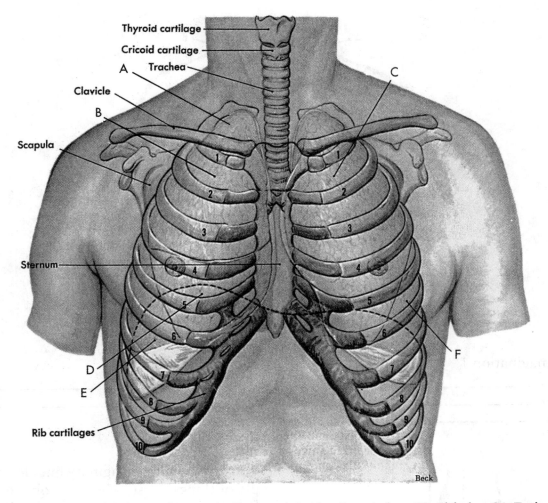

Thyroid cartilage
Cricoid cartilage
Trachea
A
Clavicle
B
Scapula
Sternum
D
E
Rib cartilages
C
F
Beck

Projection of the lungs and trachea in relation to the rib cage and clavicles. *(From Anthony CO, Thibodeau GA: Textbook of anatomy and physiology, ed 12, St Louis, 1987, Mosby.)*

15. Where are your lungs?

   A. _____
   B. _____
   C. _____
   D. _____
   E. _____
   F. _____

Pneumopnuggets

When you put your stethoscope just below the clavicle (in the front!) you are listening over the upper lobes. You can also see that the lower lobes aren't really on the front of the chest at all! They're a little on the side, but mostly in the back. If you know your locations, your auscultation improves. If you look at the location of the apexes, you will see they are *above* the clavicle! When someone inserts a subclavian line, the lung can be punctured in the process.

Copyright © 2003, 1999 Mosby, Inc. All rights reserved.

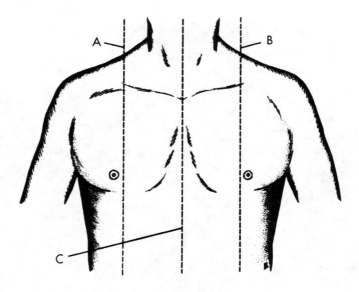

Imaginary lines on the anterior chest wall.

16. Imagination 1
    A. _____
    B. _____
    C. _____

17. Imagination 2
    A. _____
    B. _____

Pneumopnuggets

You can use these imaginary lines for a couple of things. First, when you obtain a 12-lead ECG for a patient, you use the lines to line up the electrodes and to count ribs. The lines also are good if you notice something unusual (such as a scar or a lesion) and want to document its location.

Imaginary lines on the lateal chest wall.

Copyright © 2003, 1999 Mosby, Inc. All rights reserved.

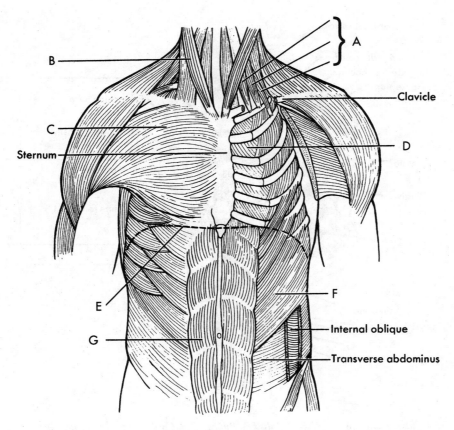

B

A

Clavicle

C

Sternum

D

E

F

Internal oblique

G

Transverse abdominus

The muscles of ventilation.

18. Pump me up

A. _____

B. _____

C. _____

D. _____

E. _____

F. _____

G. _____

Pneumopnuggets

Watch closely when someone breathes. Start with someone healthy, such as a child.

See the belly move out on inspiration. That's diaphragmatic breathing. See the relaxed exhalation. That's normal. A good place to see people breathe incorrectly (besides the hospital) is a shopping mall. Many people use their accessory muscles to breathe. The chest, especially the upper chest, moves on inspiration, but there is no outward excursion of the abdomen. When you experience distress, or exercise really hard, you will see the abdominal muscle group come into play to force exhalation. Sharpen your assessment skills by watching the *anatomy* of breathing!

Copyright © 2003, 1999 Mosby, Inc. All rights reserved.

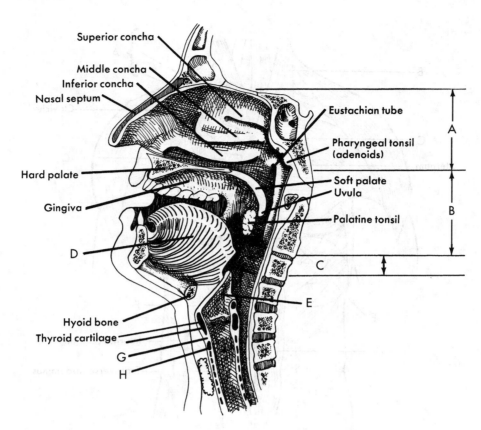

Structures of the upper airway and oral cavity. *(From Ellis PD, Billings DM: Cardiopulmonary resuscitation: Procedures for basic and advances life support, St Louis, 1980, Mosby.)*

19. What's up, doc?

A. _____
B. _____
C. _____
D. _____
E. _____
F. _____
G. _____
H. _____

Pneumopnuggets

Look at the nasopharynx. You'll be sticking tubes in there. It's fun if you know your anatomy. Notice that the nasopharynx goes straight back a short distance then drops down into the oropharynx. When you insert a catheter or airway, don't go straight back (very far), aim downward. Stay in the midline along the septum, or you'll ram the turbinates. In this cross-sectional view, it's easy to see how that big fat tongue could block the airway if it were to fall back.

Copyright © 2003, 1999 Mosby, Inc. All rights reserved.

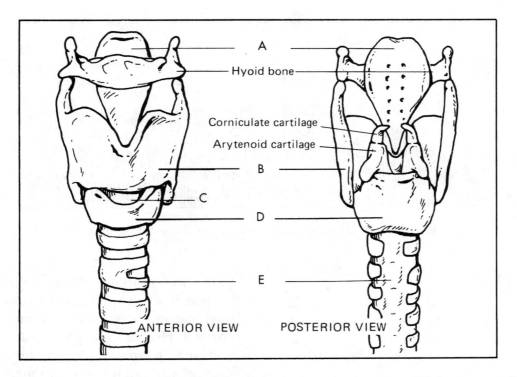

Anterior and posterior views of the laryngeal cartilages and trachea. *(From Martin DE, Youtsey JW: Respiratory anatomy and physiology, St Louis, 1988, Mosby.)*

20. "Adam's apple"
    A. _____
    B. _____
    C. _____
    D. _____
    E. _____

Pneumopnuggets

The thyroid cartilage sticks out on guys. So find a guy, and go for the throat. Palpate the thyroid cartilage. Feel the front and the sides. Now move your finger down (just a little) from the big bump on the front. Feel the soft spot? That's the cricothyroid membrane. (You may learn how to do a cricothryotomy in school.) The cartilage just below that is the cricoid, the only complete ring of the trachea. Keep going and feel the rings of the trachea. Gently (!) grasp the entire box in your fingers and wiggle back and forth. It's supposed to be mobile! Now ask your victim, I mean friend, to swallow while you keep your fingers on the thyroid cartilage. What happens?

Copyright © 2003, 1999 Mosby, Inc. All rights reserved.

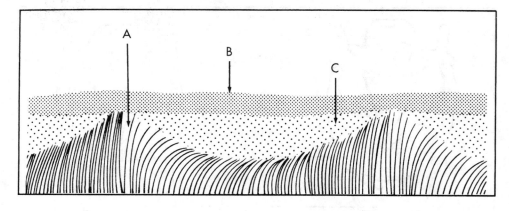

(From Martin DE, Youtsey JW: Respiratory anatomy and physiology, St Louis, 1988, Mosby.)

21. See cilia
    A. _____
    B. _____
    C. _____

Pneumopnuggets

Your airway makes more than 100 mL of mucus every day.

Where does it all go? Without good ciliary function where would it go? Drugs (such as those in cigarette smoke) can impair ciliary function. Hot or toxic gases (such as those produced in smoking) can destroy cilia. Diseases also can involve the cilia.

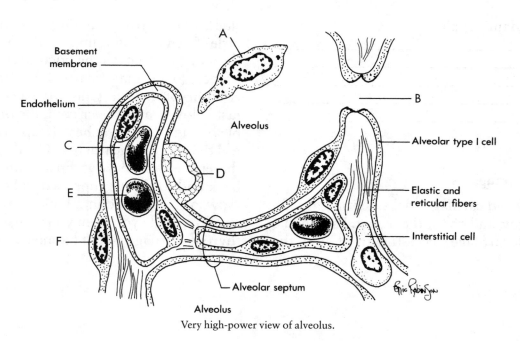

Very high-power view of alveolus.

22. You can call me Al
    A. _____
    B. _____
    C. _____
    D. _____
    E. _____
    F. _____

Copyright © 2003, 1999 Mosby, Inc. All rights reserved.

Pneumopnuggets

These buggers are small! The distance from alveoli to blood is only approximately 0.2 μm. (Remember, there are 1000 micrometers in a millimeter.) Oxygen has less than 1 second to cross this distance and combine with the red blood cells. So anything, such as the fluid from pulmonary edema, that increases this distance impairs gas exchange.

There are approximately 300 million alveoli in an adult lung. If you were to flatten them out, the area would be the size of a tennis court. (A pretty delicate one.)

▶ LOBES AND SEGMENTS

Students are always dismayed when they have to learn postural drainage and find out the lungs have 5 different lobes and 18 individual segments. It's not so hard when you know there are some duplicates and break the whole thing down into little pieces. Fill in the chart below. You can make your own version and fill it in until you get them memorized. This will help you with postural drainage. Notice that the left lung has only 8 segments, even though they are numbered them 1 through 10. Refer to Table 7-6 for help.

Right Lung
Right Upper Lobe
1. _____
2. _____
3. _____

Right Middle Lobe
4. _____
5. _____

Right Lower Lobe
6. _____
7. _____
8. _____
9. _____
10. _____

Left Lung
Left Upper Lobe
Upper Portion
1 + 2. _____

3. _____

Lower Portion (Lingula)
4. _____
5. _____

Left Lower Lobe
6. _____
7 + 8. _____

9. _____
10. _____

▶ MEET THE OBJECTIVES

We've covered most of the material in Chapter 7. Here are a few more ideas that are important to know about the respiratory system.

23. Name the nerves that innervate the diaphragm, intercostal muscles, and larynx. State the origin of these nerves and describe what will happen if they are damaged.
    A. _____
    B. _____
    C. _____

Copyright © 2003, 1999 Mosby, Inc. All rights reserved.

24. List the four divisions of the upper air-way and describe their main functions.

Division	Function
A. _____	_____
	_____
B. _____	_____
	_____
C. _____	_____
	_____
D. _____	_____
	_____

25. Describe the pathway gas follows as it is conducted through the lower airway. Use Table 7-7 on p. 177 as a guide.

► CHAPTER HIGHLIGHTS

Fill in the blanks to identify eight key points from Chapter 7.

26. The _____ houses and protects the lungs.

27. The _____ is the primary muscle of ventilation.

28. The upper respiratory tract _____ and _____ inspired air and protects the lungs against _____ substances.

29. The lower respiratory tract _____ gases from the upper airway to the respiratory _____ of the lung.

30. The airways branch into _____, which are made up of _____ in both the left and right lungs.

31. The respiratory bronchioles and _____ provide a large _____ area that facilitates gas exchange.

32. Fetal _____ and _____ differ markedly from those functions in the postnatal period.

33. Closure of the _____ and ductus _____ are important events in the transition from intrauterine to extrauterine life.

► CASE STUDIES

Case 1

A cruel respiratory instructor forces the students to learn the anatomy of the lung. Completely by coincidence, the instructor slips while running with scissors, and the sharp shears puncture the right side of his chest. The students gather around their fallen facilitator to discuss the anatomical consequences of this tragedy.

34. What would happen to the lung on the affected side?

Copyright © 2003, 1999 Mosby, Inc. All rights reserved.

35. What would happen to the pleural space on the affected side?

36. What is this condition called?

37. What is the management of this condition?

39. What is OSA, and how is it managed?

40. What is the similarity between snorers and unconscious victims who need resuscitation?

41. How would you approach management of the airway of an unconscious person?

Case 2

An RCP is working the night shift at a large urban medical center. As she makes her rounds, she hears loud snoring coming from a patient's room. Even though snoring is a commonly heard sound at night, the RCP stops to investigate.

38. What anatomical change results in snoring?

▶ WHAT ABOUT THOSE BOARD EXAMS?

Respiratory anatomy is not on the boards, but the kinds of applications we've been using in this chapter are part of the test. For example, you'll probably see several questions about pneumothorax.

▶ FOOD FOR THOUGHT

I hope you had fun with your lungs. Lung function is pretty miraculous when you think about all the parts that have to be working together to make ventilation and respiration successful. What happens to these structures when disease is present?

Copyright © 2003, 1999 Mosby, Inc. All rights reserved.

42. What happens to the airways and alveoli when a patient is having an acute episode of asthma?

43. What changes occur in the airways and alveoli in emphysema?

▶ **INFORMATION AGE**

A quick search of the web produces more than 80,000 hits on "pulmonary anatomy." These range from simple overviews:
www.methodisthealth.com/pulmonary/ anatomy.htm

to more complex information from the excellent Virtual Hospital website:
www.vh.org/adult/provider/radiology/ LungAnatomy/RightLung/ RtLungSegAnat.html

While you're at the Virtual Hospital website take a look at all the resources offered. VH.org one of the sites on my top ten list.

Copyright © 2003, 1999 Mosby, Inc. All rights reserved.

The Cardiovascular System

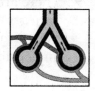

"We are all alike, on the inside."

Mark Twain

▶ THE HEARTBEAT OF AMERICA

Your heart beats, on average, about 38 million times in 1 year. (I wish I could get a fuel pump for my car that works that well.) No matter how well the respiratory system works to exchange gas with the blood, it would be meaningless without the heart's pushing that blood out to the organs via the vascular system. Those blood vessels are the best transportation network in the world, constantly reacting to the need for more or less flow of nutrients to the tissues.

▶ LANGUAGE OF THE HEART

Because cardiovascular function is closely connected to the respiratory system, you will meet up with it again and again in the course of your training. The words you learn today will help you throughout your career. Match the terms to the definitions listed below as they apply to respiratory care.

_____ 1. Afterload
_____ 2. Automaticity
_____ 3. Baroreceptors
_____ 4. Cardiac output
_____ 5. Chemoreceptors
_____ 6. Pericardium
_____ 7. Preload
_____ 8. Stenosis

A. Membranous sac that surrounds the heart
B. Stroke volume multiplied by heart rate
C. Ventricular stretch provided by end-diastolic volume
D. Biological sensors that monitor arterial blood pressure
E. Pathological narrowing or constriction
F. The force the ventricle pumps against
G. Biological sensors that monitor arterial blood oxygen
H. Ability to initiate a spontaneous electrical impulse

▶ MEET THE OBJECTIVES

Chapter 8 presents five objectives for learning. How well do you know your cardiovascular system?

Copyright © 2003, 1999 Mosby, Inc. All rights reserved.

9. There are four valves in the heart. Patients commonly suffer disorders of the mitral valve. What is the effect of mitral stenosis on the lung?

10. Explain how specialized tissue allows the muscle cells in the ventricle to contract in a coordinated and efficient manner.

11. Compare and contrast local control of blood vessels with central control mechanisms.

12. Describe how the cardiovascular system responds to exercise and blood loss by balancing blood volume and vascular resistance.

13. Match the mechanical events to their corresponding electrical events in the normal cardiac cycle. (*Hint:* Take a look at Figure 8-14)

	Electrical Event	*Mechanical Event*
A.	_____	_____
B.	_____	_____
C.	_____	_____

▶ CHAPTER HIGHLIGHTS

Fill in the blanks to identify six key points from Chapter 8.

14. The _____ system consists of the heart and vascular network, which maintain _____ by regulating the distribution of blood flow in the body.

15. Cardiac _____ is primarily determined by preload, _____, contractility, and _____ _____.

16. Central control of the vascular system is primarily maintained by the _____ division of the _____ nervous system.

17. The heart and vascular systems ensure that tissues receive sufficient blood to meet their _____ needs.

18. Just as faucets control the flow of water into a sink, the _____ control blood flow into the capillaries.

19. Specialized myocardial tissue, such as the _____ fibers, conduct impulses rapidly to ensure synchronous contraction of the ventricles.

Copyright © 2003, 1999 Mosby, Inc. All rights reserved.

► CASE STUDIES

Case 1

Cora Sone, a 57-year-old patient, is admitted to the coronary care unit with a diagnosis of mitral stenosis. The patient is breathing rapidly and complains of shortness of breath. Her pulse oximetry readings reveal hypoxemia. Auscultation reveals inspiratory crackles in the posterior lower lobes.

20. What is mitral stenosis?

21. What mechanical events are occurring to cause pulmonary edema and stiffening of the lung tissue?

22. What action should the RCP take at this time?

Case 2

A respiratory care student is giving an aerosolized bronchodilator to Keith Kane, a 27-year-old patient with asthma. Breath sounds reveal bilateral wheezing. The pulse oximeter shows 98% saturation on room air. The student notices the heart rate rising from 82 to 98 beats/min during therapy.

23. What are the effects of sympathetic and parasympathetic stimulation on the sinus node in the heart?
    A. _____
    B. _____

24. Describe the two ways that drugs produce bronchodilation.
    A. _____
    B. _____

25. On the basis of this information, why would you expect increased heart rate to be a common side effect of drugs that cause bronchodilation? How much can the heart rate increase before you would consider terminating the treatment?

► WHAT DOES THE NBRC SAY?

Cardiac anatomy, like respiratory anatomy, does not have a particular place on the national exams. That doesn't mean it's not important. We use this material as a foundation for clinical applications such as hemodynamics and electrocardiography. Advanced Cardiac Life Support certification courses expect you to know cardiac concepts before you try to understand emergency cardiovascular pharmacology.

Copyright © 2003, 1999 Mosby, Inc. All rights reserved.

▶ FOOD FOR THOUGHT

26. What four mechanisms combine to aid in promoting venous return to the heart?
    A. _____
    B. _____
    C. _____
    D. _____

27. What is meant by the "thoracic pump"? What effect does positive pressure ventilation, such as intermittent positive pressure ventilation (IPPV), have on venous return to the chest?

▶ INFORMATION AGE

CTSnet.org is a site sponsored by the cardiac and thoracic surgical societies. It contains basic and in-depth information. As there are for pulmonary anatomy, there are tons of other websites on this topic. The Internet is a good place to look for specialized information on the heart and heart disease.

Copyright © 2003, 1999 Mosby, Inc. All rights reserved.

Ventilation

"Keep breathing."
Sophie Tucker

Chapter 9 is only 20 pages long. Twenty pages that are loaded with heavy-duty information. Our challenge is to sort out what is important to remember, learn the basic principles, and make the knowledge connect to what is clinically important. If you're like me, you'll have to read this chapter two or three times to get the big picture.

▶ FIRST THINGS FIRST

I want to start off by emphasizing the difference between ventilation and respiration.

Remember that the primary purpose of the lung is to supply the body with oxygen and remove wastes in the form of carbon dioxide (CO_2). _____ is the process of moving air in and out of the lungs. When CO_2 builds up in the body, the pH of blood decreases, and a state of _____ results. We can measure the amount of air that moves in and out with a device called a _____. The pressure changes in the chest are measured with a body box, or _____.

Finally the actual rate of air flow is measured with a _____. Much of respiratory care is aimed at reducing the _____ of breathing and restoring adequate ventilation. The process of _____, on the other hand, is the exchange of gas between blood and other tissues. This involves complex chemical and physiological events at the cellular level. We'll dive into this subject more in Chapter 10.

A number of factors affect our ability to move air in and out at a reasonable oxygen cost. These can be factors outside the chest such as _____, fluid buildup in the abdomen, which impairs diaphragmatic movement. Or they could be the result of spinal disorders such as _____, a twisted and curved spine, or _____ _____, a severe stiffening of the spine. Problems also arise inside the lung itself. Conditions such as pulmonary fibrosis make the lung stiffer, or less _____.

▶ PICTURE THIS . . .

Air moves in and out of the chest because of pressure gradients. Label the following diagram to help improve your understanding of these pressure changes. Write out the definition of each gradient.

Copyright © 2003, 1999 Mosby, Inc. All rights reserved.

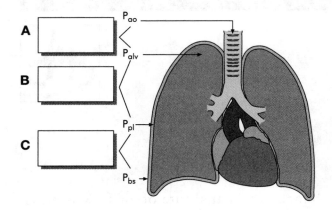

Pressures, volumes, and flows involved in ventilation. *(From Martin L: Pulmonary physiology in clinical practice: The essentials for patient care and evaluation, St Louis, 1987, Mosby.)*

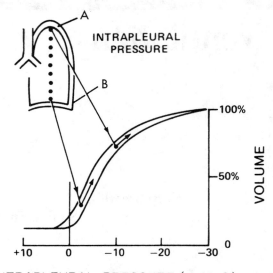

INTRAPLEURAL PRESSURE (cmH_2O)

Causes of regional differences in ventilation down the lung. *(From West JB: Respiratory physiology: The essentials, Baltimore, 1990, Williams & Wilkins.)*

1. Trans what?
   A. _____
      _____
   B. _____
      _____
   C. _____
      _____

2. Where has all the ventilation gone?
   A. _____
   B. _____

3. Where does the bulk of ventilation go during a normal breath in an upright person?

Pneumopnuggets

Our ability to generate the necessary pressure changes requires muscle power. Muscles need glucose, oxygen, and nerve innervation (among other things) to work properly. Any clinical condition that requires larger pressure gradients to move air (such as asthma) makes the muscles work harder. As when you work out, a pulmonary patient can experience muscle fatigue from increased work of breathing (WOB).

▶ MAY I HAVE ANOTHER ...?

Fill in the missing pressures for the apex and base of the lung.

Pneumopnuggets

You can use this information clinically. Patients with serious unilateral, or one-sided, lung disease (such as bad pneumonia) have poor ventilation on the affected side. Positioning the patient so the good lung is dependent preferentially increases ventilation in that lung and away from the bad lung. Remember: *Down with the good lung!*

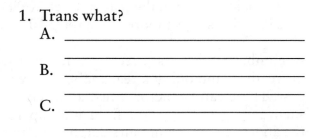

Copyright © 2003, 1999 Mosby, Inc. All rights reserved.

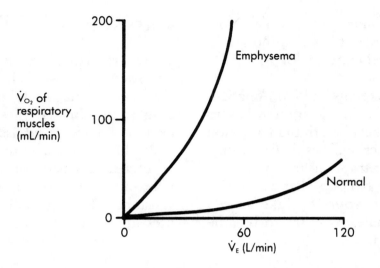

Relation of oxygen cost to expiratory minute ventilation for a healthy subject and for a patient with emphysema. *(From Slonim NB, Hamilton LH: Respiratory physiology, ed 5, St Louis, 1987, Mosby. After Churchill EJM, Westlake EK, Cherniack RM: J Appl Physiol 11:303, 1957.)*

► WORK OF BREATHING

It's time to talk about the bottom line. Work of breathing has a definite energy cost. We can measure the metabolic cost in terms of oxygen consumed, and we can reduce the work for patients through our interventions. A healthy person consumes approximately 250 mL of oxygen per minute. Only 5% of this oxygen is needed to power the muscles of ventilation. The cost increases approximately 1 mL for each liter of additional ventilation. Look at what happens to this cost when a patient has emphysema.

Four factors contribute to WOB: compliance, resistance, active exhalation, and breathing pattern. Let's look at each of these separately and talk about strategies for improvement.

► COMPLIANCE

Compliance is a measure of lung elasticity, or stretchability. It is defined as

Change in volume (liters) ÷ Change in pressure (cm H_2O)

A healthy lung is pretty stretchy, and compliance is 0.2 L for every cm H_2O of pressure generated.

However, the lungs sit inside the thorax, which has its own compliance. Completely coincidentally, the compliance of the chest wall also is 0.2 L/cm H_2O. You have to remember that the lung wants to recoil in and the chest wants to spring out, so they are pulling in opposite directions. Mathematically this is like a cancellation, so the net result is a compliance of 0.1 L/cm H_2O for healthy lungs in a healthy chest. However, if the lungs are overinflated or underinflated, the relation changes. You can understand this phenomenon by trying a simple experiment.

Experiment

Get an ordinary balloon. Blow it up a tiny bit. This is your underinflated lung. Blow it up some more. Hard to do, right? Now

Copyright © 2003, 1999 Mosby, Inc. All rights reserved.

blow it up some more. Pretty easy. Now inflate the balloon until it is almost full. Blow in some more! Hard to do!

Lungs are a little like this balloon. A patient who has a very low lung volume has to work harder to take a breath than a person with a normal functional residual capacity. A person with air trapping (as in emphysema) is like the balloon that is overinflated. *Try this for yourself:* Take a deep breath. Don't exhale. Now try to breathe in. You get the idea.

Bottom Line

You can move 500 mL of air with 5 cm H_2O pressure. Pretty good!

Questions

4. What interventions can we apply to the lung to increase the amount of residual air (and compliance) in a patient's lungs when the lungs are underinflated? (*Hint:* You won't find this one in Chapter 9. Try Chapter 36.)

5. What simple breathing techniques can we apply during exhalation to decrease the amount of residual air in a patient's lungs when the lungs are overinflated? (*Hint:* optimal breathing patterns for obstructive airway diseases)

▶ RESISTANCE

There are two kinds of resistance: tissue and frictional. Tissues have to move when the chest expands. Obesity (outside the lung) and fibrosis (inside the lung) are examples of increased tissue resistance. The really big problem is the frictional resistance created when you move air through your pipes (80% of all resistance). Airway resistance (Raw) is defined as the driving pressure it takes to create a flow of gas. Or to put it mathematically: Raw = Change in pressure (cm H_2O) ÷ Change in flow rate (L/min). Your upper airway causes most of this resistance. Normal value is 0.5 to 2.5 cm H_2O per liter per second of flow. Conditions such as asthma narrow the airways and greatly increase resistance. You can understand this with another simple experiment.

Experiment

Get a straw and a coffee stirrer (the hollow kind). Breathe in and out slowly through the stirrer. Now the straw. Which one is easier? Now try putting your lips together and sucking in the air really fast. Feel the work?

Bottom Line

The inner diameter of the airway determines the amount of resistance.

(Remember old what's his name's law?) If the bronchi decrease from 2 mm to 1 mm in diameter, the resistance increases *16 times!* Your muscles have to generate a much higher pressure to achieve ventilation if the airway is narrow.

Copyright © 2003, 1999 Mosby, Inc. All rights reserved.

Questions

6. What important changes occur in the airway of an asthmatic patient to increase resistance? (*Hint:* This one isn't in the chapter either! You'll have to look up the pathophysiology of asthma in Chapter 20.)

7. What kind of medications can RCPs use to reduce airway resistance in asthma?

► ACTIVE EXHALATION

Normal exhalation is passive. The power comes from energy you store by stretching the lung and chest during inspiration. When you actively exhale, you have to use your abdominal muscles and internal intercostals. Remember that additional muscle work takes additional energy. You can observe patients using their abdominal muscles when they are in distress and trying to get the air out quicker, or through narrowed airways. Try this for yourself.

Experiment

Place your hands on your belly. Breathe in. Exhale normally. Breathe in again. This time, push firmly in with your hands as you exhale. Air moves faster, right?

Release your hands, and breathe in again. This time, bear down with your abs and blow out hard and fast until your lungs are empty. Feels like work!

Bottom Line

Actively exhaling has a price. When patients do this, they are exercising or in distress.

Questions

8. What does it mean when you see active exhalation in your patient?

9. What happens to persons with spinal cord injuries who can't use their abdominal muscles? (*Hint:* What other important respiratory activity is performed with these muscles?)

► VENTILATORY PATTERN

The way you breathe can change the amount of work. In healthy people, a big, deep breath increases the elastic part of WOB. Fast breathing increases the frictional work.

Healthy people adjust their tidal volume and respiratory rate to minimize WOB during exercise. Our patients exhibit altered

Copyright © 2003, 1999 Mosby, Inc. All rights reserved.

patterns, too. Patients with fibrosis (loss of elasticity) breathe with a rapid, shallow pattern to reduce the mechanical work of distending the lung. Patients with obstructive diseases such as asthma and emphysema need to reduce their rate to reduce work, because they have increased frictional resistance.

Experiment

Tie something tightly around your upper chest. I use a bathrobe tie. The tie restricts chest movement. Try breathing faster with shallow breaths. Now try to breathe slowly and deeply. Which way feels better? Now, untie yourself and get out your straw or coffee stirrer. Breathe rapidly and shallowly through the tube. Now take slow, deep breaths. Which way feels better? (This is as close as I could get to simulating these two types of conditions.)

Bottom Line

You can learn a lot by observing someone's breathing pattern.

Questions

10. What is the optimal pattern of breathing for patients with obstructive airways diseases?

11. I don't have any more questions, do you?

▶ DEAD SPACE

My teachers in respiratory school always said I had cerebral dead space.

I guess they meant things went in and out of my brain without exchange of anything vital! Dead space is, plainly put, wasted ventilation. It is gas that does not participate in exchange with the blood. You normally waste the first third of each breath, or about 1 mL per pound of ideal body weight. Alveolar dead space occurs when gas enters the alveoli, but no blood comes to pick up the oxygen. A pulmonary embolus (e.g., blood clot, fat clot, air bubble) blocks blood flow to alveoli and causes an increase in dead space. Too much (50%-60% of each breath) dead space results in inability to maintain adequate ventilation through spontaneous breathing. The patient needs mechanical ventilation until the problem improves.

Copyright © 2003, 1999 Mosby, Inc. All rights reserved.

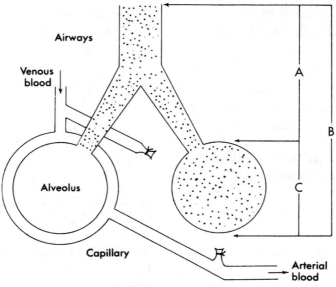

Three types of dead space.

► MAY I SEE A PICTURE PLEASE?

12. Label the types of dead space in this diagram.
    A. _____
    B. _____
    C. _____

Questions

13. What is the normal range for anatomic dead space?

14. What type of breathing pattern is seen with markedly increased dead space?

15. What is the difference between *hyperventilation* and *hyperpnea*?

► MATHEMAGIC

In Chapter 5, I mention that math is part of our board examination process and a clinical reality. Don't use a calculator to solve these problems!

16. Calculate exhaled minute ventilation for a patient who has a tidal volume of 800 mL and a frequency of 8 breaths/min.

    Formula _____
    Calculation _____
    Answer _____

Copyright © 2003, 1999 Mosby, Inc. All rights reserved.

17. Calculate anatomic dead space for a patient who is 6 feet tall and weighs 180 pounds.

Formula _____
Calculation _____
Answer _____

18. Calculate alveolar minute ventilation using the data from Questions 1 and 2.

Formula _____
Calculation _____
Answer _____

▶ WHAT ABOUT THOSE BOARD EXAMS?

The NBRC (and everyone else) expects you to be able to calculate exhaled minute volume and alveolar minute volume and to apply the information. Here's a sample.

19. The minute ventilation for a 68-kg (150 lb) patient who has a respiratory rate of 12 breaths/min and a tidal volume of 600 mL would be
    A. 4800 mL
    B. 5400 mL
    C. 6000 mL
    D. 7200 mL

20. The estimated alveolar minute ventilation for an 82-kg (180 lb) patient who has a respiratory rate of 10 breaths/min and a tidal volume of 500 mL would be
    A. 3200 mL
    B. 3500 mL
    C. 4800 mL
    D. 5000 mL

21. Which of the following ventilator settings would provide the optimal alveolar ventilation?

	Rate	Volume
A.	10	600
B.	12	500
C.	15	400
D.	20	300

▶ INFORMATION AGE

Strangely enough, **training.seer.cancer.gov** has a dynamic section on anatomy and physiology of the entire body. Included in the respiratory system pages, **training.seer.cancer.gov/module_anatomy/unit9_1_resp_intro.html,** is an entire section on mechanics of ventilation as well as lots of other goodies. Of course you can use this site to look at any body system or to learn more about cancer. Pretty nifty!

Copyright © 2003, 1999 Mosby, Inc. All rights reserved.

Gas Exchange and Transport

"To Air is human, to Respire divine."
Paul Thackara, RRT

In Chapter 10 we're going to go for it and jump in the deep end (of physiology, that is). I know you'll find this challenging at first, but when you have mastered the basics of gas transport; you're going to feel exhilarated! It's going to feel great to get a grasp of how gas exchange works and how respiratory care practitioners apply physiology to patient care.

▶ ALL ABOARD

Let's get on the hemoglobin-oxygen train and take a little ride. First you're going to learn the different names for all those forms hemoglobin (Hb) takes when it combines. It's natural for this complex molecule to want to be in a relationship. Hemoglobin meets oxygen (O_2). When they get together, the new name is _____. Their newfound affinity is likely to end when they meet up with the _____ effect at the tissue level. So, hemoglobin takes up with CO_2 and we get _____. The fickle heme drops off CO_2 at the lung when they run into the _____ effect. Life can go on like this, unless our conjugated protein meets up with a really unusual gas such as carbon monoxide (CO). This combination is called _____ and really lasts because hemoglobin's affinity for CO is _____ times greater than its affinity for O_2.

▶ WHY BE NORMAL?

Not all hemoglobins are created equal. Some are downright unnatural. Abnormal hemoglobins are given letter designations. Hemoglobin S, whose common name is _____ _____ hemoglobin, not only carries on poorly with O_2 but also can cause red blood cells to deform and clump together into thrombi. Babies are born with hemoglobin _____, which causes a _____ shift of the curve and makes babies more prone to cyanosis. Sometimes heme is altered in other ways. When the iron compound is oxidized, we get _____, which causes the blood to turn a brownish color. Nitrite poisoning can cause this transformation of our gas-loving protein.

▶ OXYGEN TRANSPORT

You Can Call Me Al

Before O_2 can go to the tissues, it has to get into the alveoli. There is a useful formula for calculating the partial pressure of O_2 (P_{AO_2}) in those little grape-like clusters. True, this equation has never won any popularity contests with students, but it is clinically useful (and can show up on those board exams). So, put on your thinking

Copyright © 2003, 1999 Mosby, Inc. All rights reserved.

caps, and we'll show 'em who's in charge here! The fancy formula looks like this:

$$P_{AO_2} = F_{IO_2} (P_B - P_{H_2O}) - P_{aCO_2} \left(F_{IO_2} + \frac{1 - F_{IO_2}}{R} \right)$$

We usually simplify this to read:

$$P_{AO_2} = F_{IO_2} (P_B - 47) - P_{aCO_2}/0.8$$

Or in English . . .

The partial pressure of O_2 in the alveoli is equal to the inspired O_2 percentage times the barometric pressure minus water vapor pressure.

Why? Dalton's law gives us the first part (Partial pressure = Concentration × Total pressure). Because water vapor in the lung acts as a gas, it takes up space. That's space O_2 can't occupy.

Next: Subtract arterial CO_2 times a factor.

Why? What we want to know is how much CO_2 is in the alveoli (CO_2 takes up space, too.) Hard to measure. *Solution:* Use a converted arterial value in its place. You don't really need to do this when the patient is breathing a high F_{IO_2}, such as 60% or more.

At this point my students usually ask

Who Cares?

All of this sounds like pulmonary laboratory stuff, except for the fact that we can find out how *efficiently* the lungs transfer O_2 into the blood by comparing *alveolar P_{O_2} to arterial P_{O_2}!* This relation is called the *A – a gradient.* A normal A – a gradient is about 5 to 10 mm Hg on room air, or about 10%.

▶ **MATHEMAGIC**

1. Calculate alveolar O_2 tension for a person breathing room air. Assume that barometric pressure is 760 mm Hg, F_{IO_2} is 21%, and P_{aCO_2} is 40 mm Hg.

Formula _____
Solution _____
Answer _____

2. If the patient in problem 1 has an arterial P_{O_2} of 90 mm Hg, what is the A – a gradient?

Formula _____
Solution _____
Answer _____

3. Calculate alveolar O_2 tension for a person breathing 60% O_2 (P_B is 760 mm Hg, CO_2 40 mm Hg)

Formula _____
Solution _____
Answer _____

4. If the patient in problem 3 has an arterial P_{O_2} of 90 mm Hg, what is the A – a gradient?

Formula _____
Solution _____
Answer _____

Both patients have identical P_{aO_2} values of 90 mm Hg. If you only look at P_{O_2}, or look only at O_2 saturation, they would seem to be the same.

But: The A – a gradients are very different. The second patient is having serious problems getting O_2 from the lung into the blood. In fact, the patient breathing 60% O_2 should have a P_{aO_2} of 349 mm Hg ($P_{AO_2} - 10\%$).

Copyright © 2003, 1999 Mosby, Inc. All rights reserved.

"By the Pricking of My Thumbs..."

Everyone loves a good rule of thumb. If you're in a big hurry and don't have a calculator at the bedside, you can try this shortcut. To estimate alveolar P_{O_2} for a patient breathing room air, multiply F_{IO_2} by 5 ($5 \times 20 = 100$). For 40% or more, multiply by 6 ($40 \times 6 = 240$). *Remember,* this only works when the CO_2 value is normal. Besides, what RCP doesn't have a calculator at the bedside?

Barriers to Diffusion

5. Do not pass go until you pass through the three barriers to diffusion:
   A. _____
   B. _____
   C. _____

Pneumopnuggets

The partial pressure of a gas is the main driving force across the alveolar-capillary membrane. Respiratory care practitioners routinely increase the driving pressure of O_2 by increasing the P_{AO_2}. Carbon dioxide has a much lower driving pressure, but is about 20 times more soluble than O_2, so it has little difficulty in making the journey. In some cases time can limit diffusion because of increased blood flow. Fever and septic shock are clinical examples.

Let's Get Moving!

Once it gets into the blood, O_2 is transported in only two ways. First, it dissolves in the plasma. To calculate dissolved O_2, multiply P_{aO_2} by 0.003.

$$\text{Dissolved } O_2 = P_{aO_2} \times 0.003$$

Easy!

The second way that O_2 is transported is as oxyhemoglobin: 1.34 mL of O_2 binds to each gram of hemoglobin (per 100 mL of blood). If all hemoglobin carried O_2, this would be simple, but it doesn't. Remember the anatomic shunt? Hemoglobin saturation is usually less than 100%.

$$\text{Combined } O_2 = 1.34 \times Hb \times \% \text{ Saturation}$$

Put them together and what have you got?

$$O_2 \text{ Content} = P_{aO_2} \times .003 + 1.34 \times Hb \times \% \text{ Saturation}$$

▶ MATHEMAGIC

Not this again. *Au contraire,* my friends. Although computers in the hospital can calculate content for you, the NBRC thinks you should be able to do this yourself (and without a calculator!).

6. Calculate O_2 content for patient 1, who has a Hb of 15 g, S_{aO_2} of 97%, and P_{aO_2} of 100 mm Hg.

Formula _____
Solution _____
Answer _____

7. Calculate O_2 content for a patient 2, who has a Hb of 15 g, S_{aO_2} of 80%, and P_{aO_2} of 50 mm Hg.

Formula _____
Solution _____
Answer _____

8. Last one. Calculate O_2 content for patient 3, who has a Hb of 10 g, S_{aO_2} of 97%, and P_{aO_2} of 100 mm Hg.

Formula _____
Solution _____
Answer _____

Copyright © 2003, 1999 Mosby, Inc. All rights reserved.

Now compare the results. Patient 2 has pretty poor values, but a good hemoglobin. Patient 3 has good values, but a poor hemoglobin. Who has better oxygenation?

The Moral of the Story

Looking at pulse oximetry values or any other simple indices of oxygenation, such as PaO_2, doesn't tell the whole story. You *always* have to consider hemoglobin. A patient may need blood for management of poor O_2 content. Remember that there may be enough hemoglobin, but it may not be able to combine with O_2, as in carbon monoxide poisoning.

▶ THROW ME A CURVE

The last piece of the oxygenation puzzle (for now at least) is to look at the relation between O_2 and hemoglobin. This relation is described by the *oxyhemoglobin dissociation curve*. Look at the curve shown on p. 240 in Figure 10-9. The flat upper part of the curve means that you can have a large drop in PaO_2 and only get a small drop in saturation. In fact, PaO_2 can drop from 600 mm Hg to 60 mm Hg, and the saturation will only drop from 100% to 90%! The steep part of the curve is equally important, physiologically speaking. A small increase in PaO_2 gives you a large increase in saturation. If you increase the PaO_2 from 27 mm Hg to 60 mm Hg, the saturation will rise from 50% all the way to 90%. Normally, a given PaO_2 produces predictable hemoglobin saturation. Fill in the correct values for partial pressure of O_2 and saturation (with a normal pH) on the chart at right:

PaO_2	SaO_2
9. 40 mm Hg	_____
10. _____	_____
11. 60 mm Hg	_____
12. _____	97%

But the curve doesn't always stay in the same place!

Fill in the correct answers for how the curve will shift on the chart below:

Factor	*Shift*
13. Acidosis	_____
14. Hypothermia	_____
15. High 2,3-diphos-phoglycerate (2,3-DPG)	_____
16. Fever	_____
17. Hypercapnia	_____
18. Carboxyhemoglobin	_____

The shift of the curve to the right facilitates O_2 unloading to the tissues, but a given PaO_2 has a lower hemoglobin saturation. A left shift does the opposite.

▶ CARBON DIOXIDE TRANSPORT

Carbon dioxide is transported three ways in the blood. As does O_2, CO_2 dissolves right into the plasma. This factor is more important than dissolved O_2, because it transports a fair amount of CO_2. As is O_2, CO_2 is carried by hemoglobin. Unlike the amount of O_2, the amount of CO_2 is relatively small.

Copyright © 2003, 1999 Mosby, Inc. All rights reserved.

Most CO_2, approximately 80%, is transported in the form of bicarbonate. Sorry, no math problems for you to do right now. But do remember this equation:

$$CO_2 + H_2O = H_2CO_3 = HCO_3^- + H^+$$

This reaction is called *hydrolysis,* because it involves combining CO_2 with water. Carbonic acid is formed first, but it quickly ionizes into bicarbonate and hydrogen ions.

Remember, the reaction can move in both directions. Most hydrolysis occurs inside red blood cells because of the presence of an enzyme (carbonic anhydrase) that speeds up the reaction rate.

Carbon dioxide level is inversely proportional to alveolar ventilation. If you increase alveolar ventilation, CO_2 decreases. Normal Pa_{CO_2} is 35 to 45 mm Hg. A high CO_2 level means that the patient is not ventilating adequately. We draw arterial blood gases when we want to accurately assess ventilation. A high CO_2 in the blood indicates hypoventilation. Because CO_2 has an acidifying effect on the blood, the pH of the blood decreases when the CO_2 level rises. The normal lower limit of pH is 7.35. The normal upper limit is 7.45. Low values reflect acidosis, whereas increased pH represents an alkaline state.

► BAD GAS EXCHANGE

Oxygen delivery and CO_2 removal are where it's at, physiologically speaking. The following questions test your knowledge of the causes of poor gas exchange.

19. Inadequate delivery of O_2 to the tissues is known as _____.

20. _____ is the medical name for a low level of O_2 in the blood.

21. Physiologic _____ occurs when blood passes through areas of the lung that have no ventilation.

22. Ventilation-_____ imbalances are the most common cause of low blood O_2 in patients with lung disease.

23. Patients with pulmonary fibrosis have a _____ defect that results in low blood O_2 levels.

24. Low blood pressure results in _____ and poor tissue O_2 delivery.

25. Myocardial infarction is an example of _____, a localized reduction in blood flow to tissues that can result in tissue death.

26. Increased _____ space ventilation may result in increased levels of CO_2 in the blood.

27. Drug overdose may result in inadequate _____ ventilation due to central nervous system depression.

28. Patients with severe COPD are unable to maintain adequate ventilation because of ventilation-_____ imbalances.

► BOARD EXAMS

The NBRC thinks you should be good at assessing gas exchange and managing abnormalities. Here are some examples:

Copyright © 2003, 1999 Mosby, Inc. All rights reserved.

29. Blood gas analysis reveals the following results:

    pH   7.50
    Pa_{CO_2} 30 mm Hg
    Pa_{O_2} 110 mm Hg

    These data indicate the presence of
    A. Metabolic acidosis
    B. Acute hyperventilation
    C. Acute hypoventilation
    D. Chronic obstructive pulmonary disease

30. Calculate oxygen content for a patient with the following data:

    Hb   10g
    Pa_{O_2} 80 mm Hg
    Sa_{O_2} 95%

    A. 12.73 mL O_2/dL
    B. 12.97 mL O_2/dL
    C. 13.40 mL O_2/dL
    D. 13.64 mL O_2/dL

31. Calculate Pa_{O_2} for a patient with the following data:

    P_B 747 mm Hg
    F_{IO_2} .21
    Pa_{O_2} 95 mm Hg
    Pa_{CO_2} 40 mm Hg
    Sa_{O_2} 97%

    A. 97 mm Hg
    B. 103 mm Hg
    C. 107 mm Hg
    D. 117 mm Hg

▶ CASE STUDIES

Case 1

Kelsey O., a 29-year-old homemaker is brought to the emergency department after exposure to smoke during a house fire. She is breathing at a rate of 30 breaths/min. Her heart rate is 110 beats/min. Blood pressure is 160/110 mm Hg. She reports having a headache and nausea. The pulse oximeter is reading a saturation of 99%.

32. Why are pulse oximetry readings unreliable in this setting?

33. What is wrong with this patient?

34. What action would you take at this time?

Case 2

James Westbrake is brought back to the unit after major surgery for injuries sustained in a motorcycle accident. He has been given a massive blood transfusion to replace loss from both the trauma and the surgical procedure. The pulse oximeter is reading 96% on room air, but the nurse has requested that you evaluate because of the patient's clinical condition. You find him sitting up and breathing 32 times per minute. He has tachycardia and tachypnea and reports difficulty breathing. Breath sounds are clear on auscultation.

Copyright © 2003, 1999 Mosby, Inc. All rights reserved.

35. The patient's clinical signs are consistent with what gas exchange abnormality?

36. What is one of the potential problems with banked blood?

37. Name some of the other possible causes of Mr. Westgate's distress.

38. What diagnostic procedure could you recommend?

Case 3

Jeannie Corpus is admitted with a diagnosis of pneumonia. Arterial blood gas analysis reveals a pH of 7.55, Pa_{CO_2} of 25 mm Hg, Pa_{O_2} of 75 mm Hg, and an Sa_{O_2} of 94%. She reports feeling short of breath.

39. Interpret these blood gas values in terms of gas exchange.

40. What other laboratory information plays a key role in helping determine O_2 content?

41. What is absolute anemia, and how is it treated?

Case 4

Kim Yung has been brought by paramedics to the emergency department after an accidental overdose of narcotics at a party. Mr. Yung is unconscious and has a respiratory rate of 8 breaths/min. The pulse oximeter shows a saturation of 85%.

42. Why would CO_2 be elevated in this patient?

Copyright © 2003, 1999 Mosby, Inc. All rights reserved.

43. Why is the O_2 saturation so low?

▶ FOOD FOR THOUGHT

Is your brain full yet? Dysoxia is a form of hypoxia in which cells do not take up O_2 properly.

44. What is the classic example of dysoxia?

45. When does tissue O_2 consumption become dependent on O_2 delivery?

46. Why does lactic acid form when tissues are hypoxic?

▶ INFORMATION AGE

I got really excited when one of our paramedic students showed me this site on the oxyhemoglobin dissociation curve: **www.ventworld.com/resources/oxydisso/oxydisso.html**

This unique tool allows you to enter variables such as increased temperature or decreased CO_2 that will actually show you what happens to the dissociation curve. SUPER!

Of course this is only one of the fun and educational things at: **ventworld.com**

Ventworld claims to be the Internet's premier site on mechanical ventilation. It certainly has a wealth of information. It is sponsored by a corporation but has extensively used expert RCPs. Ventworld is a good example of an exception to our rule about being wary about .com sites on the Internet.

Copyright © 2003, 1999 Mosby, Inc. All rights reserved.

Fluids and Electrolytes

"I am a prohibitionist. What I propose to prohibit is the reckless use of water."
Bob Edwards

Imagine yourself swimming in a warm ocean lagoon. The salty water is filled with life. Currents move you, and waves propel you through this complex ecologic system. Now think about the inside of your body. Warm, wet, and filled with salts. An intricate environment in which life depends on the relationships of fluids and electrolytes. Chapter 11 reviews various types of solutions, the mechanisms that control fluid movement, acid-base basics, and the role of major electrolytes in body function.

▶ DROWNING IN WORDS

You'll need to have some new vocabulary to keep you afloat in the sea of salts and solutions. Looks like a crossword puzzle is needed here! See the puzzle on p. 72.

Copyright © 2003, 1999 Mosby, Inc. All rights reserved.

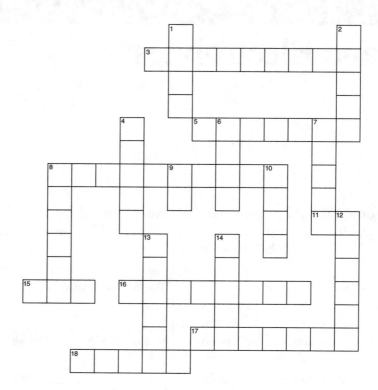

ACROSS

3. Solutions with maximum amount of solutes
5. Refers to potassium in the blood
8. Plasma is one example of this type of solution
11. Chemical name for calcium
15. Another name for colloid solution
16. Refers to sodium in the blood
17. Positively charged ions
18. _____ covalent solutions are produced by molecular compounds in water that produces ions

DOWN

1. Gives hydroxyl ions when placed in solution
2. Presence of abnormally large amount of fluid in the intercellular tissue space of the body
4. _____ tonic, a solution with more than 0.9% NaCl
6. Yields hydrogen ions when placed in solution
7. Electrovalent physiological solution
8. Substance dissolved in solvent
9. Chemical name for sodium
10. Table salt's chemical name
12. Negatively charged particles
13. Red bloods cells in _____, are an example of a suspension
14. Fluid in the interstitial spaces

▶ WATER, WATER EVERYWHERE . . .

The human body is mostly water. Water makes up as much as 80% of your weight. Because water is relatively heavy, the easiest way to track gain and loss is by weighing the patient. Clinicians also monitor intake and output (I and O) of water very closely.

Now you need to open your textbook and look up some information about this subject.

Copyright © 2003, 1999 Mosby, Inc. All rights reserved.

1. Rank the relative amount of water in the following persons. Put "1" by the group with the lowest amount of water and "5" by the group with the largest percentage of body water.

_____ Men
_____ Newborns
_____ Children
_____ Women
_____ Obese persons

2. Name the two major compartments for body distribution of water. List subdivisions and give the relative amount (%) of water in each area.

Compartment	%H₂0
A. _____	_____
B. _____	_____
1. _____	_____
2. _____	_____

► WHERE HAS ALL THE WATER GONE, LONG TIME PASSING . . .

A lot of water leaves your body every day through sensible and insensible losses. Give examples of these water losses and an average daily amount.

Source	Amount
3. Sensible	_____
A. _____	_____
B. _____	_____
C. _____	_____
4. Insensible	_____
A. _____	_____
B. _____	_____

You can also lose water through additive losses such as sweating, diarrhea, and vomiting.

5. Describe the loss of water that occurs through fever.

6. Lost water is regained through two primary sources. List these sources and give amounts.

Source	Amount
A. _____	_____
1. _____	_____
2. _____	_____
B. _____	_____

► ACID-BASE BASICS

If your body were a playground, acids and bases would be the seesaw ride! You don't have to be a chemistry major to play. Acids are substances that release H^+ when placed in a watery solution. Another definition is that acids are substances that are proton donors. Bases release hydroxyl ions (OH^-) or accept protons. Pure water is the reference point for determining acidity or alkalinity. Any solution with more H^+ than water is considered an acid. A solution with less H^+ is considered alkaline, or basic. A logarithmic scale, called the pH scale, is used to indicate the relative amount of acidity or alkalinity of a substance. Water is assigned a value of 7.0 on the pH scale. Because the scale is logarithmic, a substance with a pH of 6 is 10 times more acidic than water. The human body exists in a narrow range of pH values. Normally, our arterial blood has a pH of 7.35 to 7.45. A prolonged pH below 7.0 or above 7.60 usually is fatal! Chapter 12 gets into clinical applications and interpretations of acid-base balance.

Copyright © 2003, 1999 Mosby, Inc. All rights reserved.

► ELECTRIFYING INFORMATION

Electrolytes are chemicals that dissociate into ions when placed into solution, thus becoming capable of conducting electricity. Positively charged ions are called *cations,* and negative particles are called *anions.* Seven major electrolytes in the body are essential to life. Electrolytes are naturally regulated by the kidney (mostly) and can be manipulated by oral or intravenous intake in the healthcare setting. Let's see if you know your electrolytes.

7. List the seven major electrolytes and their primary purpose in the body.

Electrolyte	Symbol	Purpose
A. _____	_____	_____
B. _____	_____	_____
C. _____	_____	_____
D. _____	_____	_____
E. _____	_____	_____
F. _____	_____	_____
G. _____	_____	_____

You will also need to know the average normal plasma value for these electrolytes. Match the value to the chemical in the list below.

8. _____ Bicarbonate	A. 140 mEq/L
9. _____ Calcium	B. 24 mEq/L
10. _____ Chloride	C. 4.0 mEq/L
11. _____ Magnesium	D. 5.0 mEq/L
12. _____ Phosphorus	E. 100 mEq/L
13. _____ Potassium	F. 2.0 mEq/L
14. _____ Sodium	G. 140 mEq/L

Electrolytes are so important that a patient will exhibit some pretty interesting signs and symptoms if the levels of these powerful substances become too high or low.

Complete the chart below to match up disorders, causes, and symptoms of electrolyte disturbances.

	Imbalance	Cause	Symptom
15.	_____	Sweating	_____
16.	Hypo-kalemia	_____	_____
17.	_____	Star-vation	Diaphrag-matic weakness
18.	Hyper-calcemia	_____	_____
19.	_____	Chronic renal disease	_____

Notice the similarities in the symptoms of many of these imbalances. What's a clinician to do? When you see muscle weakness, abnormal fatigue, ECG disturbances, or metabolic acid-base disorders, *take a look at the electrolytes!*

► CASE STUDIES

Case 1

John Dough, a 68-year-old man with congestive heart failure (CHF), is being treated with a combination of diet and diuretics. Mr. Dough returns from a trip to New Orleans reporting difficulty breathing and swollen ankles. He is admitted to the coronary care unit for observation and treatment. Auscultation reveals bilateral inspiratory crackles in the lung bases. Respiratory frequency is 28 breaths/min. Heart rate is 110 beats/min with dysrythmias.

Copyright © 2003, 1999 Mosby, Inc. All rights reserved.

20. Patients with CHF usually are placed on what special type of diet? Why?

21. Diuretics commonly cause loss of what specific electrolyte that affects cardiac function? How will this electrolyte be replaced in the hospital? At home?

22. As an RCP, what action will you take to further assess cardiopulmonary status? What is likely to be your initial treatment of this patient?

23. What is the cause of this patient's crackles?

Case 2

Andy Wilson is a 68-year-old, homeless alcoholic man found in respiratory distress by the paramedics and brought to your emergency department. Mr. Wilson is mal-nourished. Auscultation reveals bilateral inspiratory crackles in the lung bases. Respiratory frequency is 28 breaths/min. Heart rate is 110 beats/min.

24. What protein accounts for the high osmotic pressure of plasma? Why is Mr. Wilson lacking in this substance?

25. Explain why this patient has crackles.

26. As an RCP, what action will you take to further assess cardiopulmonary status? What is likely to be your initial treatment of this patient?

▶ MATHEMAGIC

Respiratory care practitioners frequently work with weight/volume solutions and perform dilution calculations. Dilution calculations are used in drug preparation and in the pulmonary laboratory. You will be expected to perform some of these calculations on your board examinations. Remember, no calculators!

Copyright © 2003, 1999 Mosby, Inc. All rights reserved.

27. Albuterol is prepared in a 5% solution (weight/volume). How many grams of albuterol are dissolved in 100 mL to make this solution?

Formula _____
Solution _____
Answer _____

28. Respiratory care practitioners don't usually administer 100 mL of drugs to their patients. Instead, they give 1 mL or less. How many milligrams of albuterol would be present in 1 mL of the 5% solution in problem 20?

Formula _____
Solution _____
Answer _____

29. After drawing up 1 mL of a 5% solution of albuterol into a syringe, the RCP places the bronchodilator into a nebulizer along with 2 mL of saline solution for dilution. The total solution is now 3 mL in the nebulizer. What is the new concentration of the drug?

Formula _____
Solution _____
Answer _____

▶ WHAT ABOUT THOSE BOARD EXAMS?

The NBRC would give this chapter three gold stars for emphasis on important test material. Here are some sample questions in the same format as your tests.

30. A patient with severe hypokalemia is receiving an intravenous infusion of potassium to correct this serious disorder. What should you monitor?
    A. SpO_2
    B. Respiratory frequency
    C. Mental status
    D. ECG rhythm

31. Which of the following signs and symptoms would you expect to observe in a patient with hypokalemia?
    I. Metabolic acid-base disturbance
    II. Muscle twitching
    III. ECG abnormality
    A. I only
    B. I and II only
    C. I and III only
    D. I, II, and III

32. All of the following would be consistent with administration of a large amount of intravenous saline solution *except*:
    A. Increased pulmonary vascular markings on the chest radiograph
    B. Presence of crackles on auscultation
    C. Increased urine output
    D. Increased hematocrit

33. A respiratory care practitioner delivers isotonic saline solution to a patient through a nebulizer. What concentration of saline solution is the practitioner delivering?
    A. 0.0%
    B. 0.45%
    C. 0.90%
    D. 1.0%

▶ FOOD FOR THOUGHT

Administration of fluids with varying tonicities by both IV and aerosol routes is common.

Copyright © 2003, 1999 Mosby, Inc. All rights reserved.

34. What happens to cells in the presence of a hypertonic solution?

35. What happens to cells when a hypotonic solution is given?

36. What name is given to the movement of water across a semipermeable membrane?

▶ **INFORMATION AGE**

Here's a popular site that provides simple, understandable explanations of . . . everything:
www.howstuffworks.com

Copyright © 2003, 1999 Mosby, Inc. All rights reserved.

Acid-Base Balance

"The universe is full of magical
things patiently waiting for our wits
to grow sharper."

Eden Phillpots

If our bodies are factories that use oxygen and glucose to manufacture energy, then they are also producers of waste in the form of water, heat, and CO_2. An RCP must understand the roles of the lungs and the kidneys in removing waste, how buffering systems work, and how to interpret the results of ABG analysis. Drawing, analyzing, and, most of all, interpreting blood gas findings is one of the hallmarks of our profession. Learning this skill will require some memorization and lots of practice.

▶ INTERPRET WHAT?

There's no point in building your knowledge without a foundation. Before you can learn to use acid-base information clinically, you will have to know your terminology. Match the following terms to their definitions:

1. _____ Acidemia
2. _____ Volatile acid
3. _____ Anion gap
4. _____ Hyperventilation
5. _____ Metabolic acidosis
6. _____ Alkalemia
7. _____ Kussmaul's breathing
8. _____ Hypoventilation
9. _____ Fixed acid
10. _____ Respiratory alkalosis
11. _____ Metabolic alkalosis
12. _____ Standard bicarbonate
13. _____ Base excess
14. _____ Respiratory acidosis
15. _____ Buffer

A. Acid that can be excreted in gaseous form
B. Decreased H^+ concentration in the blood
C. Ventilation that results in decreased CO_2
D. Respiratory processes resulting in increased H^+
E. Acid excreted by the kidney
F. Abnormal ventilatory pattern in response to metabolic acidosis
G. Nonrespiratory processes resulting in decreased H^+
H. Difference between electrolyte concentrations
I. Respiratory processes resulting in decreased H^+
J. Increased H^+ concentration in the blood
K. Nonrespiratory processes resulting in increased H^+
L. Chemical substance that minimizes fluctuations in pH
M. Plasma concentration of HCO_3^- corrected to normal CO_2
N. Difference between normal and actual buffers available
O. Ventilation that results in increased CO_2

Copyright © 2003, 1999 Mosby, Inc. All rights reserved.

► **WHERE HAS ALL THE ACID GONE?**

I know I was surprised when I found out that the lungs excrete more acid each day than the kidneys do! Answer the following questions to find out if you understand the buffering process.

16. Draw a diagram of the process called isohydric buffering.

17. Explain how the lungs can compensate for increased production of fixed acids.

18. Buffers are composed of what two components?

19. What happens when you add the acid hydrogen chloride (HCl) to sodium bicarbonate ($NaHCO_3^-$)?

20. Describe the two general types of buffering systems in the body and give examples of each system and what they buffer in the body.

21. Does ventilation actually remove H^+ from the body? Support your answer with information from the text.

22. Why are buffers in the kidney essential for secretion of excess H^+?

► **BALANCING ACT**

When you're healthy, the lungs, kidney, and buffers work together to keep your pH normal so that enzyme systems can function and homeostasis is maintained. The system responds pretty rapidly to local or systemic changes. As long as the ratio of HCO_3^- buffer to dissolved CO_2 is 20:1, your pH will be about 7.40. A variety of conditions can cause the balance to shift. Increases in ventilation result in respiratory alkalosis. Increases in HCO_3^- (or other base buffers) result in metabolic alkalosis. These changes are referred to as *acute* if they take place

Copyright © 2003, 1999 Mosby, Inc. All rights reserved.

over a short time. If the changes become chronic, the body tries to compensate to bring the pH back to normal. Of course the respiratory system responds rapidly to metabolic disturbances, but the kidney takes time to adjust the HCO_3^-. Answer these questions to test your understanding of simple acid-base disturbances.

23. List the normal range of values for pH, $Paco_2$, and HCO_3^-. (You have to memorize these values!)

	Low Normal	High Normal
A. pH	_____	_____
B. $Paco_2$	_____	_____
C. HCO_3^-	_____	_____

24. Write out the Henderson-Hasselbach equation.

25. Complete the primary acid-base and compensation chart below.

Disorder	Primary Defect	Compen- sation
A. Respiratory acidosis	_____	_____
B. Respiratory alkalosis	_____	_____
C. Metabolic acidosis	_____	_____
D. Metabolic alkalosis	_____	_____

26. What is the rule of thumb for determining the expected increase in HCO_3^- for any acute increase in CO_2?

27. How much will HCO_3^- increase with a chronic increase in CO_2?

▶ A METHOD TO THE MADNESS

There is a simple four-step method for interpreting blood gas values.

▶ **Evaluate pH**
  1. >7.45 = Alkalosis
  2. <7.35 = Acidosis
  3. 7.35-7.45 = Normal (or fully compensated)

▶ **Evaluate respiratory status ($Paco_2$)**
  1. <35 = Alkalosis
  2. >45 = Acidosis

▶ **Evaluate metabolic status (HCO_3^-)**
  1. >26 = Alkalosis
  2. <22 = Acidosis

▶ **Evaluate compensation**
  1. Complete: pH is normal with abnormal CO_2 and HCO_3^-

Copyright © 2003, 1999 Mosby, Inc. All rights reserved.

(Even with complete compensation, pH tends to be on the side of the primary disorder, 7.40.)

2. Partial: pH is abnormal but not as much as expected

▶ TRY IT, YOU'LL LIKE IT!

Interpret the following blood gas results. I'll help you with the first one.

pH, 7.30; $Paco_2$, 60 mm Hg; HCO_3^-, 26 mEq/L

The pH is below 7.35, so the overall state is acidosis. The $Paco_2$ is above 45 mm Hg, which represents *acidosis*. The pH and the $Paco_2$ agree! We have *respiratory acidosis*. The HCO_3^- has risen 2 mEq/L above normal. This elevation is most likely due to the increased CO_2 (remember, bicarb goes up 1 unit for each 10–mm Hg acute increase in CO_2). So we have *acute (uncompensated) respiratory acidosis*.

Now it's your turn:

28. pH, 7.34; $Paco_2$, 60 mm Hg; HCO_3^-, 32 mEq/L

29. pH, 7.36; $Paco_2$, 60 mm Hg; HCO_3^-, 34 mEq/L

Stop right there! We're going to continue interpreting blood gas results in our case studies and board exam review questions.

▶ WELCOME TO THE GAP!

Metabolic acidosis can be life-threatening, so we need to try to establish the cause. One way to do this is through the history. For example, we know the patient took an aspirin overdose. Another method for determining the type of metabolic acidosis is by looking at the difference between positive and negative ions. Of course, you need the electrolyte values to do this calculation. Here's how you do it:

$$\text{Sodium (Na}^+) - \text{Chloride (Cl}^-) + \text{Bicarbonate (HCO}_3^-) \text{ or } 140 - (105 + 24) = 11$$

A normal range for the gap is 9 to 14 mEq/L. Potassium usually is ignored. When the body loses bicarb through diarrhea, chloride increases, and the gap stays normal. When bicarb is used to buffer excess fixed acids, the gap increases.

30. Name the three common causes of anion gap metabolic acidosis.
    A. _____
    B. _____
    C. _____

31. What are the signs of respiratory compensation for metabolic acidosis?

Copyright © 2003, 1999 Mosby, Inc. All rights reserved.

32. What are the neurological symptoms of severe acidosis?

▶ MATHEMAGIC

There are several math calculations in this chapter. You have to use a calculator to solve some of them.

Bicarbonate Blues

33. Calculate the new HCO_3^- level (assume 24 mEq/L as the starting point) for an acutely elevated $Paco_2$ of 50 mm Hg (assume it started at 40 mm Hg).

Formula _____
Solution _____
Answer _____

34. Calculate the new HCO_3^- level (assume 24 mEq/L as the starting point) for an acutely elevated $Paco_2$ of 70 mm Hg (assume it started at 40 mm Hg).

Formula _____
Solution _____
Answer _____

35. Calculate the new HCO_3^- level (assume 24 mEq/L as the starting point) for a chronically elevated $Paco_2$ of 70 mm Hg (assume it started at 40 mm Hg).

Formula _____
Solution _____
Answer _____

Hassle?

36. Calculate pH if HCO_3^- is 30 mEq/L and $Paco_2$ is 40 mmHg.

Formula _____
Solution _____
Answer _____

37. Calculate pH if HCO_3^- is 24 mEq/L and $Paco_2$ is 40 mmHg.

Formula _____
Solution _____
Answer _____

38. Calculate pH if HCO_3^- is 24 mEq/L and $Paco_2$ is 60 mmHg.

Formula _____
Solution _____
Answer _____

Gap?

39. Calculate anion gap if Na^+ is 144 mEq/L, Cl^- is 100 mEq/L, and HCO_3^- is 22 mEq/L.

Formula _____
Solution _____
Answer _____

Copyright © 2003, 1999 Mosby, Inc. All rights reserved.

40. Calculate anion gap if Na^+ is 135 mEq/L, Cl^- is 105 mEq/L, and HCO_3^- is 26 mEq/L.

Formula _____
Solution _____
Answer _____

► CASE STUDIES

The following case studies systematically take you through the major acid-base disorders. Let's start with some simple, acute states. Remember to evaluate using the four-step process.

Case 1

Mrs. Miller takes too much diazepam (Valium) and is found soon thereafter in a coma breathing slowly and shallowly. Arterial blood gas results reveal pH, 7.25; Pa_{CO_2}, 70 mm Hg; and HCO_3^-, 29 mEq/L.

41. How would you interpret these ABG results?

42. What is the primary cause of the disorder?

Case 2

Mr. Miller is worried about Mrs. M's condition. He describes dizziness and tingling in his hands. His ABG results reveal pH, 7.60; Pa_{CO_2}, 20 mm Hg; and HCO_3^-, 23 mEq/L.

43. How would you interpret these ABG results?

44. What is the primary cause of the disorder?

Case 3

Little Jimmy Miller has been sick with the stomach flu. Arterial blood gas results reveal pH, 7.60; Pa_{CO_2}, 40 mm Hg; and HCO_3^-, 36 mEq/L.

45. How would you interpret these ABG results?

46. What is the primary cause of the disorder?

Copyright © 2003, 1999 Mosby, Inc. All rights reserved.

Case 4

Teenager Debbie Miller has not been taking her insulin. Arterial blood gas results reveal pH, 7.25; Pa_{CO_2}, 40 mm Hg; and HCO_3^-, 14 mEq/L.

47. How would you interpret these ABG results?

48. What is the primary cause of the disorder?

Of course, blood gases don't stay simple for long. Partial or complete compensation can occur.

Case 5

Grandpa Miller has smoked for years, and now he has COPD. Arterial blood gas results reveal pH, 7.35; Pa_{CO_2}, 50 mm Hg; and HCO_3^-, 34 mEq/L.

49. How would you interpret these ABG results?

50. What is the source of compensation?

Case 6

As soon as Debbie Miller's brain realizes the acute nature of her illness, compensation begins. Arterial blood gas results now reveal pH, 7.35; Pa_{CO_2}, 25 mm Hg; and HCO_3^-, 12 mEq/L.

51. How would you interpret these ABG results?

52. What is the source of compensation?

Case 7

Grandma Miller has CHF. She takes furosemide (Lasix) to reduce extra water in her body. Arterial blood gas results now reveal pH, 7.46; Pa_{CO_2}, 45 mm Hg; and HCO_3^-, 32 mEq/L.

Copyright © 2003, 1999 Mosby, Inc. All rights reserved.

53. How would you interpret these ABG results?

A. I only
B. III only
C. I and II only
D. I and III only

56. Interpret the following ABG results:

FiO_2	0.21
pH	7.36
$Paco_2$	37 mm Hg
HCO_3^-	22 mEq/L
Pao_2	95 mm Hg

A. Acute respiratory alkalosis
B. Acute metabolic alkalosis
C. Compensated respiratory alkalosis
D. Normal ABG results

54. What is a possible cause of the primary disorder?

57. During CPR, blood gases are drawn. The results are as follows:

FiO_2	1.0
pH	7.15
$Paco_2$	55 mm Hg
HCO_3^-	12 mEq/L
Pao_2	210 mm Hg

▶ WHAT ABOUT THOSE BOARD EXAMS?

Blood gas (acid-base) analysis is one of the largest areas in all of the exams. The Entry Level examination focuses on simple interpretations, but the Registry examinations ask for higher order thinking. Here are some examples.

55. A 17-year-old girl is brought to the emergency department by paramedics. Her mother states she has a diabetes. Room air ABG analysis reveals:

pH	7.26
$Paco_2$	16 mm Hg
HCO_3^-	8 mEq/L
Pao_2	110 mm Hg

This information indicates which of the following?

I. Partly compensated metabolic acidosis.
II. This Pao_2 is not possible on room air.
III. Respiratory alkalosis is present.

What action should be taken to correct the acid-base abnormality shown here?

A. Increase the rate of ventilation
B. Decrease the FiO_2
C. Administer sodium bicarbonate intravenously
D. Add positive end-expiratory pressure (PEEP) to the ventilation system

58. The results of an arterial blood gas analysis are

FiO_2	.21
pH	7.55
$Paco_2$	25 mm Hg
HCO_3^-	24 mEq/L
Pao_2	105 mm Hg

Copyright © 2003, 1999 Mosby, Inc. All rights reserved.

These data indicate which of the following?
- A. Metabolic acidosis
- B. Metabolic alkalosis
- C. Uncompensated hyperventilation
- D. Uncompensated hypoventilation

59. A 72-year-old man with a history of renal failure is seen in the emergency department. The respiratory care practitioner notes that the patient is taking 28 very deep breaths per minute. Which of the following accurately describes this breathing pattern?
- A. Cheyne-Stokes breathing
- B. Ataxic breathing
- C. Kussmaul's breathing
- D. Eupneic breathing

► EXERCISE YOUR MENTAL MUSCLES

In later chapters you will be called on to use your newfound blood gas interpretation skills to make many clinical decisions about patient care. *If you're having difficulty interpreting acid-base status, you should take time to solidify these skills now!* Here are some suggestions:

1. *Get access to blood gas interpretation software.* Your instructors probably have a program that will give you sample after sample to interpret.

2. *Make flash cards.* Take some 3- by 5-inch cards. Write high, normal, and low values for pH, Pa_{CO_2}, and HCO_3^-. Make two extra cards for pH that represent compensation. Use 7.36 for compensated acidotic states and 7.44 for alkalotic states. On the back of each card write out the name of the state. For example, on the Pa_{CO_2} 50 mm Hg card, write "respiratory acidosis." Get the idea? Now proceed through the combinations using the four-step method of interpretation. Pretty soon you will be an ace!

► *Drill, drill, drill until you have mastered basic blood gas interpretation!*

► FOOD FOR THOUGHT

Blood gas disorders can become really complicated at times. Just like life. In some cases, a patient has one disorder superimposed on another. Take the continuing saga of Grandpa Miller.

Grandpa Miller acquires a lung infection after visiting his daughter in the hospital. Arterial blood gas results now reveal pH, 7.46; Pa_{CO_2}, 35 mm Hg; Pa_{O_2}, 57 mm Hg; and HCO_3^-, 34 mEq/L.

60. How would you interpret these ABG results?

61. Why did the blood gas change from case 5?

► INFORMATION AGE

Go to Virtual Hospital at **www.vh.org/ adult/provider/internalmedicine/bloodgases/ index.html** for more useful material from this excellent site.

Copyright © 2003, 1999 Mosby, Inc. All rights reserved.

If you'd like to get into something different and more in depth try "What's New in Blood Gas Interpretation" at the Mt. Sinai Medical Center site:
www.mtsinai.org/pulmonary/ noninvasive/intro.htm

You can get a seemingly endless parade of information on the Internet when you ask your search engine for "blood gas interpretation."

Copyright © 2003, 1999 Mosby, Inc. All rights reserved.

Regulation of Breathing

"The brain is a wonderful organ.
It starts working the moment
you get up in the morning and
doesn't stop until you get
to the office."

R. Frost

You are getting sleepy, very sleepy . . . you didn't stop breathing did you? In just one year as an adult, you will breathe more than *seven million times!* Most of those breaths will be automatically initiated by your brainstem. Just like clockwork. Good thing, eh? (I have trouble remembering where I put my car keys.) It makes sense that RCPs would need to know how this system works and what happens when it doesn't. Chapter 13 is a fitting end to the section on anatomy and physiology, because it summarizes the control mechanisms that regulate the respiratory system.

▶ READING, WRITING, AND REGULATING

The brain and nervous system have a language all their own. Learning these terms will make it easier to understand concepts in this chapter. (And you can impress your friends with your linguistic abilities!)

Copyright © 2003, 1999 Mosby, Inc. All rights reserved.

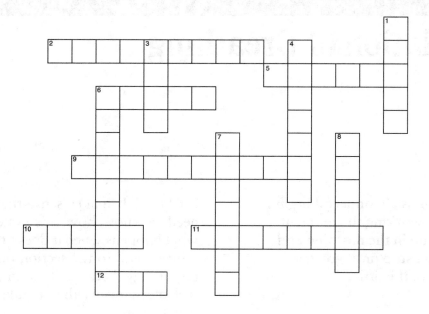

ACROSS

2. Chemo _____, respond to changes in oxygen and pH to signal the need to breathe
5. + Breuer = parasympathetic inflation reflex
6. Absence of breathing
9. Receptors in the carotid bodies
10. 5 deep breaths...apnea...five deep breaths... apnea?
11. Coughing, sneezing, laryngospasm, bronchospasm, and more when you stimulate these receptors!
12. Fluid that bathes the brain instead of blood

DOWN

1. Important cranial nerve involved in sensory and motor reflexes
3. The other center in the brainstem
4. Big Boss of the brainstem
5. Breathing pattern characterized by prolonged inspiratory gasps
7. Primary chemoreceptors
8. + Stokes = gradually increasing, then decreasing volumes with apneic episodes

▶ WHERE'S THE ACTION?

Input into how we breathe comes from many areas. Conscious thought, receptors throughout the body, and reflexes all play important roles. The job of the medulla is to organize the information and send messages to the motor fibers that innervate the muscles of the airway and chest (a sort of mental air-traffic controller). The medulla is located in the brainstem just above the spinal cord. If you cut the brainstem (don't try this at home) below the medulla, all ventilatory effort ceases. Another structure, the pons, sits on top of the medulla.

Copyright © 2003, 1999 Mosby, Inc. All rights reserved.

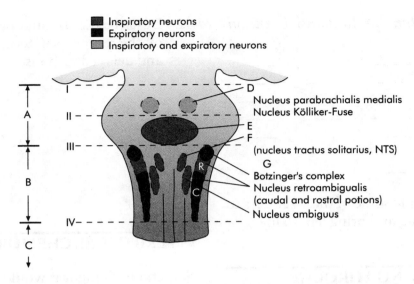

Dorsal view of the brainstem. Dashed lines I to IV refer to transections at different levels. *(From Beachey W: Respiratory care anatomy and physiology: Foundations for clinical practice, St Louis, 1998, Mosby.)*

1. Label the parts of the central-controlling bodies.
   A. _____
   B. _____
   C. _____
   D. _____
   E. _____
   F. _____
   G. _____

2. Briefly explain the role of the two primary respiratory groups in the medulla.

3. Compare and contrast the two primary centers in the pons.

4. What diseases or conditions might affect the performance of the respiratory controllers in the brainstem?

▶ **AUTOMATIC PILOT**

Respiratory reflexes are involuntary nervous responses located in airways, muscles, and tissues that influence breathing by sending information directly to the medulla (mostly via the vagus nerve). You'll need to be able to identify the most important reflexes, so here goes. Each reflex goes with a particular stimulus and has a response from receptors in a specific location.

Copyright © 2003, 1999 Mosby, Inc. All rights reserved.

Reflex	Stimulus	Response	Location
5. Hering-Breuer	___	___	___
6. Deflation	___	___	___
7. Head	___	___	___
8. Vagovagal	___	___	___
9. C fiber	___	___	___
10. Proprio-ceptor	___	___	___

Later on let's apply some of these reflexes to the clinical setting and bring 'em to life.

▶ BETTER LIVING THROUGH CHEMISTRY

Regulating ventilation ensures that tissues are exposed to just the right amount of O_2, CO_2, and H^+. Blood carries these substances to specialized nerve structures called *chemoreceptors* that are strategically placed in the brainstem, carotid bodies, and arch of the aorta. All these chemoreceptors respond in some way to decreased levels of O_2 and pH or an increased level of CO_2 in the blood (and vice versa).

▶ CENTRAL CHEMORECEPTORS

Central chemoreceptors sit in the medulla taking a bath in the cerebrospinal fluid (CSF). They are not in direct contact with blood because of the blood-brain barrier, a semipermeable membrane that surrounds the brain.

11. Explain the process that allows CO_2 to stimulate the central receptors.

12. Describe the stimulating effects of CO_2 on the receptors in terms of immediate and delayed responses.

▶ PERIPHERAL CHEMORECEPTORS

Somebody thought it would be a good idea to monitor the chemical composition of blood leaving the heart and heading toward the brain. Pretty smart!

13. Describe the peripheral receptor response to decreased arterial O_2 levels.

14. What specific range of PaO_2 values causes the greatest response?

15. How does altitude modify the receptor's response to hypoxemia?

Copyright © 2003, 1999 Mosby, Inc. All rights reserved.

16. Describe the peripheral receptor response to hypercapnia and acidemia. How is it different from the central response?

▶ NO ONE UNDERSTANDS ME!

I want to introduce you to one of the most misunderstood concepts in the pathophysiology of lung disease. When you understand this one, you'll really be able to amaze the doctors, nurses, and respiratory instructors (not to mention your mom and dad).

Here goes something. . . . Some patients, especially those with COPD, become chronically hypoxic and hypercapnic. This happens when a high arterial CO_2 level persists. The kidneys compensate in a process that restores pH. Some of the HCO_3^- diffuses into the head and corrects the pH of the CSF. The central receptors are fooled into thinking everything is fine. Because these patients are low on O_2, the hypoxic stimulus drives ventilation.

So far, so bad. When someone intervenes and gives this type of patient O_2, the patient may experience an acute rise in arterial CO_2. The simple explanation is that the patient is no longer driven by the peripheral receptors to breathe because of low O_2 levels. Although this is true, it is too simple an explanation. Increased O_2 also worsens the ventilation/perfusion ratio ($\dot{V}\dot{Q}$) in the lungs by increasing blood flow to poorly ventilated areas and through absorption atelectasis. Ventilation is decreased in low $\dot{V}/\dot{Q}$ areas, and increased in high $\dot{V}/\dot{Q}$

regions. The result is increased arterial P_{CO_2}. (My students always ask "so what?" at this point.)

The point is that CO_2 in high concentration in the blood is bad for you. It further decreases drive to breathe by depressing the central nervous system. So, don't give the patient too much O_2, but **never withhold O_2 from a hypoxic patient!**

17. What concentration of O_2 is usually given to chronically hypercapnic patients?

18. What is the best way to monitor oxygenation in these patients?

19. Why do low concentrations of O_2 usually result in adequate improvement?

▶ OUCH!

If the brain is physically or physiologically injured, abnormal breathing patterns occur. When you observe these patterns, you know something is wrong with the controller.

Copyright © 2003, 1999 Mosby, Inc. All rights reserved.

20. Describe Cheyne-Stokes breathing (use words or draw a picture). State two important causes of this distinctive pattern.

21. How does Biot's breathing differ from Cheyne-Stokes in terms of pattern and origin?

22. Describe apneustic breathing. What does this pattern indicate?

23. What are the two central neurogenic breathing patterns? State three events that could cause these patterns.

► CASE STUDIES

Case 1

Bobby Donor rides his motorcycle without a helmet. He sustains a closed head injury during an accident that results in a subdural hematoma. The paramedics intubate Bobby with an endotracheal tube.

24. What is the goal of ventilation during the early period after acute closed head trauma?

25. Why would you limit the use of this technique after 24 hours?

Case 2

Grandpa Miller (see Chapter 12) is back in the hospital. Grandpa became short of breath at home, and his family increased his O_2 from 2 L/min to 6 L/min. When he arrives at the hospital, Mr. Miller is somnolent (sleepy) and difficult to arouse. The ABG results reveal pH, 7.25; Pa_{CO_2}, 75 mm Hg; Pa_{O_2}, 90 mm Hg; HCO_3^-, 37 mEq/L on 6 L by nasal cannula.

Copyright © 2003, 1999 Mosby, Inc. All rights reserved.

26. What changes should you make in Grandpa's therapy? Why?

27. What target PaO_2 would be more appropriate for this patient? Why?

► WHAT ABOUT THOSE BOARD EXAMS?

The NBRC won't exactly ask you direct questions about the information in this chapter, but the exams do have related questions. Variations on this theme are as follows:

28. A patient who has had COPD for many years is admitted for an acute episode of dyspnea. An arterial blood gas is drawn on room air with these results:

pH	7.50
$PaCO_2$	48 mm Hg
PaO_2	44 mm Hg
HCO_3^-	36 mEq/L
SaO_2	84%

What therapy do you recommend at this time?
A. 28% Venturi mask
B. 35% Venturi mask
C. Nasal cannula delivering 5 L/min
D. Simple mask delivering 10 L/min

29. A cooperative elderly patient with chronic asthma visits her pulmonologist's office. You observe the following findings:

Pulse	94 beats/min
Respiratory rate	28 breaths/min
Temp	36.5° C
Blood pressure	135/90 mm Hg
FIO_2	0.21
pH	7.33
$PaCO_2$	70 mm Hg
PaO_2	35 mm Hg
HCO_3^-	34 mEq/L

What action would you take at this time?
A. Administer bronchodilator therapy with a metered-dose inhaler (MDI)
B. Administer oxygen via 24% Venturi mask
C. Administer oxygen via cannula at 6 L/min
D. Administer oxygen via nonrebreathing mask

30. A patient with COPD and a history of hypercapnia is receiving oxygen via simple mask in the recovery room after admission for pneumonia. On transfer to the medical floor, he is found to be increasingly drowsy and difficult to arouse. The nurse requests that you give the patient a breathing treatment with a bronchodilator. The most appropriate action would be to
A. Administer the breathing treatment as requested
B. Obtain an arterial blood gas sample
C. Change the oxygen to 2 L/min via nasal cannula
D. Change the oxygen to 40% via Venturi mask

There are many variations of this type of question regarding chronic hypercapnia and O_2 administration on both the Entry Level and the Registry examinations!

Copyright © 2003, 1999 Mosby, Inc. All rights reserved.

You may also expect questions such as the following:

31. A patient is being mechanically ventilated after craniotomy. During a suctioning procedure, the intracranial pressure monitor shows a sudden increase in ICP. The patient becomes restless and agitated. What is the most appropriate immediate action for the respiratory care practitioner in this situation?
    A. Increase the F_{IO_2} on the ventilator to deliver 100% oxygen
    B. Recommend administration of a sedative
    C. Increase rate and volume of ventilation with a resuscitation bag
    D. Ask the nurse to page the physician "STAT"

▶ EXPERIMENT

This exercise will seem simple, but it will help you understand control of breathing. It's even better if you have a pulse oximeter, O_2, and a nonrebreathing mask.

Remember to be safe: Sit down when you do this, and have a partner.

Put the oximeter probe on your finger. Breathe normally. Now inhale deeply and hold your breath. Time how long you can hold your breath. Next, inhale and exhale deeply several times. Fill your lungs, and time how long you can hold your breath.

32. How long could you hold your breath the first time: _____? What about the second try: _____?

33. What were the pulse oximeter readings before _____, during _____, and at the end of breath-hold _____?

34. Compare the results and explain the differences in breath-hold time and why you had to breathe. What is the meaning of the "pulse ox" readings?

Now, breathe 100% O_2 for several minutes. At the end of the time, hyperventilate while breathing the O_2. Now hold your breath.

35. What happened to the time of breath-hold?

36. Given a vital capacity of 5 L and an O_2 consumption of 250 mL/min, what is the theoretical maximum breath-hold time of a normal adult?

If you really want to try this experiment at its best, see your instructor about breathing from a high-flow continuous positive airway pressure (CPAP) system at 100% O_2, or use a ventilator!

▶ FOOD FOR THOUGHT

The reflexes and receptors that control breathing are important. So is the input of conscious thought. The higher brain centers have a definite effect on how we breathe.

Copyright © 2003, 1999 Mosby, Inc. All rights reserved.

37. Why do we take a patient's respiratory rate without telling him or her we are doing it?

38. Name as many factors as you can that involve the higher brain centers' increasing the rate of ventilation. (*Hint:* How do you breathe when a police car pulls up behind you and turns on the flashing lights?)

► **INFORMATION AGE**

Springfield Community College has a site with good basic information: **distance.stcc. edu/AandP/AP/AP2pages/respiration/ control.htm**
www.pitt.edu/~paccm/pdfs/ introtothelung/controlofbreathing.pdf

This is a comprehensive 25-page discussion of the subject designed for medical students. This one is in *pdf* format, which means you need Adobe Acrobat Reader to look at it. Acrobat is a free download that you might as well get anyway, because you'll need it to look at a lot of things on the Web. The advantage to this software is that you'll get your information in a text format that is easy to read and easy to print!

Copyright © 2003, 1999 Mosby, Inc. All rights reserved.

Bedside Assessment

"As I grow older, I pay less attention
to what men say. I just watch
what they do."

Andrew Carnegie

Patient assessment is the compass we steer by in the clinical setting. Chapter 14 helps you learn the basics, but only practice will give you mastery. Your ability to evaluate using your senses will make all the difference in your career. This material is so important I've packed this chapter full of questions, cases, and more questions!

▶ WORD POWER

Chapter 14 starts off with an impressive list of nearly 40 new words for you to learn. Power up your medical terminology by reading the chapter and solving this crossword puzzle.

Copyright © 2003, 1999 Mosby, Inc. All rights reserved.

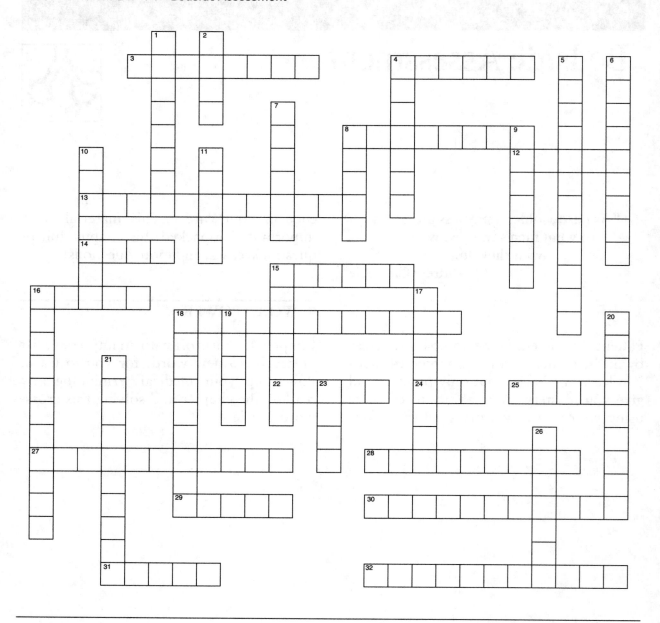

▶ START AT THE VERY BEGINNING...

Successful assessors develop a systematic way of evaluating patients. Except in life-threatening emergencies, most practitioners begin by interviewing the patient. The interview may be short or long depending on the situation. The increasing use of protocols requires us to conduct more in-depth interviews. Let's review the essentials of interviewing and history taking.

1. What information would you gather before entering the patient's room?

Copyright © 2003, 1999 Mosby, Inc. All rights reserved.

ACROSS

1. Bluish discoloration of the skin
4. Mucus from the tracheobronchial tree
8. Discontinuous abnormal breath sounds
12. Prefix for fast
13. _____ emphysema is air under the skin
14. Look for distended veins here
15. Mucus that comes out the mouth
16. Medical term for slow
18. Extra, or abnormal sounds
22. _____ pressure, the difference between systolic and diastolic blood pressure
24. Level of consciousness
25. Designed to expel mucus
27. _____ alternans occurs when you go back and forth between the diaphragm and the accessory muscles!
28. You have this if your breathing is labored when you lie down
29. Auscultation reveals breath _____
30. Body temperature below 32 Celsius
31. Stay at least 2-4 feet away to give the patient a personal _____ space during the interview
32. Sweaty stuff

DOWN

1. _____ pressure, when the heart contracts
2. Dys, ortho, hypo, tachy—are all prefixes that go with this one
4. Abdominal _____, occurs when the diaphragm is tired and the belly sinks in with each breath
5. Abnormal voice sounds heard over consolidation
6. Slow respiratory rate
7. _____ of monkeys (also a chest shape associated with air trapping)
8. Treasure, pigeon, or barrel
9. High-pitched continuous upper airway sound
10. Patient's perception of difficult breathing
11. Foul smelling
15. Another name for fainting
16. Heart rate below 60
17. Got pus?
18. Pattern of end-stage muscle fatigue
19. _____ signs
20. Rapid breathing pattern
21. Coughing up blood
23. Primary organ of gas exchange
26. I've got the fever

---

2. Describe how to *start* the ideal interview. Be sure to discuss space, privacy, and introductions.

3. Circle the *better approach* from each set of choices in the following list:
   A1. "Hi, Bob, good morning."
   A2. "Good morning, Mr. Johnson."
   B1. Stand at the foot of the bed.
   B2. Sit in a chair at the bedside.
   C1. Make room for your notes on the bedside table.
   C2. Keep your clipboard on your lap.
   D1. "Do you need anything right now?"
   D2. "I'll tell your nurse to check on you."
   E1. "I'll be back to see you in 1 hour."
   E2. "I'll return in a while to check on you."

▶ ARE YOU ASKING THE QUESTIONS RIGHT?

The way you ask questions determines your relationship with the patient and the amount and quality of the information you gather.

Copyright © 2003, 1999 Mosby, Inc. All rights reserved.

4. Circle the *better approach* from each set of choices in the following list:
   A1. "What are you coughing up?"
   A2. "You didn't cough up blood, did you?"
   B1. "I understand you don't like your breathing treatments."
   B2. "Why don't you like these treatments?"
   C1. "How is your breathing today?"
   C2. "Is your breathing better today?"

5. When are "closed" questions most useful? Give an example.

▶ **SIGNS AND SYMPTOMS OF CARDIOPULMONARY DISEASE**

I don't know about you, but five things come to mind when I think of common symptoms of heart and lung disease. I'm sure there are more, but if these situations stand out in your mind, you can use them to your benefit as part of the interviewing process.

▶ *"I feel short of breath."*

6. Describe the dyspnea (Borg) scale. Why would this be useful?

7. How else can you identify the degree of dyspnea a patient feels?

▶ *"Cough it up, honey!"*

8. What are the possible causes of these common types of cough?

Cough	Causes
A. Dry cough	_____
B. Loose, productive cough	_____
C. Acute, self-limiting cough	_____
D. Chronic cough	_____

9. What is the difference between mucus and sputum?

10. What are the three characteristics of sputum that should be documented and reported to the physician?

Copyright © 2003, 1999 Mosby, Inc. All rights reserved.

11. Define *nonmassive* hemoptysis and give three common causes.

12. Define *massive* hemoptysis and give three possible causes.

▶ *"It hurts when I take a deep breath!"*

13. What is the most serious kind of non-pleuritic chest pain?

14. How does pleuritic chest pain differ from nonpleuritic pain?

▶ *"Hot stuff!"*

15. Marked elevation of temperature has what effect on metabolic rate, O_2 consumption, CO_2 production, and breathing pattern?

16. Along with fever, what are two signs that are highly suggestive of respiratory infection?

▶ **MEDICAL HISTORY**

Whether you personally take medical histories or not, you need to be familiar with the standard format used in this process that is *always* conducted at some point (usually early on) during a patient's admission to the formal healthcare setting.

17. What do the initials "CC" and "HPI" stand for? List at least five important areas described in the HPI.

Copyright © 2003, 1999 Mosby, Inc. All rights reserved.

18. What do the initials "PMH" stand for? List at least five important areas described in the PMH.

General appearance is assessed during the first few seconds of *every* encounter with a patient. During your first encounter, you might look at the patient's body as a whole, facial expression, anxiety level, positioning, and personal hygiene.

19. Describe the significance of the findings for each of the areas of general appearance listed below.

Finding	Significance
A. Weak, emaciated, and diaphoretic	_____
	_____
	_____
B. Appears anxious	_____
	_____
	_____
C. Sitting up, leaning with arms on table	_____
	_____
	_____

▶ IS ANYONE HOME?

What's the difference between stuporous and lethargic? Obtunded and comatose? Alert and confused? These aren't completely subjective terms, and you will see them used frequently in the medical record. After taking a look at the overall appearance, you need to determine the level of consciousness. For starters, the patient is either obviously conscious or not when you look at him or her. If the patient is conscious, you have to find out the level of alertness. If the patient does not seem obvi-ously conscious, you need to find out how depressed the sensorium is and describe this with commonly accepted terms.

20. What does the phrase "oriented × 3" mean?

21. Compare and contrast the terms "lethargic" and "obtunded."

22. What is the difference between a "stu-porous" patient and a "comatose" patient?

23. What is the first thing an RCP should evaluate in cases of depressed level of consciousness?

Special rating systems such as the Glasgow Coma Scale are used to further identify the degree of coma. You need to keep in mind that special circumstances, such as deaf-ness, can make assessment more difficult.

Copyright © 2003, 1999 Mosby, Inc. All rights reserved.

► VITAL INFORMATION

Temperature, pulse, respiratory rate (RR), and blood pressure (BP) are the traditional vital signs. Inexpensive, useful, and easy to obtain. (Pulse oximetry readings are being called the "fifth vital sign" because they are taken so often.) Vital signs offer great clues about response to therapeutic interventions, but they're not as simple as you might think considering how often they are measured. Let's start with the basics.

24. Fill in the correct normal adult values (or terms) in the chart below.

Sign	Average Normal	Low	High
A. Temperature	_____	_____	Hyperthermia
B. _____	_____	72/min	_____
C. Respiratory rate	_____	12 /min	_____
D. Systolic blood pressure	_____	90 mm Hg	_____
E. _____	_____	_____	90 mm Hg

25. Name the four common sites for temperature measurement. Give a *disadvantage* of each site.

    Site   *Disadvantage*
A. _____ _____
B. _____ _____
C. _____ _____
D. _____ _____

26. Match these pulsating terms to their throbbing definitions!

A. _____ Tachycardia
B. _____ Bruits
C. _____ Amplitude
D. _____ Paradoxical pulse
E. _____ Pulsus alternans
F. _____ Bradycardia

1. Palpable vibrations in pulse
2. Strength of pulse
3. Pulse less than 60 beats/min
4. Drop in amplitude with inspiration
5. Pulse greater than 100 beats/min
6. Alternating strong and weak pulses

27. Match the flowing respiratory patterns to their whooshing definitions! (*Hint:* I cheated! Try the glossary!)

A. _____ Tachypnea
B. _____ Eupnea
C. _____ Orthopnea
D. _____ Trepopnea
E. _____ Hyperpnea
F. _____ Bradypnea

1. Difficulty breathing in a supine position
2. Abnormally low respiratory rate
3. Deep breathing
4. Normal breathing pattern
5. Abnormally high respiratory rate
6. Labored breathing in an upright position

Copyright © 2003, 1999 Mosby, Inc. All rights reserved.

28. How can you prevent patients from becoming aware that you are taking their respiratory rate (and from consciously altering it)?

29. What condition can result in syncope in a hypovolemic patient? How can you prevent this from happening? How is it managed medically?

    A. Condition _____
    B. Prevention _____
    C. Treatment _____

30. What does it mean when patients have a larger (>6-8 mm Hg) than normal drop in systolic pressure during inspiration?

► EXAMINING THE CHEST AND LUNGS: THE BIG FOUR

This is like learning the Ten Commandments, but there are only four:

Thou shalt inspect the chest.
Thou shalt palpate the chest.
Thou shalt percuss the chest.
Thou shalt auscultate the chest.

Sounds so easy when you put it that way, doesn't it? Before you start to assess, make sure you have enough **light**, enough **privacy**, enough **time**, and enough **quiet**. *Of course, you can't always get what you want!* Chapter 14 describes the *ideal* evaluation of a patient. You have to adapt to meet the circumstances every time!

See Me

There's a lot you can see when you take a quick look at the patient. Practice looking. Let's find out if you know what to look for in a patient with respiratory problems.

31. Write a description of the following six abnormal chest shapes.

Abnormal Shape	Description
A. Barrel	_____
	_____
	_____
	_____
	_____
B. Kyphosis	_____
	_____
	_____
	_____
	_____
C. Kyphoscoliosis	_____
	_____
	_____
	_____
	_____
D. Pectus carinatum	_____
	_____
	_____
	_____
	_____

Copyright © 2003, 1999 Mosby, Inc. All rights reserved.

E. Pectus
   excavatum
   _____
   _____
   _____
   _____

F. Scoliosis
   _____
   _____
   _____
   _____
   _____

E. Increased
   intracranial
   pressure (ICP)
   _____
   _____
   _____
   _____

F. Metabolic
   acidosis
   _____
   _____
   _____
   _____
   _____

32. Breathing patterns are important too. Describe the pattern that goes with the following six conditions.

Condition	Pattern of Breathing
A. Asthma	_____
	_____
	_____
	_____
	_____
B. Atelectasis	_____
	_____
	_____
	_____
	_____
C. Chest trauma	_____
	_____
	_____
	_____
	_____
D. Epiglottitis	_____
	_____
	_____
	_____
	_____

▶ EXPERIMENT

To get good at this, you might try the mall. Yes, the mall. If you sit with a nice cup of espresso, you can see chest shape, breathing pattern, and all the rest. Compare adult patterns with those of children. Compare the chest shape of an elderly person with that of a young adult. After you try this exercise, answer the following questions.

33. Did you observe anyone breathing with the diaphragm? How could you tell?

34. Did you observe the use of accessory muscles? How could you tell?

Copyright © 2003, 1999 Mosby, Inc. All rights reserved.

35. How does the chest shape of a young adult differ from that of a senior?

36. What unusual chest shapes did you observe? Anyone using portable O_2?

Feel Me

Palpation is the art of touching the chest wall. Palpation is an art (and a useful one) because it's so subjective. You have to get a feel for it. Don't practice this at the mall!

37. Explain the difference between vocal, tactile, and rhonchial fremitus.

38. Describe the difference in fremitus between emphysema and pneumonia.

39. How does subcutaneous emphysema form? What is the feeling of air under the skin called?

▶ **EXPERIMENT**

You should learn palpation in the laboratory of your program. Because disrobing is necessary, gowns and privacy are needed (as is professionalism). Assess tactile fremitus by asking your classmate to repeat the word "ninety-nine" while you palpate under the clavicles, between the shoulder blades, along the sides, and over the lower lobes. Measure chest expansion as demonstrated in Figure 14-5 in your text. Now answer these questions.

40. Describe the temperature of your partner's skin.

41. Were there any areas of abnormal fremitus? Why? Why not?

Copyright © 2003, 1999 Mosby, Inc. All rights reserved.

42. Estimate the amount of chest expansion in centimeters. What is normal adult expansion?

Touch Me

Or tap me. Diagnostic percussion of the chest is another art form that is rarely practiced these days. Still, it can be useful in detecting important abnormalities, and your board examiners expect you to be able to interpret the results of percussion findings!

43. Complete the chart below by identifying the percussion notes for these conditions.

Condition	Percussion Note
A. Emphysema	_____
	_____
	_____
	_____
	_____
B. Atelectasis	_____
	_____
	_____
	_____
	_____
C. Pleural effusion	_____
	_____
	_____
	_____
	_____

D. Pneumothorax _____
_____
_____
_____
_____

E. Pneumonia _____
_____
_____
_____
_____

44. What are the limitations of percussion? What can't you feel?

▶ **EXPERIMENT**

You should do this in the lab while you are performing the palpation and auscultation exercises. Place your left middle finger on the intercostal space on the side of the chest. Rapidly strike it with the index finger or middle finger of your right hand. Do this on both sides of the chest. Repeat over the lower lobes in the back. Have your partner take a really deep breath and hold it while you tap. Have your partner exhale fully, then tap.

Try tapping over something solid like the scapula. Try tapping over the abdomen. Tap on your own head. Is it hollow? It takes practice to get good at percussion. **Don't include this procedure in a routine examination of a patient** unless other observations suggest an appropriate problem. Have an expert present when you try this in the clinical setting.

Copyright © 2003, 1999 Mosby, Inc. All rights reserved.

45. What happened to the resonance when your partner inhaled deeply? Exhaled?

Hear Me

This is it. This is the big one. Auscultation seems so easy, and identifying breath sounds so difficult. Follow Steve's Ten Commandments to improve your technique.

    I. Sit the patient up whenever you can.
   II. Turn off the TV, radio, and other external sources of noise.
  III. Ask the patient to breathe slowly and deeply through the mouth.
  IV. Listen to skin whenever you can.
   V. Listen to the lower lobes first.
  VI. Listen to one full inspiration and exhalation in each spot.
 VII. Listen to both sides in each spot.
VIII. Auscultate lower, middle, and upper portions of the lung.
  IX. Listen to the front and the back of the chest.
   X. Compare right and left lungs. Compare upper and lower lobes.

Simple, right? Now you try it.

▶ EXPERIMENT

You should try this in the laboratory before going to the bedside. You can listen at home, too. The more normal sounds you auscultate, the better you will be at recognizing abnormal sounds. All you need is your stethoscope, a partner (you can even start on yourself), and a quiet place to listen. Adjust the earpieces so they are pointing slightly forward, not straight into your ears. (Check to make sure the diaphragm, not the bell, is "on" if your scope is adjustable). Now listen.

1. Place your partner in a sitting position (or high Fowler's).

2. Ask your partner to breathe in and out slowly through the mouth.

3. Listen on skin over the posterior lower lobes (below the shoulder blade).

4. In and out, right side and left side.

5. Listen on the side of the chest (still lower lobes).

6. Listen between the shoulder blades (not over the spine).

7. Listen on the front to the middle lobe and lingula (anterior, below nipple).

8. Listen on the front below the collarbone (above nipples).

9. Listen over the trachea.

Look in *Egan's* on p. 326 Figure 14-7. You can auscultate 20 or more places on the chest, but we don't usually do this much auscultation in the clinical setting. It takes too long for a routine evaluation. Always listen to upper, middle, and lower, front and back. When you hear abnormal sounds or are examining a critically ill patient, you should expand your assessment.

Now that you've read the chapter and practiced, try answering these questions.

Copyright © 2003, 1999 Mosby, Inc. All rights reserved.

46. Fill in the chart below with descriptions of your favorite breath sounds.

Breath Sound	Pitch	Intensity	Location
A. Vesicular	_____	_____	_____
B. Bronchial	_____	_____	_____
C. Bronchovesicular	_____	_____	_____

47. Compare the mechanisms and causes of coarse, low-pitched crackles and fine end-inspiratory crackles.

48. Contrast monophonic and polyphonic wheezes in terms of mechanism, phase of ventilation, and conditions that produce these different musical sounds.

49. How do rhonchi differ from crackles ?

► EXTREMITY EXAM

You will almost always want to take a look at the patient's fingers. For one thing, the findings go hand in hand with those of pulse oximetry. Cardiopulmonary disease can alter the fingers and other extremities.

50. How do you test for capillary refill? (Test your own while you're at it.) What is a normal capillary refill time?

51. Where should you check for edema caused by right heart failure? Why?

52. Compare and contrast the significance of peripheral cyanosis and central cyanosis.

► CASE STUDIES

Case 1

George Brush is an alert 67-year-old politician admitted for dyspnea and hemoptysis. While interviewing the patient, you find that he has been coughing up small amounts of thick, blood-streaked mucus several times per day for the last few days. Mr. Brush has a history of 100 pack-years of cigarette smoking. Physical examination reveals barrel chest, use of accessory muscles, and digital clubbing.

Copyright © 2003, 1999 Mosby, Inc. All rights reserved.

53. Mr. B's history and chest configuration suggest what primary pulmonary disorder?

54. Along with enlargement of the ends of the fingers, what sign helps you recognize clubbing?

55. What does the presence of clubbing suggest in this case?

56. Why do you think Ms. Stewart's mental status has deteriorated?

57. What other "vital sign" should be evaluated?

58. Which abnormal vital sign has the most clinical significance in this case?

Case 2

Marla Stewart is a 47-year-old homemaker admitted for a systemic infection 3 days after cutting herself in the kitchen while preparing chicken. She reports dyspnea and has a fever. Her vital signs are pulse, 110 beats/min; respiratory rate, 28 breaths/min; and blood pressure 76/58 mm Hg. The nurse's notes reveal that Ms. Stewart was alert on admission, but she is now confused and anxious. Her extremities are warm, and capillary refill is normal.

Case 3

You are called to the medical ward to evaluate John Hopkins, a 29-year-old medical student who was admitted for shortness of breath and is now reporting chest pain. Mr. Hopkins tells you the pain came on suddenly and is worse when he inhales. Your interview reveals that this pain is on the right side and feels like a sharp, stabbing sensation. Temperature is normal, but blood pressure, heart rate, and respiratory rate are elevated. Palpation reveals crepitus over the right lateral chest wall.

Copyright © 2003, 1999 Mosby, Inc. All rights reserved.

59. What other physical assessments would be useful in determining the nature of the problem?

60. What immediate treatment should you initiate in this situation?

61. What diagnostic test would be helpful in determining the cause of the pain?

62. What does the finding of crepitus on palpation indicate?

started yesterday and has been gradually getting worse. Auscultation reveals decreased breath sounds in both bases with end-inspiratory crackles.

63. What is the most likely cause of the dyspnea?

64. What test is indicated to confirm the diagnosis?

65. What respiratory care interventions are indicated?

▶ WHAT ABOUT THOSE BOARD EXAMS?

Killer. What more can I say? Entire sections of each exam are devoted to patient assessment. The NBRC exam matrix is filled with "assess by inspection," "assess by palpation," "assess by auscultation," and "interview the patient." Even the most conservative estimate would be 12 questions on this subject alone! When you combine this portion of the test with other questions that require you to use assessment information to make

Case 4

Harry Garcia, a 59-year-old rock star, is recovering from open heart surgery performed 2 days ago. Mr. Garcia is alert and oriented × 3. He reports dyspnea and a dry cough. Vital signs reveal a pulse of 104 beats/min and a respiratory rate of 32 breaths/min with a shallow pattern. Mr. Garcia tells you that the difficulty breathing

Copyright © 2003, 1999 Mosby, Inc. All rights reserved.

decisions, you can expect a minimum of 10% of the Entry Level examination to be on the material in Chapter 14. I know you will be looking at this subject more closely later on as you prepare for your boards. For now, let me give you some sample questions.

66. During a chest examination of an intubated patient, the respiratory care practitioner palpates vibrations on exhalation over the upper chest. What action should be taken at this time?
    A. The patient should be given a bronchodilator
    B. The patient should be suctioned
    C. The patient should be given supplemental oxygen
    D. The patient should be placed on mechanical ventilation

67. A patient's medical record indicates he has orthopnea. Which of the following best describes this condition?
    A. Difficulty breathing at night
    B. Difficulty breathing when upright
    C. Difficulty breathing on exertion
    D. Difficulty breathing when lying down

68. A child is brought to the emergency department because of severe respiratory distress. On entering the room, the respiratory care practitioner hears a high-pitched sound when the child inhales. This is most likely
    A. Wheezing
    B. Stridor
    C. Rhonchi
    D. Crackles

69. A respiratory care practitioner is asked to evaluate a patient for oxygen therapy. The practitioner notices that the patient is sleepy but arouses when questioned. This level of consciousness is best described as
    A. Confused
    B. Obtunded
    C. Stuporous
    D. Lethargic

70. Which of the following breath sounds is most likely to be heard during acute exacerbation of asthma?
    A. Wheezes
    B. Crackles
    C. Stridor
    D. Rhonchi

71. All of the following physical findings are consistent with pneumonia *except*
    A. Dull percussion note
    B. Presence of inspiratory crackles
    C. Bronchial breath sounds over the affected area
    D. Bradypnea

72. Which of the following findings suggest(s) that a patient is oriented?
    I. Awareness of the correct date
    II. Ability to correctly state his or her own name
    III. Awake when you enter the room
    A. I only
    B. I and II only
    C. I and III only
    D. I, II, III

73. During an interview, the patient states he has been coughing up thick, foul-smelling sputum. This finding is most consistent with
    A. A bacterial infection of the lung
    B. A diagnosis of lung cancer
    C. Obstructive lung disease
    D. Pulmonary tuberculosis

Copyright © 2003, 1999 Mosby, Inc. All rights reserved.

74. A respiratory care practitioner is inspecting the chest of a child with respiratory distress. The practitioner notes that the child has a large concave depression of the sternum. This finding should be documented as
    A. Barrel chest
    B. Pectus carinatum
    C. Pectus excavatum
    D. Kyphoscoliosis

75. All of the following physical findings are consistent with complete upper airway obstruction *except*
    A. Inability to speak
    B. Stridor
    C. Supraclavicular retractions
    D. Flaring of the nostrils

76. While assessing a patient who is dyspneic and tachypneic, a respiratory care practitioner notices bluish discoloration of the lips and oral mucosa. The practitioner should document which of the following in the medical record?
    A. Presence of cyanosis
    B. Presence of hypoxemia
    C. Presence of increased work of breathing
    D. Presence of orthopnea

▶ FOOD FOR THOUGHT

My brain is full, how about yours?

▶ INFORMATION AGE

While searching for good information on assessment, I found this awesome website of a pulmonologist at the University of Manitoba. The site is for pulmonary residents, but it's loaded with good material for the RCP or student. There is a fine section on assessment, and there are loads of small on-line presentations that are easy to use. **www.ssharma.com**

It's a gold mine for students (teachers too)! You should stop reading right now and get on-line to look at this website. Thank you, Dr. Sharma.

Copyright © 2003, 1999 Mosby, Inc. All rights reserved.

ECG and Lab Assessment

"There is only one thing worse
than hardness of heart and that
is softness of head."
Theodore Roosevelt

Chapter 15 to follow Chapter 14! A lot of students struggle with this, but I know you'll feel capable when you finish these exercises.

In the clinical setting, laboratory assessment directly follows the interview and physical assessment. The NBRC Clinical Simulation Examination often follows a similar format. So it seems natural for

▶ A PICTURE IS WORTH...

I don't see any really new words we haven't already covered, so why not go right to the picture? Label all of the heart parts and conduction clues.

Copyright © 2003, 1999 Mosby, Inc. All rights reserved.

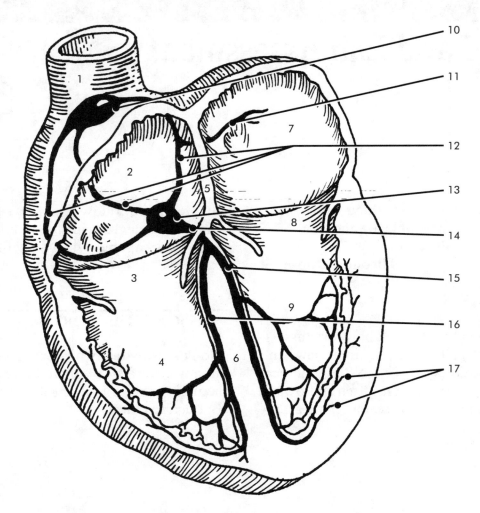

Anatomy of the electrical conduction system of the human heart.

Heart Parts

1. _____

2. _____

3. _____

4. _____

5. _____

6. _____

7. _____

8. _____

9. _____

Conduction Clues

10. _____ The natural "pace-maker" of the heart

11. _____ Conducts impulses through the atria

12. _____ Carries impulses across the right atrium

13. _____ The "backup pace-maker"

14. _____ Why not "hers"?

15. _____ Carries impulse to the left ventricle

Copyright © 2003, 1999 Mosby, Inc. All rights reserved.

16. _____ Carries impulse to the right ventricle

17. _____ Fingerlike projections that penetrate the ventricles

---

▶ MORE PICTURES?

Let's perfect basic identification. Label these four common waves and indicate the event they represent.

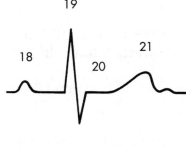

Normal configuration of ECG waves. *(From Wilkins RL, Krider SJ, Sheldon RL: Clinical assessment in respiratory care, ed 3, St Louis, 1995, Mosby.)*

	Wave	*Represents*
18.	_____	_____
19.	_____	_____
20.	_____	_____
21.	_____	_____

22. Where is atrial repolarization?

23. What is the maximum duration of the PR interval?

24. What pathological abnormality results in a depressed or elevated ST segment?

▶ MAKING MEASUREMENTS

Electrocardiographic paper is made up of tiny boxes or grids that allow you to measure time on the horizontal axis and millimeters of deflection on the vertical axis. A darker line occurs every 5 boxes.

25. What is the normal paper speed for an ECG?

Copyright © 2003, 1999 Mosby, Inc. All rights reserved.

26. The time (horizontal) represented by 1 small box is _____ seconds and by 1 large box is _____ seconds.

27. One millivolt of electrical energy produces a deflection of _____ small boxes, or _____ large boxes.

▶ START AT THE VERY BEGINNING...

Because many RCPs obtain ECGs for patients or take care of monitored patients, you will need to be able to evaluate the rhythms you see to maintain safe patient care. Successful assessors have developed a systematic way of evaluating the ECG.

▶ Step 1: Evaluate the Rate

You can evaluate the rate manually or rely on the electronic data. There are time marks every 3 seconds. So the number of QRS complexes in 6 seconds can be multiplied by 10. When the rate is regular, you can divide 300 by the number of large boxes between 2 QRS complexes.

Try It, You'll Like It!

Count the rate in Pattern 1 using both manual methods.

28. The number of QRS complexes in this 6-second strip is _____. Multiply by 10 to get a rate of _____.

29. There are _____ heavy lines between complex A and complex B; 300 divided by this number is _____. That's the average rate.

Does every P wave have a QRS complex after it? That indicates a sinus rhythm.

30. A rate less than 60 beats/min is called sinus _____.

31. A rate greater than 100 beats/min is called sinus _____.

▶ Step 2: Measure the PR Interval

Count the number of small boxes between the start of the P wave and the start of the QRS complex. Remember the normal value of less than 0.20 seconds (5 small boxes). A P wave followed by a QRS complex but separated by a prolonged PR interval represents a

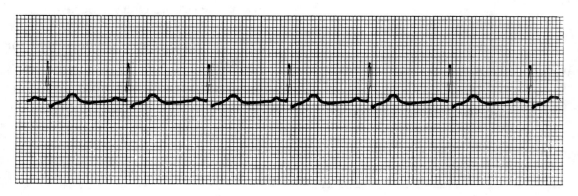

Pattern 1.

Copyright © 2003, 1999 Mosby, Inc. All rights reserved.

delay at the atrioventricular (AV) node. This condition is called *first-degree heart block.* Treatment usually is not needed. We just monitor for worsening block.

Try It, You'll Like It!

Measure the PR interval in Pattern 2.

32. The time from the P wave to the QRS complex is _____ seconds.

33. What arrhythmia does this represent?

34. The duration of the QRS complex is _____ seconds.

▶ Step 3: Evaluate the QRS Complex

The normal QRS complex is no more than 0.12 seconds (3 small boxes) wide. Wide QRS complexes are abnormal and do not result in good ventricular contractions.

Try It, You'll Like It!

Measure the QRS complex in Pattern 3.

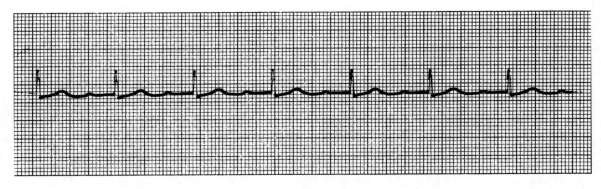

Pattern 2.

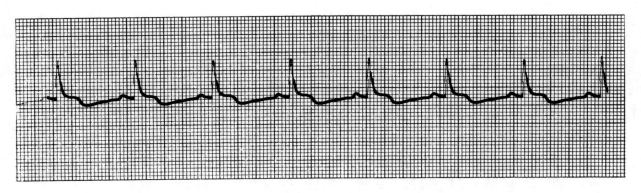

Pattern 3.

Copyright © 2003, 1999 Mosby, Inc. All rights reserved.

▶ Step 4: Evaluate the T Wave

Normal T waves are upright and rounded. Inverted T waves represent poor blood flow to the heart muscle. Strangely shaped T waves may be caused by hyperkalemia.

35. The T wave in Pattern 1 is upright/inverted (*circle one*).

▶ Step 5: Evaluate the ST Segment

A normal ST segment is basically flat. Isoelectric. Elevated or depressed ST segments are bad! They represent oxygenation problems and are seen in conditions such as myocardial infarction (MI) (that's a heart attack).

Try It, You'll Like It!

Evaluate the ST segment in the Pattern 4 ECG.

36. The ST segment in this pattern is elevated/flat/depressed (*circle one*).

▶ Step 6: Identify the R-R Interval

You are looking for a regular relationship. If the R waves are not the same distance apart, you have an irregular rhythm.

Try It, You'll Like It!

Evaluate the R-R interval in the Pattern 5 ECG.

37. The R-R interval in this pattern is regular/irregular (*circle one*).

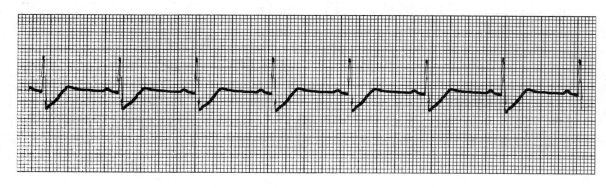

Pattern 4.

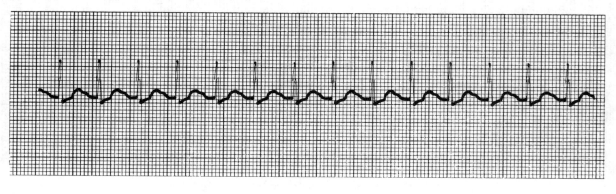

Pattern 5.

Copyright © 2003, 1999 Mosby, Inc. All rights reserved.

▶ RECOGNIZING ARRHYTHMIAS

Now that you have the basic idea, let's take a look at the major dysrhythmias that you will encounter. This is pattern recognition, so look for the "picture" each rhythm shows.

Normal Sinus Rhythm

Upright P wave. Normal PR interval. Each P wave is followed by a normal QRS complex. R-R intervals are regular, and the rate is 60 to 100 beats/min. No treatment is needed for this rhythm.

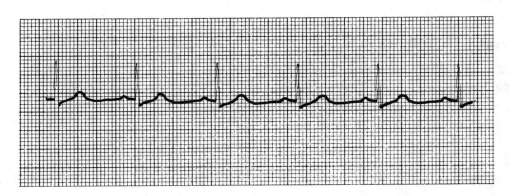

Pattern 6.

Sinus Bradycardia

Upright P wave. Normal PR interval. Each P wave is followed by a normal QRS complex. R-R intervals are regular, *but the rate is less than 60 beats/min.* This is *absolute brady-* *cardia.* It is a problem only if the blood pressure drops. You might see this rhythm during suctioning as a result of vagal stimulation. Stop suctioning! Intravenous atropine is a treatment for this arrhythmia.

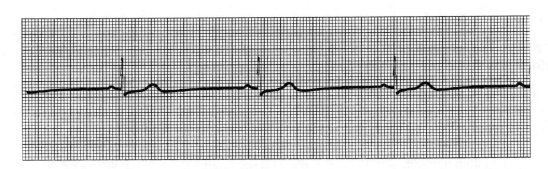

Pattern 7.

Sinus Tachycardia

Upright P wave. Short PR interval. Each P wave is followed by a normal QRS complex. R-R intervals are regular, *but the rate is more than 100 beats/min!* This is *sinus* *tachycardia.* Tachycardia is the first sign of hypoxemia in most patients. Consider whether you are doing something to cause it, such as suctioning. Pattern 5 is an example of sinus tachycardia.

Copyright © 2003, 1999 Mosby, Inc. All rights reserved.

First-Degree Heart Block

Upright P wave. *Prolonged* PR interval. Each P wave is followed by a normal QRS complex. R-R intervals are regular. This rhythm is a problem only if signs and symptoms such as low blood pressure and chest pain come with it. First-degree block can be caused by drugs or MI. Pattern 2 is an example.

Second-Degree Heart Block

Our block is moving lower down the conduction pathway. Not good! There are two types.

Second-Degree Type I

This one is called Wenckebach or Mobitz type I. The P waves have a progressively prolonged transmission (prolonged PR interval) followed by a P wave with no QRS complex. There usually is a repeated pattern, such as three P waves and one lost QRS complex.

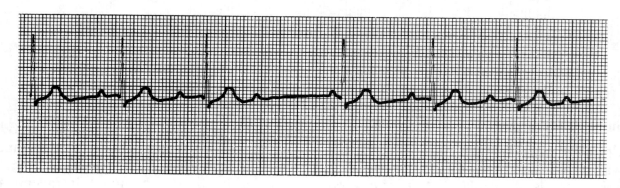

Pattern 8.

Second-Degree Type II

Mobitz Type II. Definitely not a good sign. This block is worse than type I. You will see some P waves conducted (followed by a QRS complex) and some P waves with no following QRS complex.

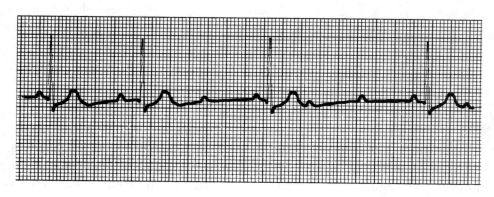

Pattern 9.

Copyright © 2003, 1999 Mosby, Inc. All rights reserved.

Third-Degree Heart Block

Also called complete heart block, this rhythm is definitely life-threatening. No impulses from the sinoatrial (SA) node are conducted. Because the ventricles have their own intrinsic rate, you will see the atria paced by the SA node (P waves) and the ventricles (QRS complex) pacing themselves. These QRS complexes often are wide. Blood pressure is poor, and an artificial pacemaker is needed.

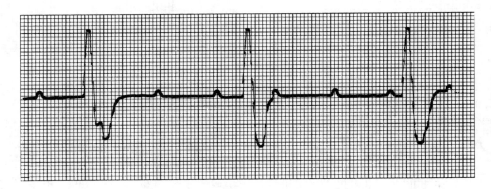

Pattern 10.

A Little Story

An easy way to keep the blocks straight is a love story gone wrong.

A couple gets married. At first, they have a normal sinus rhythm. She (P wave) is at home, and he (QRS complex) comes home on time (Pattern 11, *A*). After a while, he is spending more time with his secretary after work. She (P wave) is at home, he is coming home late. A first-degree block (Pattern 11, *B*). Eventually, while she (P wave) is at home, he (QRS complex) comes home later, then later, and one night, he does not come home (missed QRS complex) (men!). A second-degree type I block (Pattern 11, *C*). She (P wave) is rightfully furious and tells him to mend his ways or else. He (QRS complex) starts coming home on time but goes back to his old ways and does not come home. A second-degree type II block (Pattern 11, *D*). After this final insult, she (P wave) is at home, and he (QRS complex) is at home, but they are sleeping in separate bedrooms and have nothing to do with each other. Third-degree block (Pattern 11, *E*)! A pacemaker (or a divorce lawyer) is needed in this situation.

Copyright © 2003, 1999 Mosby, Inc. All rights reserved.

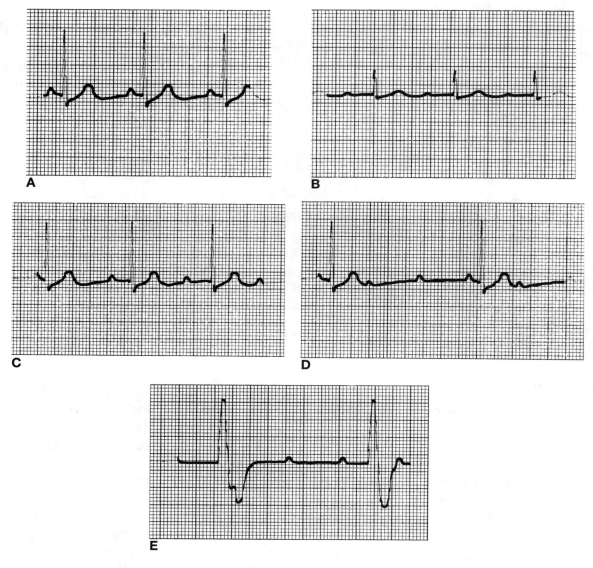

Pattern 11.

Atrial Dysrhythmias

Atrial fibrillation is erratic quivering of the atria that does not deliver a good preload to the ventricles. Also, clots can form in the atria. Sometimes the ventricle responds to fibrillation with a rapid rate. No P wave is seen, but the QRS complexes probably look normal. Atrial dysrhythmias are managed with drugs, such as digitalis, or electrical treatments. Notice the R-R intervals.

Copyright © 2003, 1999 Mosby, Inc. All rights reserved.

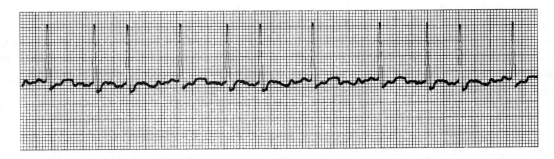

Pattern 12.

Atrial flutter is a very rapid (250 beats/min) atrial rate. You can spot it every time by noting the "sawtooth" or "picket fence" pattern of the atrial discharge. This condition is managed with drug or electrical treatments.

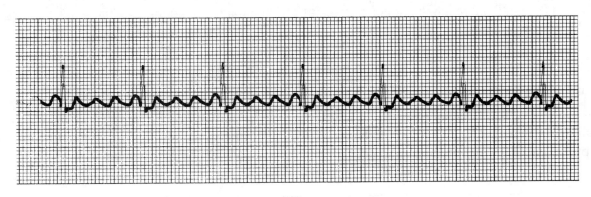

Pattern 13.

Premature Ventricular Contractions

PVCs. You will want to notice these abnormal QRS complexes because they are often caused by hypoxemia. In other words, if you are suctioning and the patient experiences PVCs, STOP! Oxygenate the patient. Other causes include stress, caffeine, and nicotine. No big deal. Intravenous lidocaine is the therapy for excessive PVCs (usually more than six per minute).

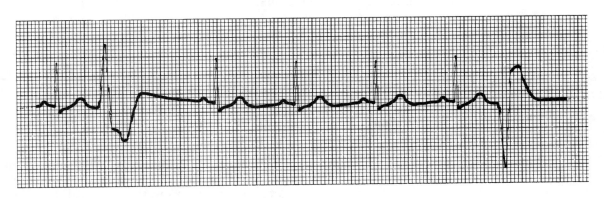

Pattern 14.

Copyright © 2003, 1999 Mosby, Inc. All rights reserved.

Ventricular Tachycardia

Tachycardia, of course, is a rate greater than 100 beats/min. But this rhythm shows no P waves and has a wide QRS complex. The patient usually does not have a pulse.

This condition is life threatening! Stop, call for help, check for a pulse, and act appropriately. Lidocaine (or amiodarone) or defibrillation is needed.

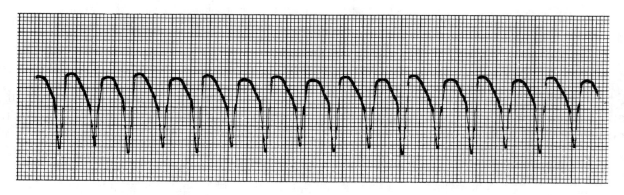

Pattern 15.

Ventricular Fibrillation

The only rhythm worse than ventricular fibrillation is a flat line (asystole). There is no pulse, cardiac output, or blood pressure.

Only defibrillation helps, but you can do CPR and give oxygen and drugs until defibrillation can be performed.

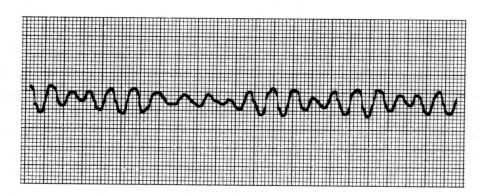

Pattern 16.

Practice recognizing the important arrhythmias. After a while, these basic patterns will be easy to spot, just like a Van Gogh painting, and you won't have to think too hard.

► LABBA DABBA DOO!

Certain laboratory test results are very useful to the RCP. You will need to learn the normal values and what abnormal results mean if you want to pass your boards or to get the big picture in the hospital. Let's start with complete blood cell count (CBC).

Copyright © 2003, 1999 Mosby, Inc. All rights reserved.

White

38. What does a large elevation in white blood cell (WBC) count suggest?

    A.

    B.

39. Name three common causes of low WBC count.

    A.

    B.

    C.

40. What specific type of WBC count is elevated in bacterial pneumonia? Viral pneumonia?

    A.

    B.

Red

41. What term describes a low red blood cell (RBC) count? What is the management of this disorder?

    A.

    B.

Copyright © 2003, 1999 Mosby, Inc. All rights reserved.

42. What is a normal hemoglobin level, and why are RCPs especially interested in hemoglobin levels?
    A.

    B.

43. What blood abnormality is caused by chronic hypoxemia?

44. Before performing ABG analysis, you would be wise to check which two values?

▶ LYTES, CAMERA, ACTION

Respiratory care practitioners are interested in electrolyte values because electrolytes affect acid-base balance and muscle function. Electrolytes are discussed in Chapter 11. See how much you remember.

45. What is the normal range for serum potassium?

46. Why is potassium of particular interest in patients being weaned from mechanical ventilation?

47. What value on the venous chemistry panel represents bicarbonate?

48. What other test is indicated when a chemistry panel shows abnormal anion gap?

49. What are the two tests that together indicate renal function?

Copyright © 2003, 1999 Mosby, Inc. All rights reserved.

▶ ENZYMES

Enzymes are present everywhere in the body. They make reactions happen (remember carbonic anhyd*rase?*). Specific enzymes are released when tissues are damaged. Myocardial infarction is a good example.

50. Name the two common liver enzymes that might be elevated in patients with hepatitis. Give the old names (what most people remember, like your old teachers!) and the new names.

    Old   *New*
    A. _____   _____
    B. _____   _____

51. Elevation of what specific enzyme found only in the heart is suggestive of MI?

▶ SPUTUM IS OUR BREAD AND BUTTER!

You will probably be asked to obtain many sputum specimens during your career. Sputum samples are needed when lung infection is suspected. Gram stain, culture, and sensitivity testing are almost always performed, but only if you get the right stuff!

52. Why would the laboratory reject your beautiful sputum specimen?

53. What is the purpose of growing the bacteria on a culture plate?

▶ CASE STUDIES

Case 1

Young Joan, a student, is suctioning a patient orally with tonsil suction. The monitor shows sinus bradycardia. Blood pressure is falling. Alarms are sounding.

54. What should Joan do?

55. What physiologic mechanism is responsible for the drop in rate?

Copyright © 2003, 1999 Mosby, Inc. All rights reserved.

Case 2

Young Annie, a student, is suctioning a patient through the endotracheal tube. The monitor shows sinus tachycardia with frequent PVCs. Alarms are sounding. The patient is agitated.

56. What should Annie do?

57. What physiologic mechanism is responsible for the increased rate and arrhythmias?

Case 3

While performing a ventilator check on a patient in the coronary care unit, Young Shawnna, a student, observes the rhythm on the monitor has changed from atrial fibrillation to ventricular fibrillation.

58. What should Shawnna do first?

59. Name at least three responses indicated to manage this rhythm.

▶ WHAT ABOUT THOSE BOARD EXAMS?

Actual pictures of ECG rhythms usually appear in the Clinical Simulation Examination and occasionally on the other written exams. Cardioversion and defibrillation are on the Written Registry Examination. You need to supplement the text with more information to understand these subjects. The Advanced Cardiac Life Support material from the American Heart Association is a good resource. The Entry Level examination doesn't have too much on the heart, only basics. Here are sample questions from Chapter 15 that you might run into.

60. Sputum culture and sensitivity would be indicated for which of the following conditions?
    A. ST segment elevation
    B. Pleural effusion
    C. Pneumothorax
    D. Bronchitis

61. A patient arrives in the emergency department vomiting. Blood gas results reveal metabolic alkalosis. On the basis of this information, you would also suggest
    A. A stat chest radiograph
    B. Electrolyte analysis
    C. Blood cultures
    D. Urinalysis

Copyright © 2003, 1999 Mosby, Inc. All rights reserved.

62. While receiving a nebulized bronchodilator treatment in the telemetry unit, a patient experiences an episode of pulseless ventricular tachycardia. Immediate management of this rhythm is
    A. Administration of oxygen
    B. Administration of intravenous epinephrine
    C. Defibrillation
    D. Placement of a chest tube

▶ FOOD FOR THOUGHT

You want more? Try these.

63. A young adult male patient has symptoms of hypoxemia and signs of pneumonia. What are several possible reasons the WBC count is severely depressed?

64. What type of person might have absolute bradycardia without symptoms and would not need any treatment?

65. Newer enzyme tests are available. What is troponin (TNI or TnT)?

▶ INFORMATION AGE

You can learn more about troponin at: **www.labtestsonline.org/understanding/ analytes/troponin/glance.html**

The hottest new issue in cardiac medicine is inflammation. Inflammation can cause vascular and cardiac damage in persons who have normal cholesterol levels. Inflammation can result in cardiac disease in otherwise healthy persons. For more on the C-reactive protein test for inflammation look at **focus.hms.harvard.edu/2002/ Nov22_2002/pathology.html**

Copyright © 2003, 1999 Mosby, Inc. All rights reserved.

Analysis and Monitoring of Gas Exchange

"Vision is the art of seeing the invisible."
Jonathan Swift

Analyzing and monitoring gas exchange is one of the most important areas of the respiratory care profession. Chapter 12 covers interpreting the acid-base balance of ABGs. Naturally, there's more to it than that. Chapter 16 covers the equipment used to analyze blood and much more. For example, there are noninvasive methods for monitoring gas exchange, such as capnometry and pulse oximetry. So whether you're talking about clinical practice or thinking about credentialing examinations, you're going to need a firm grasp on this slippery subject.

▶ LIFE'S A GAS

You'll have to learn the specialized terminology of invasive and noninvasive monitoring if you want to get the most mileage out of this material. Solve this crossword puzzle to test your understanding of the key terms in Chapter 16.

Copyright © 2003, 1999 Mosby, Inc. All rights reserved.

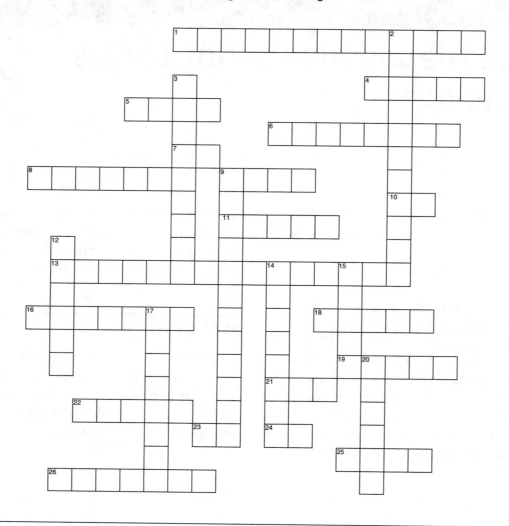

► FIRST THINGS FIRST . . .

First, you have to make a choice between analysis and monitoring. Analysis usually means obtaining a sample of body fluid and putting it in some type of lab analyzer to get results. Properly obtained, these measurements have a high degree of accuracy. Unfortunately, they are like a snapshot of a single event. Monitoring usually is done at the bedside and is a continuous process. More like watching a video. Next, you have a choice of invasive or noninvasive techniques. Invasive techniques are probably more accurate, but they also have a greater risk of harm to the patient. They are a good way to establish a base-line. Noninvasive methods often are used for monitoring and are especially useful when used with invasive techniques. Conclusion? No one method is best. Your role as a clinician is to get the right balance. My role is to help you figure out how to do that.

► MEET THE OBJECTIVES

You've read the chapter, and now you're feeling a little overwhelmed. I don't blame you! Answer the following questions, and you will get a grip on the good stuff. Relax, get some coffee or soda. This is going to take a little time.

Copyright © 2003, 1999 Mosby, Inc. All rights reserved.

ACROSS

1. Oxygen analyzer that measures the flow of electrons between negatively and positively charged poles.
4. _____ of care, testing blood at the bedside instead of in the lab.
5. Systematic errors in measurement.
6. Artery in the arm that's not your first choice.
7. _____ vivo, inside the body.
8. Big artery in the groin that is used for drawing blood when other choices fail.
9. Allen's, for example.
10. _____ vivo, outside the body.
11. Never do this with a used needle.
13. Pulse oximeters use this principle to detect arterial pulsation.
16. Device that provides ongoing information to clinicians.
18. Oxygen analyzing electrode.
19. Preanalytical ones, bubble in sample for example.
21. _____ invasive monitoring doesn't hurt!
22. Modify this test and perform before radial puncture.
23. Quality control.
24. Oximeter used to measure carbon monoxide in the blood.
25. Point-of-_____: method of testing blood at the bedside.
26. Measure blood values in the laboratory.

DOWN

2. External quality control testing program.
3. Alternative to arterial sampling in infants.
9. Clot buster.
12. Sensor that works on optical detection instead of electrochemical properties.
14. Oxygen analyzer that doesn't use a battery.
15. Non-invasive oximeter commonly used to measure hemoglobin's saturation with oxygen.
17. Determine the saturation of hemoglobin with a photoelectric device.
20. Artery of choice for puncture or cannulation.

Copyright © 2003, 1999 Mosby, Inc. All rights reserved.

1. In your own words, explain how an electrochemical analyzer converts the number of O_2 molecules (P_{O_2}) into a measurable reading.

2. There are two common types of electrochemical analyzers. Name them.
   A. _____
   B. _____

3. Explain the differences between the two types of analyzers in terms of principle of operation and response time.

4. Describe the two-step process for calibrating an O_2 analyzer.

5. What is the standard of reference for gas exchange analysis? What does this mean?

6. List four reasons why the radial artery is the preferred site for ABG sampling.
   A. _____
   B. _____
   C. _____
   D. _____

7. Describe the modified Allen test and the definition of a positive result.
   A.

   B.

8. Name four other sites you can use if the radial artery is unavailable or has a poor pulse.
   A. _____
   B. _____
   C. _____
   D. _____

9. How long should you wait after changing the F_{IO_2} before performing ABG analysis for a patient with healthy lungs? A patient with COPD?
   A.

   B.

Copyright © 2003, 1999 Mosby, Inc. All rights reserved.

10. What technique can help prevent hyperventilation due to pain or anxiety from altering the sample results?

11. The AARC ABG sampling guidelines describe several medications that can cause prolonged bleeding. These are anticoagulants (clot preventers) and thrombolytics (clot busters). Give two examples of each of these classes of drugs.
    A. Anticoagulants
        1. _____
        2. _____
    B. Thrombolytics
        1. _____
        2. _____

12. Name the four things you can do to avoid most preanalytical sampling errors.
    A. _____
    B. _____
    C. _____
    D. _____

13. What precaution should you take when handling any laboratory specimen?

14. What are the three primary values measured with a blood gas analyzer?
    A. _____
    B. _____
    C. _____

15. If you wanted to measure actual hemoglobin saturation, what type of analyzer would you need?

16. What is the range of accuracy for most commercially available pulse oximeters?

17. Describe three noninvasive ways you can determine the reliability of a pulse oximeter at the bedside.
    A. _____
    B. _____
    C. _____

18. According to AARC guidelines, what action should you take to verify the results when pulse oximetry is unreliable or the results do not confirm suspicions about the patient's clinical state?

Copyright © 2003, 1999 Mosby, Inc. All rights reserved.

19. Describe the three main quality assurance procedures used to maintain consistently accurate blood gas results.
    A. Automated calibration

    B. Control media

    C. Proficiency testing

20. For which patients is capillary sampling appropriate?

21. What are the two most common errors committed during capillary sampling?

22. Explain what variables are reliable and unreliable in capillary sampling compared with arterial sampling.

23. What are the primary advantages and disadvantages of transcutaneous gas monitoring over arterial sampling?
    A. Advantages
        1. _____
           _____
        2. _____
           _____
    B. Disadvantages
        1. _____
           _____
        2. _____
           _____

24. When would you choose a pulse oximeter over a transcutaneous monitor for monitoring an infant's oxygenation status?

25. When would the transcutaneous monitor be preferred over the pulse oximeter?

Copyright © 2003, 1999 Mosby, Inc. All rights reserved.

26. Describe proper placement of a cap-nometer sampling chamber or adaptor for a patient who is being mechanically ventilated.

27. What is the range of normal values for end-tidal CO_2 for healthy persons, and how do these values compare with arterial CO_2?

28. An end-tidal CO_2 of "0" may indicate a serious problem. Name two life-threatening causes of a 0 value for end-tidal CO_2.
    A. _____
    B. _____

29. While obtaining end-tidal CO_2 measurements, you notice that the baseline does not return to 0 on inspiration. Interpret this result.

30. While obtaining end-tidal CO_2 measurements, you notice that no real plateau is reached. Give two possible interpretations of this result.
    A. _____
    B. _____

Whew! I'm tired. Time to take a break.

▶ CHAPTER HIGHLIGHTS

The questions you just answered cover many of the important points; however, this chapter is really crammed with details. Here are a few more questions that highlight some of the main points we haven't already covered.

31. What are the three most common causes of O_2 analyzer malfunctions?
    A. _____
    B. _____
    C. _____

32. Blood gases provide more information than other methods of gas exchange analysis. What are the three general areas that blood gas analysis helps to assess?
    A. _____
    B. _____
    C. _____

33. What is the maximum ideal time between ABG sampling and analysis?

34. What are the two primary benefits and hazards of indwelling peripheral arterial lines?
    A. Benefits
       1. _____
       2. _____
    B. Hazards
       1. _____
       2. _____

Copyright © 2003, 1999 Mosby, Inc. All rights reserved.

35. What is point-of-care testing, and what are the potential benefits of this method of testing blood samples?

36. What is the difference between capnography and capnometry?

► CASE STUDIES

Now that you have the information, let's see if you can apply it to the following scenarios.

Case 1

Biff Hoser, a 34-year-old firefighter, is brought to the emergency department for management of smoke inhalation sustained while he was fighting a house fire. Heart rate is 126 beats/min; respirations are 28 breaths/min and labored. SpO_2 is 100% on 6 L by nasal cannula. Blood pressure is 145/90 mm Hg. Breath sounds are coarse with inspiratory crackles in both bases. Biff's face is smudged with soot, and he is coughing up sputum with black specks in it.

37. What clinical signs of hypoxemia does Mr. Hoser display?

38. Explain why the pulse oximeter is reading 100% in spite of these signs.

39. What is the most probable cause of the hypoxemia?

40. What blood test would you recommend to confirm your suspicions?

Case 2

Little Maggie Simpleton is a premature infant. She is wearing supplemental O_2. Her doctor is concerned about the effects of hyperoxia on her lungs and eyes. Maggie is being monitored with a pulse oximeter, which shows a saturation of 100%.

Copyright © 2003, 1999 Mosby, Inc. All rights reserved.

41. What range of P_{O_2} is possible with an Sp_{O_2} of 100%?

42. What type of noninvasive monitoring would you recommend in this situation?

Case 3

Grandpa Miller is an elderly patient admitted for acute exacerbation of long-standing COPD. He is wearing a nasal cannula at 2 L/min.

43. What is the simplest way to quickly assess his oxygenation status?

44. Why would you recommend ABG analysis for this patient?

Case 4

Jimmy Dornor was riding his motorcycle without a helmet when he crashed. Now he has a head injury and is receiving mechanical ventilation. His doctor asks you to make recommendations regarding monitoring of gas exchange.

45. What are the advantages of using capnometry to monitor CO_2 in this situation?

46. Where would you place the capnometer probe in the ventilator circuit?

47. During monitoring, you notice that the capnograph does not return to "0" when Jimmy inhales. What does this indicate?

Copyright © 2003, 1999 Mosby, Inc. All rights reserved.

48. A few minutes later Jimmy's exhaled CO_2 level begins to rise. So does his blood pressure. Jimmy becomes agitated. What action would you take?

49. Why do rising CO_2 levels increase ICP?

► **WHAT ABOUT THOSE BOARD EXAMS?**

The NBRC has a strong affinity for monitoring gas exchange. So should you! You will find pulse oximeters and O_2 analyzers on the Entry Level examination. Capnography and transcutaneous monitoring are covered on the Registry exams. So study mixed venous sampling, co-oximetry, blood gas analyzers, and quality control. Here's a baker's dozen of what you can expect.

50. A respiratory care practitioner is preparing to perform pulse oximetry. Which of the following would be *least* beneficial for assessing accuracy of the device?
    A. Checking the capillary refill time
    B. Assessing skin color and temperature
    C. Performing an Allen test on the patient
    D. Assessing pulse rate

51. Which of the following would you perform after obtaining an arterial blood gas sample?
    I.   Remove air bubbles from the sample
    II. Mix the sample by rotating the syringe
    III. Maintain site pressure for at least 1 minute
    IV. Add heparin to the sample
    A. I only
    B. I, II only
    C. I, II, III only
    D. I, II, III, IV

52. A pulse oximeter is being used to monitor a patient who was rescued from a fire. The SpO_2 is 90%; however, the patient is unconscious and shows signs of respiratory distress. What additional test should the respiratory care practitioner recommend?
    A. CT Scan
    B. Electrolyte measurement
    C. Co-oximetry
    D. Hemoglobin level and hematocrit

53. A polarographic oxygen analzyer fails to calibrate when exposed to 100% oxygen. The first action the respiratory care practitioner should take would be to
    A. Replace the battery
    B. Replace the membrane
    C. Replace the fuel cell
    D. Try another oxygen source

Copyright © 2003, 1999 Mosby, Inc. All rights reserved.

54. An infant is placed on a transcutaneous oxygen monitor. The transcutaneous PO_2 ($TcPO_2$) reading is 40 mm Hg less than the PaO_2 obtained from an arterial sample. All of the following could cause this problem *except*
    A. Improper calibration of the transcutaneous electrode
    B. Room air contamination of the transcutaneous electrode
    C. Inadequate heating of the skin at the electrode site
    D. Inadequate perfusion of the skin at the electrode site

55. Which of the following analyzers is calibrated to a value of 0 when exposed to room air?
    A. Clark electrode
    B. Galvanic oxygen analyzer
    C. Capnometer
    D. Geissler-type nitrogen analyzer

56. Which of the following would be most useful in assessing proper tube placement after endotracheal intubation?
    A. Transcutaneous monitoring
    B. Arterial blood gas analysis
    C. Pulse oximetry
    D. End-tidal CO_2 monitoring

57. Complications of arterial puncture include all of the following *except*
    A. Pulmonary embolus
    B. Hematoma
    C. Infection
    D. Nerve damage

58. A galvanic oxygen analyzer is being used in a check of the ventilator system to measure the delivered FIO_2. The set FIO_2 is 40%; however, the analyzer is reading 32%. Which of the following is the most likely cause of this discrepancy?
    A. The batteries in the analyzer need to be changed
    B. The electrode membrane has water condensation on its surface
    C. The analyzer needs to be calibrated
    D. The ventilator needs servicing

59. Which of the following affect the accuracy of pulse oximeter measurements?
    I. Increased bilirubin levels
    II. Decreased hematocrit levels
    III. Dark skin pigmentation
    IV. Exposure to sunlight
    A. I, II only
    B. II, III only
    C. III, IV only
    D. II, III, IV only

60. A sample for arterial blood gas analysis is drawn from a patient who is breathing room air. Analysis reveals the following results:
pH	7.45
$PaCO_2$	35 mm Hg
PaO_2	155 mm Hg

Which of the following best explains these results?
    A. Too much heparin was added to the sample
    B. An air bubble has contaminated the sample
    C. Analysis of the sample was delayed for more than 60 minutes
    D. The patient was hyperventilating during the puncture

Copyright © 2003, 1999 Mosby, Inc. All rights reserved.

61. Which of the following sites would be the best for continuous monitoring of exhaled carbon dioxide during mechanical ventilation?
    A. Exhalation valve
    B. Inspiratory side of the ventilator circuit
    C. Expiratory side of the ventilator circuit
    D. Endotracheal tube connector

62. Which of the following is true concerning the use of a transcutaneous P_{O_2} monitor?
    A. TcP_{O_2} should be checked with arterial blood samples
    B. The skin temperature control should be maintained at 37° C
    C. The site should be changed every 24 hours
    D. The low calibration point is determined with room air

▶ FOOD FOR THOUGHT

63. How would you modify your technique if you had to perform ABG analysis for a patient receiving anticoagulants?

64. What problems may occur as a result of icing ABG samples?

65. Switching probes from one brand of pulse oximeter to another is strongly discouraged. What can happen if you switch probes?

66. Why can you use a capnometer during CPR but not a pulse oximeter?

▶ INFORMATION AGE

Here's a site with a good primer on gas exchange:
www.jcu.edu/biology/RESP1.HTM

The following site compares human gas exchange with that of animals and insects:
www.emc.maricopa.edu/faculty/farabee/BIOBK/BioBookRESPSYS.html

Copyright © 2003, 1999 Mosby, Inc. All rights reserved.

CHAPTER 17

Pulmonary Function Testing

> "Most teachers would continue
> to lecture on navigation while
> the ship is going down."
>
> **James Boren**

Remember when you were little, and blowing out those candles on your birthday cake was an exciting but difficult task? That was your first PFT! (After that it all goes downhill.) If you could blow out the candles, you passed and got your wish. I wish everybody liked PFTs as much as I do, but I admit it is a tough subject. In the last few years lung testing has taken on even greater importance. Multiskilling, assessment-based protocols, increased interest in asthma, disability and legal issues, and a strong focus on credentialing examinations are just a few reasons for the resurgence of interest in the science of diagnosing and quantifying pulmonary disorders.

▶ INITIALLY . . .

A quick glance at the Key Terms in Chapter 17 should leave you breathless with desire (or despair) to know what all those abbreviations mean. It would be pretty difficult to have a conversation with a pulmonary function technologist without speaking in initialisms. Do not pass go until you can match the definition with the abbreviation or symbol.

1. _____ D_L
2. _____ ERV
3. _____ V_T
4. _____ IRV
5. _____ RV
6. _____ TLC
7. _____ VC
8. _____ IC
9. _____ FRC
10. _____ MVV
11. _____ FVC
12. _____ PEFR
13. _____ $FEF_{200-1200}$
14. _____ FEV_1
15. _____ $FEF_{25\%-75\%}$
16. _____ FEV_1/FVC

A. Volume inspired with a normal breath
B. Greatest amount of air you can breathe in 12 to 15 seconds
C. Largest amount of air the lungs can hold
D. Fastest flow rate generated at the very beginning of forced exhalation
E. Milliliters of gas the lung can transfer to the blood
F. Amount of air you can exhale after a maximum inspiration
G. Ratio of volume exhaled in 1 second to total volume exhaled
H. Average expiratory flow during the early part of forced exhalation
I. Amount of air you can inhale after a normal exhalation
J. Amount of air you can inhale after a normal inspiration

Copyright © 2003, 1999 Mosby, Inc. All rights reserved.

K. Air left in the lungs after a maximum exhalation

L. Air left in the lungs after a normal exhalation

M. Amount of air you can forcefully exhale after a maximum inspiration

N. Average expiratory flow during the middle part of forced exhalation

O. Volume of air you can forcefully exhale in 1 second

P. Amount of air you can exhale after a normal exhalation

▶ FIRST THINGS FIRST . . .

As if learning all those initialisms isn't enough, we can't really go on until you put the four lung volumes and four lung capacities into perspective with their normal values in a healthy adult. Use the box I've provided below. *Memorize this information!* It will serve you well on your board exams!

17. Fill in the names and normal values that go with each letter in the box.

Volume/Capacity	Value
A. _____	_____
B. _____	_____
C. _____	_____
D. _____	_____
E. _____	_____
F. _____	_____
G. _____	_____
H. _____	_____

Now see if you can draw the box and fill in the values on a separate sheet of paper without looking. Check your answers. Do this until you have it absolutely wired!

▶ MEET THE OBJECTIVES

Answer the following questions to find out if you have grasped the important points for each area of lung testing.

Copyright © 2003, 1999 Mosby, Inc. All rights reserved.

Lung Volume

Lung volume measurement is an important adjunct to spirometry and helps quantify and determine a diagnosis of restriction or obstruction. Specialized equipment is needed to perform these tests.

18. Which volumes cannot be measured with a spirometer?

19. Which capacities cannot be measured with a spirometer?

20. Name the three tests used to determine the volumes and capacities that can't be measured.
    A. _____
    B. _____
    C. _____

21. What is thoracic gas volume?

22. How will volumes or capacities for a patient with air trapping obtained by helium dilution or nitrogen washout differ from those obtained with a body plethysmograph?

23. What effect will an air leak have on the values obtained by helium dilution or nitrogen washout?

Spirometry

Spirometry is the most commonly performed PFT, and vital capacity (or forced vital capacity [FVC]) is the most commonly obtained value. Many types of spirometers exist, but any one that meets the standards and is working properly can be used.

24. What four variables are used to calculate normal values for spirometry?
    A. _____
    B. _____
    C. _____
    D. _____

25. What is meant by an "acceptable" FVC, and what is the minimum number of acceptable FVC maneuvers?
    A. Duration
    B. Variance of two best FVC values
    C. Satisfactory start
    D. Minimum number

Copyright © 2003, 1999 Mosby, Inc. All rights reserved.

26. Which FVC should you report? Which forced expiratory volume in 1 second (FEV_1)?
    A. FVC

    B. FEV_1

27. Which flow rate is the greatest?

28. Which flow rate represents large airways?

29. Which flow rate represents the middle range?

30. A spirometer is considered accurate if the volume is verified to be within what percentage of a known value?

31. What device is used to verify the volume of a spirometer?

32. What is the normal value for maximum voluntary ventilation (MVV)? How is this test performed?

Diffusion

Diffusing capacity (D_L) represents the ability of the lung to transfer gas into the blood. This test requires breathing a special gas mixture.

33. What gas is usually used to measure the ability of the lung to transfer gas to the blood?

Copyright © 2003, 1999 Mosby, Inc. All rights reserved.

34. What other special gas is used in this test? Why?

35. What blood test results are needed to ensure accuracy of diffusion studies?

Interpretation Fundamentals

We'll soon go to our case studies and board exam questions to test your ability to put all the information together. First, see if you have the basic ideas straight.

36. What are the two major categories of pulmonary disease classification? Fill in the chart below to compare the effects of each category. (*Hint:* See Table 17-2.)

	Category	Anatomy	Phase	Pathological Condition	Measure
A.	_____	_____	_____	_____	_____
	_____	_____	_____	_____	_____
B.	_____	_____	_____	_____	_____
	_____	_____	_____	_____	_____

37. Fill in the corresponding percentage of predicted value for the degrees of impairment.

Degree of Impairment	% Predicted Value
A. Normal	_____
B. Mild	_____
C. Moderate	_____
D. Severe	_____

38. The original normal values for pulmonary function were probably based on a 6-ft tall, 20-year-old white man. How are normal values adjusted for nonwhite patients?

Copyright © 2003, 1999 Mosby, Inc. All rights reserved.

39. Compare the FEV_1/FVC ratios you would see in normal, obstructed, and restricted patients.

    A. Normal

    B. Obstructed

    C. Restricted

► CASE STUDIES

Now that you have the information, let's see if you can apply it to the following scenarios. Use the algorithm on p. 423 (Figure 17-17), until you have the basics down pat.

Case 1

Spirometry is performed on Wendy Wheezer, a 24-year-old who reports having a "tight chest" and cough. Simple spirometry shows

Test	Actual	Predicted	% Predicted
FVC	3.2 L	4.0 L	80
FEV_1	1.6 L	3.2 L	50
FEV_1/FVC	50%	70%	

40. Interpretation?

41. What other test should be performed in light of the results and the clinical information?

Case 2

Jim is a 34-year-old respiratory care student. His instructor requires him to undergo PFT as part of a course. Here are the results:

Test	Actual	Predicted	% Predicted
FVC	3.9 L	4.8 L	81
FEV_1	3.1 L	4.1 L	76
FEV_1/FVC	79%	70%	

42. Interpretation?

43. What patient history would be helpful in interpreting these results?

Case 3

Mr. A. B. Stosis is a 60-year-old shipyard worker. He reports dyspnea on exertion and dry cough. Here are his spirometry results:

Copyright © 2003, 1999 Mosby, Inc. All rights reserved.

Test	Actual	Predicted	% Predicted
FVC	2.0 L	4.0 L	50
FEV_1	1.5 L	3.4 L	44
FEV_1/FVC	75%	70%	

44. Interpretation?

45. What additional tests would be helpful?

46. What additional history would be helpful?

Case 4

Miss D. Zeeze arrives at her doctor's office reporting dyspnea on exertion. Spirometry and lung volume results are as follows:

Test	Actual	Predicted	% Predicted
FVC	1.5 L	3.0 L	50
FEV_1	0.75 L	2.5 L	30
FEV_1/FVC	50%	70%	
Total lung capacity (TLC)	2.6 L	3.8 L	68

47. Interpretation?

48. What additional history would be helpful?

Case 5

Paul Puffer is a 70-year-old man with a 100 pack-year smoking history. He reports a dry cough and dyspnea on exertion. Results of lung tests are as follows:

Test	Actual	Predicted	% Predicted
FVC	2.9 L	4.4 L	65
FEV_1	1.3 L	3.7 L	35
FEV_1/FVC	59%	70%	
TLC	6.6 L	5.5 L	120
Functional residual capacity (FRC)	4.5 L	2.2 L	
Residual volume (RV)	3.7 L	1.1 L	
Diffusing capacity of the lung for carbon monoxide (D_{LCO})	16%	25%	64

Copyright © 2003, 1999 Mosby, Inc. All rights reserved.

49. Interpretation (be complete)?

50. What disease state do the lung volumes and history suggest?

51. Why is the vital capacity lower than predicted?

There are lots more case studies in Chapter 17 in your textbook.

▶ WHAT ABOUT THOSE BOARD EXAMS?

I estimate that up to 10% of the Written Registry exam questions are on the subject of PFT! That could be the difference between passing and . . . .

The Entry Level examination matrix says: "Perform and interpret the results of spirometry before and/or after bronchodilator." The matrix goes on to mention performing and/or interpreting FEV_1 and pulmonary function values. I guess you have to know this stuff pretty well! Try your hand at some questions in the good old NBRC style.

52. Which of the following tests would be helpful in assessing the effects of cigarette smoking on the smaller airways?
    A. FVC
    B. FEF_{25-75}
    C. FEV_1
    D. $FEF_{200-1200}$

53. A patient's physician asks you to recommend a pulmonary function test to help assess the effects of a possible tumor in the trachea. Which of the following would you recommend?
    A. Spirometry with volume-time curves
    B. Spirometry before and after bronchodilator use
    C. Lung volume studies via nitrogen washout
    D. Spirometry with flow-volume loops

54. A pulmonary function technologist tests a spirometer by injecting 3.0 L of air from a large-volume syringe. The spirometer measures a result of 2.94 L. Which of the following is true regarding this situation?
    A. The results are within normal limits
    B. The spirometer has a leak
    C. The air was injected too slowly
    D. The BTPS corrections were not made properly

55. Which of the following values could be incorrectly calculated?

Test	Actual	Predicted	% Predicted
FVC	4.4 L	4.8 L	92
FEV_1	3.5 L	4.1 L	80
FEV_1/FVC	80%	70%	
TLC	5.2 L	5.5 L	
FRC	2.0 L	2.4 L	
Expiratory reserve volume (ERV)	1.2 L	1.2 L	
RV	1.0 L	1.2 L	

Copyright © 2003, 1999 Mosby, Inc. All rights reserved.

A. TLC
B. FVC
C. FRC
D. RV

56. Which of the following pulmonary measurements is usually the smallest?
   A. Inspiratory capacity
   B. Vital capacity
   C. Functional residual capacity
   D. Total lung capacity

57. The following results were obtained with spirometry of an adult female smoker with chronic bronchitis. What is the correct interpretation?

Test	Actual	Predicted	% Predicted
FVC	3.9 L	4.8 L	81
FEV_1	3.1 L	4.1 L	76
FEV_1/FVC	79%	70%	

   A. Results indicate a mild diffusion defect
   B. Results are within the normal range
   C. A mixed obstructive/restrictive defect is present
   D. Results show obstructive lung disease

58. What percentage increase in forced spirometric volumes or flow rates after a bronchodilator is administered is the *minimum* indication that reversible airway obstruction is present?
   A. 5%
   B. 10%
   C. 15%
   D. 20%

59. Which of the following can be measured during spirometric testing?
   A. Residual volume
   B. Tidal volume
   C. Total lung capacity
   D. Functional residual capacity

60. An increased total lung capacity combined with a decreased diffusing capacity is strongly indicative of which of the following conditions?
   A. Emphysema
   B. Pneumonia
   C. Pulmonary fibrosis
   D. Pleural effusion

▶ FOOD FOR THOUGHT

Of course there is more! We have just scratched the surface of a complex area of testing. Entire textbooks are devoted to PFT! Here are a few more questions to fill up the corners of your brain.

61. What effect does smoking have on the results of a diffusion test? Why?

62. What lung volume or capacity is useful in predicting normal values for incentive spirometry?

Copyright © 2003, 1999 Mosby, Inc. All rights reserved.

63. Calculate your normal values for FVC, FEV_1, and forced expiratory flow, mid-expiratory phase ($FEF_{25\%-75\%}$) using Figure 17-13 in *Egan's*. Do it using the nomogram and the regression equation.

	FVC	FEV_1	$FEF_{25\%-75\%}$
A. Nomogram		_____	_____
B. Equation		_____	_____

Show your work for the regression equation (be sure to use a calculator!)

Formula _____

Calculation _____

_____

▶ INFORMATION AGE

I have some software my students can use to practice interpretation of pulmonary function values. If you want to go on the Internet, Virtual Hospital gets a gold star for its award-winning PFT site. Practice tests and more at:

www.vh.org/adult/provider/internalmedicine/Spirometry/Spirometry Home.html

Copyright © 2003, 1999 Mosby, Inc. All rights reserved.

Synopsis of Thoracic Imaging

> "In the field of observation, chance favors the prepared mind."
>
> L. Pasteur

Thoracic imaging provides a window for the practitioner to view structures and events inside the chest that we normally cannot see. The chest radiograph is especially important to the RCP for confirming placement of tubes and for diagnosis of conditions such as pneumothorax. You should also understand the usefulness of other common imaging techniques you will encounter in clinical practice, such as computed tomography (CT) and magnetic resonance imaging (MRI).

▶ WORD WIZARD

The chest _____ is commonly called a chest film or chest x-ray. It is one of the most common methods for evaluating the lungs and other structures in the thorax. Air-filled lung tissue appears mostly dark on the film because it is easily penetrated. This quality is called _____. The dense bone tissue of ribs appears white. Dense matter that is not easily penetrated is referred to as having _____. Soft tissues such as blood vessels appear gray because they have an intermediate density. Abnormal conditions can be seen as densities in the wrong location. Accumulation of fluid in the pleural space, or _____, appears white and can obscure the angle where the ribs meet the diaphragm. Alveoli appear white when filled with pus or blood. On a chest film these areas are called pulmonary _____. Air in the pleural space, or _____, is another example of abnormal density. This condition appears as a black area with none of the usual gray markings of blood vessels in the lung tissue.

▶ STEP-BY-STEP

Every primer on chest radiograph interpretation recommends you develop a systematic method for approaching interpretation. I remember to this day making an excellent evaluation of a chest film in the ICU for some students, only to realize I had interpreted the wrong film (still blushing). So my first step is to make sure I am looking at the right film (patient) with the time and date I need. If you are handling an actual film, as opposed to a digitized one, make sure it is placed on the viewer correctly. The "left" side of the film (usually where the heart is) should be facing your right hand side. As if the patient were standing facing you! A marker is normally placed on the film to indicate the left side.

Copyright © 2003, 1999 Mosby, Inc. All rights reserved.

1. What structures offer clues to help identify whether the patient is straight or rotated?

2. What appearance in the lung fields suggests overexposure of the chest film?

3. What appearance of the vertebral bodies suggests underexposure?

4. What effect does underexposure have on the appearance of lung tissue?

5. Systematic observation divides the chest anatomy into what three areas?
   A. _____
   B. _____
   C. _____

6. The pleura appear at the edge of the chest wall (although the pleura themselves usually are difficult to see). What are the two major pleural abnormalities detected on the chest film?
   A. _____
   B. _____

7. After trauma, you should examine the ribs for what abnormality?

8. Why is lung tissue difficult to evaluate?

9. What is the maximum size of the heart shadow on a posteroanterior (PA) projection?

10. What important muscle of ventilation should be evaluated in the chest film?

Copyright © 2003, 1999 Mosby, Inc. All rights reserved.

▶ IDENTIFYING ABNORMALITIES

The second part of Chapter 18 covers evaluation of abnormalities in the three major anatomic portions on chest images. After you read the material, answer the following questions that highlight the important points.

Evaluation of the Pleura

11. What is the costophrenic angle?

12. What sign will help you recognize the presence of fluid in the pleural space? Describe this sign.

13. What view is most sensitive for detecting pleural fluid? How is the patient positioned to obtain this view?

14. When is sonography (ultrasound) indicated in the evaluation of pleural abnormalities?

15. What other imaging procedure may be helpful?

16. Air in the pleural space is always abnormal. Name the three common causes of this condition.
    A. _____
    B. _____
    C. _____

17. What breathing maneuver will help identify a small pneumothorax on a chest film?

18. Tension pneumothorax is immediately life-threatening. Name at least two x-ray signs of tension pneumothorax.
    A. _____
    _____
    B. _____
    _____

Copyright © 2003, 1999 Mosby, Inc. All rights reserved.

19. What is the management of tension pneumothorax?

Evaluation of Lung Parenchyma

20. What are the two components of the lung parenchyma?
    A. _____
    B. _____

21. How will alveolar infiltrates appear on the chest film?

22. What is the difference between the radiographic appearance of pneumonia and that of pulmonary hemorrhage?

23. What causes airways to become visible, and what is this sign called?

24. Honeycombing, nodules, and volume loss are all x-ray hallmarks of what type of lung disorder?

25. Describe the silhouette sign. Discuss the difference between a right lower and right middle lobe infiltrate as seen on a chest film.

26. List three important indirect signs of volume loss, or atelectasis, seen on the chest radiograph.
    A. _____
    B. _____
    C. _____

27. You can count on your ribs to tell you about lung volumes. In the following chart, fill in the number of anterior ribs you would see above the diaphragm according to the degree of lung inflation.

	Lung Volume	Anterior Ribs
A.	Poor inspiration	_____
B.	Good effort	_____
C.	Hyperinflation	_____

Copyright © 2003, 1999 Mosby, Inc. All rights reserved.

28. Ribs aren't the only way to assess COPD with hyperinflation. List the two primary and three secondary x-ray signs of emphysema.
    A. Primary
       1. _____
       2. _____
    B. Secondary
       1. _____
       2. _____
       3. _____

29. Compare the sensitivity of chest radiography with that of CT for detection of obstructive airway disease.

Catheters, Lines, and Tubes

30. The endotracheal tube is made of soft plastic. Why is the chest film useful in ascertaining correct tube position after intubation?

31. Where is the distal tip of an ideally placed endotracheal tube in relation to the carina?

32. Where will the endotracheal tube usually end up if it is placed too far into the trachea?

33. What pulmonary complication can be identified on a chest film when a central venous pressure catheter is placed through the subclavian vein?

34. A pulmonary arterial catheter (Swan-Ganz) that is seen to extend too far into the lung fields of a chest x-ray may have what unwanted results?

The Mediastinum

35. Where does the mediastinum lie within the chest?

Copyright © 2003, 1999 Mosby, Inc. All rights reserved.

36. What imaging technique is most favored for assessing mediastinal masses?

39. What physical assessments could confirm the information in the chest film?

► CASE STUDIES

Case 1

You are asked to perform postural drainage and clapping on Jane Dough, a patient with a large right-sided pulmonary infiltrate. Evaluation of the chest radiograph shows a patchy white density with air bronchograms in the right lung. The right border of the heart is visible in the film.

37. On the basis of your knowledge of the silhouette sign, in which lobe is the infiltrate located?

38. What diagnosis does the presence of air bronchograms suggest?

Case 2

Grandpa Miller arrives in the emergency department with acute exacerbation of long-standing COPD. A decision is made to intubate him. It is difficult to auscultate breath sounds, and chest movement is minimal; however, your impression is that breath sounds are more diminished on the left. A chest x-ray shows the tip of the endotracheal tube 1 cm above the carina. The left lung field is slightly smaller than the right. Both diaphragms appear flat, and you are able to count eight anterior ribs above the diaphragms.

40. Where should the tip of the tube be in relation to the carina?

41. With regard to the endotracheal tube, what action should you take?

Copyright © 2003, 1999 Mosby, Inc. All rights reserved.

42. What is the significance of the flattened diaphragms and number of ribs seen above the diaphragm?

3. Position of the diaphragm
4. Presence of hyperinflation
5. Presence of pleural fluid
6. Presence of pulmonary infiltrates
7. Position of chest tubes and pulmonary arterial catheters

You will also be asked to "review the lateral neck radiograph to determine"

1. Presence of epiglottitis and subglottic edema
2. Presence of foreign bodies
3. Presence of airway narrowing

The main difference between the two exams is the difficulty level and depth of the questions. There's more! How many questions will you see on this topic? A review of available practice exams suggests one to three questions on the Certification Examination and as many as five on the Written Registry Examination. Each examination can vary considerably, but you are *guaranteed* to be tested on this material in some way! Try these on for size.

▶ WHAT ABOUT THOSE BOARD EXAMS?

I have carefully reviewed the NBRC examination matrices and come to the conclusion that no one textbook contains all the x-ray information indicated to be part of the examinations! Chapter 18 covers some of this material, and you will find much of the rest in later chapters on lung diseases and pediatric and neonatal respiratory care.

I'll give you some sample questions based on the material covered in this chapter, but you will need to carefully review each examination matrix to identify all the areas you need to know. Both the Certification and the Written Registry examinations require you to "Review the chest radiograph to determine the position of endotracheal or tracheostomy tube." You must also know when to "recommend a chest radiograph" and when to "review existing data in the patient record" such as the "results of chest radiographs." The examinations agree on content, including asking you to "review the chest radiograph to determine"

1. Presence of pneumothorax or subcutaneous air
2. Presence of consolidation or atelectasis

43. A patient has dyspnea and tachycardia after thoracentesis performed to manage pleural effusion. Evaluation of this patient should include
    A. CT
    B. MRI
    C. Chest radiography
    D. Bronchoscopy

44. A pneumothorax would appear on a chest x-ray as
    A. A white area near the lung base
    B. A white area that obscures the costophrenic angle
    C. A dark area without lung markings
    D. A dark area with honeycomb markings

Copyright © 2003, 1999 Mosby, Inc. All rights reserved.

45. The medical record of an intubated patient indicates that the morning chest film shows opacification of the lower right lung field with elevated right diaphragm and a shift of the trachea to the right. These findings suggest
   A. Left-sided pneumothorax
   B. Right-sided pleural effusion
   C. Right main intubation
   D. Right-sided atelectasis

46. On a chest x-ray, the tip of the endotracheal tube for an adult patient should be
   A. 2 cm above the vocal cords
   B. 2 cm above the carina
   C. At the carina
   D. 2 cm below the carina

47. A patient is believed to have a pleural effusion. Which of the following radiographic techniques would be most useful in making a confirmation?
   A. Computed tomography
   B. Decubitus x-ray projection
   C. Magnetic resonance imaging
   D. AP x-ray projection

Chest film interpretation appears as part of the information in questions that are not specifically about x-rays (same as blood gases). *Remember:* Chest x-rays are diagnostic, not therapeutic! If a patient is circling the drain because of tension pneumothorax, the x-ray will not be lifesaving—a chest tube will!

► FOOD FOR THOUGHT

48. Head position is very important in assessing the tip of an endotracheal tube on an x-ray. What happens to the tube if the head moves up (extension) or the chin goes down (flexion)?

► INFORMATION AGE

The National Institutes of Health (NIH) has a nice collection of x-rays: **www.nlm.nih.gov/medlineplus/ency/article/003804.htm**

Virtual Hospital also has lots of x-rays. You can download many of these pictures free and add them to your case studies and reports. Any of the search engines will give you plenty of sites to look at if you're searching for "chest x-rays." Another way to approach this topic is to search for "x-ray" + "emphysema" or whatever disease you are specifically interested in at the time.

Copyright © 2003, 1999 Mosby, Inc. All rights reserved.

CHAPTER 19

Pulmonary Infections

"Captain of the men of death . . ."
Sir William Osler

A hundred years after these words were said, pneumonia is still a leading cause of death. It is the sixth leading cause of death in the United States. There is tremendous clinical interest in ventilator-associated pneumonia right now. Respiratory care practitioners play a key role in research and prevention of this serious complication of life in the ICU. Pneumonia is simple to understand, right? There are only two types: community and nosocomial. Or is it viral and bacterial? Acute and chronic? Typical and atypical? Or perhaps aspiration pneumonia. Read on, dear student, and you will meet "the old man's friend" in its many forms.

▶ CLASSIFICATION AND PATHOGENESIS

1. What does the term *empirical therapy* mean?

2. Give the textbook definition of nosocomial pneumonia.

3. How common is hospital-acquired pneumonia?

4. List two patient populations at special risk of fatal forms of nosocomial pneumonia.
   A. _____
   B. _____

5. Name four diseases acquired by inhalation of infectious particles.
   A. _____
   B. _____
   C. _____
   D. _____

Copyright © 2003, 1999 Mosby, Inc. All rights reserved.

6. List four of the patient populations at risk of aspiration of large volumes of gastric fluid.

   A. _____

   B. _____

   C. _____

   D. _____

7. What group of respiratory patients is at special risk of aspiration of small amounts of colonized secretions?

8. Describe the role of suctioning as a cause of lower respiratory tract inoculation.

9. Give the prime example of reactivation of a latent infection.

▶ MICROBIOLOGY

10. Why is it so important to know which organisms are commonly associated with pneumonia?

11. What organism is most commonly identified as the cause of community-acquired pneumonia?

12. Name two atypical pathogens.

    A. _____

    B. _____

13. Why is no microbiological identification made in so many cases of pneumonia?

14. Name two viruses associated with pneumonia. When are they encountered?

	Virus	*Encountered*
A.	_____	_____
B.	_____	_____

Copyright © 2003, 1999 Mosby, Inc. All rights reserved.

▶ CLINICAL MANIFESTATIONS

15. Patients with community-acquired pneumonia typically have fever and what three respiratory symptoms?
    A. _____
    B. _____
    C. _____

16. What two other common respiratory problems show the same symptoms?
    A. _____
    B. _____

17. What is the classic, typical presentation of community-acquired pneumonia?

18. In intubated patients, nosocomial pneumonia usually shows up as what three changes in the patient's condition?
    A. _____
    B. _____
    C. _____

19. Describe the common x-ray abnormalities associated with pneumonia.

20. Why is the chest film of limited use in diagnosing pneumonia in critically ill patients?

▶ RISK FACTORS

21. Fill in the data for each of the following risk factors for mortality associated with community-acquired pneumonia (see Box 19-1).

Factor	Description
A. Age	_____
B. Sex	_____
C. Vital signs	_____
D. Arterial pH	_____
E. High-risk causes	_____
F. Comorbid illness	_____

22. A number of factors predispose hospital patients to pneumonia, including poor host defenses from underlying illness. Name five such "comorbidities."
    A. _____
    B. _____
    C. _____
    D. _____
    E. _____

23. List four factors that expose the lung to large numbers of microorganisms.
    A. _____
    B. _____
    C. _____
    D. _____

Copyright © 2003, 1999 Mosby, Inc. All rights reserved.

▶ DIAGNOSTIC STUDIES

24. Why is determining the predominant causative organism by sputum Gram stain, culture, and sensitivity so useful in pneumonia patients?

25. Describe the process for collecting a good specimen by expectoration.

26. Describe the satisfactory specimen.

27. Name the organism identified by each of the following specialized tests.

Test	Organism
A. Acid-fast stain	_____
B. Direct fluo-rescent stain	_____
C. Toluidine blue	_____
D. Potassium hydroxide	_____

28. When should HIV testing be recommended in cases of community-acquired pneumonia?

29. When should fiberoptic bronchoscopy be recommended in cases of community-acquired pneumonia?

30. Name four techniques useful in confirming the diagnosis of nosocomial pneumonia.
   A. _____
   B. _____
   C. _____
   D. _____

▶ THERAPY

31. What is the primary medical therapy for pneumonia?

Copyright © 2003, 1999 Mosby, Inc. All rights reserved.

32. What is the agent of choice for managing infection with the following organisms?

Organism	Agent of Choice
A. Pneumococcal infection	_____
B. *Mycoplasma*	_____
C. *Pneumocystis carinii*	_____
D. *Legionella*	_____

33. How long is a typical course of therapy for pneumonia?

34. How long does it take for the x-ray to show resolution of pneumonia in young persons? What about older patients?
    A.

    B.

▶ PREVENTION

35. Immunization is one of the primary strategies for preventing community-acquired pneumonia. Persons are immunized against which two organisms?
    A. _____
    B. _____

36. Identify three groups who should be immunized.
    A. _____
       _____
    B. _____
       _____
    C. _____
       _____

37. Identify the three "probably effective" strategies for prevention of nosocomial pneumonia.
    A. _____
    B. _____
    C. _____

38. What positioning technique is useful in preventing pneumonia in patients?

39. What is the current medication for prophylaxis of gastrointestinal bleeding that may be effective in preventing pneumonia?

▶ CASE STUDIES

Case 1

Abe Drinker is a 55-year-old man who shows up at the clinic with chills, fever, and chest pain on inspiration. Abe is coughing up rusty-colored sputum. He admits to a

Copyright © 2003, 1999 Mosby, Inc. All rights reserved.

history of heavy smoking and regular use of alcoholic beverages. Physical examination reveals heart rate, 125 beats/min; respiratory rate, 30 breaths/min; temperature, 104° F (40° C). He has inspiratory crackles in the right lower lobe. Blood gases reveal a pH, 7.34; $PaCO_2$, 50 mm Hg; PaO_2, 58 mm Hg.

40. What is the most likely diagnosis? Support your answer with clinical signs and symptoms.

41. What immediate treatment should you initiate?

42. Give at least five reasons why Mr. Drinker is at risk of dying of his condition.
    A. _____
    B. _____
    C. _____
    D. _____
    E. _____

Case 2

Mickey Souris is intubated and on a ventilator after a head injury. On the third day after craniotomy, a fever develops. During routine suctioning you notice the secretions are thick and yellow. Breath sounds are decreased in the left lower lobe.

43. What is the role of the artificial airway in development of pneumonia?

44. What test would you recommend at this time to help confirm a diagnosis?

▶ WHAT DOES THE NBRC SAY?

Interestingly enough, the NBRC doesn't say much about pneumonia. Certain lung infections may appear on the boards in the context of treatment and recognition. For example, the use of ribavirin to manage respiratory syncytial virus infection. Or inhaled pentamidine in the treatment of HIV patients with pneumonia. Isolation procedures for tuberculosis patients are a possible area of testing, as are general methods to prevent the spread of infection. You should certainly recognize when a patient has a lung infection, and *pay attention to basic microbiology.*

Copyright © 2003, 1999 Mosby, Inc. All rights reserved.

▶ FOOD FOR THOUGHT

45. What is the role of the respiratory therapist in educating at-risk populations about methods to prevent pneumonia?

46. Have you had your flu shot?

▶ INFORMATION AGE

A great site that I haven't mentioned yet is the American Lung Association (ALA) at: **www.lungusa.org**

The ALA site has lots of good information on infectious diseases such as pneumonia at: **www.lungusa.org/diseases/lungpneumoni.html**

The NIH is a site I've mentioned before that maintains a vast on-line library of information via the US National Library of Medicine. The pneumonia information is at: **www.nlm.nih.gov/medlineplus/pneumonia.html**

Of course you can use this site to look up almost anything that pertains to medicine!

Copyright © 2003, 1999 Mosby, Inc. All rights reserved.

Obstructive Lung Disease

> "Human action can be modified to some extent, but human nature cannot be changed."
>
> Abraham Lincoln

I first learned about obstructive lung disease by watching some of my family members contract it as a consequence of heavy smoking. As a child, I thought that coughing was normal! The conditions discussed in Chapter 20, COPD and asthma, are so common that you probably know someone who has them. (Lots of famous people had COPD. If Honest Abe had Marfan syndrome, he might have had lung disease.) Respiratory care practitioners spend a great deal of time working with patients with COPD. Pay special attention to the information in this chapter as you get to know the "pink puffers" and the "blue bloaters."

▶ SPUTUM POWER

Before we start on the long dark journey into the lungs, take a shot at this COPD crossword puzzle.

Copyright © 2003, 1999 Mosby, Inc. All rights reserved.

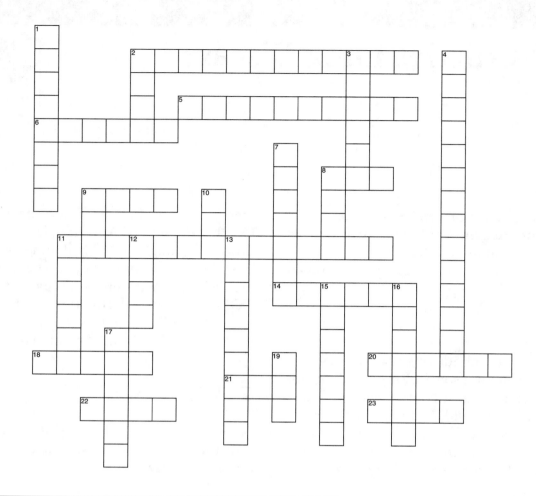

▶ CHRONIC OBSTRUCTIVE PULMONARY DISEASE

If you talk about each type of COPD as if it were "pure emphysema," you would be oversimplifying in many cases. The Venn diagram on Page 442 in *Egan's* demonstrates this nicely. Many patients have signs of mixed disease states. Asthma is classified as separate from COPD, but those with long-standing poorly controlled asthma often have signs of COPD later in life. So although it is convenient to talk about emphysema, chronic bronchitis, and asthma in the clinical setting, you will see patients who have varying degrees of pathology that represent each of these important components of the spectrum of COPD. Remember that most COPD patients have a smoking history, so you will want to explore this issue. (You can calculate pack-years by multiplying packs per day by years smoked.)

Overview

1. Chronic bronchitis is defined as a productive cough for 3 months in 2 consecutive years. What other causes of chronic cough have to be excluded?
   A. _____
   B. _____
   C. _____

Copyright © 2003, 1999 Mosby, Inc. All rights reserved.

ACROSS

1. abdominal smooth muscle contraction in the airways.
5. chronic form shows productive cough for 3 months in 2 consecutive years.
6. the only thing that increases survival of end-stage COPD patients.
8. late asthma response.
9. another four letter word for COPD!
11. results in permanent dilation of the airways.
14. this fibrosis is the most frequently lethal genetic disease of white children.
18. _____ one antitrypsin deficiency, a genetic form of emphysema.
20. where COPD stands as a killer
21. asthma you get when you exercise
22. common bedside test used to manage asthma
23. these puffers really have emphysema

DOWN

1. cystic _____, known in Europe as mucoviscidosis.
2. bloater, or patient with chronic bronchitis.
3. complex lung disease associated with wheezing and airway inflammation
4. drug that opens the airways
7. passed on from parents to children via DNA.
8. abbreviation for surgery that removes part of the emphysematous lung.
9. _____ pulmonale, the heart failure associated with hypoxemia.
10. most common way to deliver drugs to the airway
11. COPD chest shape
12. famous oxygen therapy study that proved increased survival with oxygen.
13. enlargement and destruction of the distal airways and alveoli
15. Stop it
16. the "C " in COPD
17. lung butter
19. early asthma response

---

2. Compare the incidence of chronic bronchitis with that of emphysema.

4. What is the approximate cost of healthcare associated with COPD?

3. What is the difference between the death rates for heart attack and stroke and that for COPD?

Risk Factors and Pathophysiology

5. Besides cigarette smoking (number 1 cause), name two other causes of COPD.
   A. _____
   B. _____

Copyright © 2003, 1999 Mosby, Inc. All rights reserved.

6. Describe the "susceptible smoker."

7. Explain the protease-antiprotease hypothesis of emphysema (briefly, please!).

8. Describe the three mechanisms of airflow obstruction in COPD.
   A. _____
   B. _____
   C. _____

Clinical Signs

9. Name four common symptoms of COPD.
   A. _____
   B. _____
   C. _____
   D. _____

10. Compare the onset of dyspnea in typical cases of COPD with that of α_1-antitrypsin deficiency.

11. What physical change in the chest wall occurs as a result of prolonged hyperinflation?

12. Name three other late signs of COPD.
    A. _____
    B. _____
    C. _____

13. Compare chronic bronchitis, emphysema, and α_1-antitrypsin deficiency in terms of the following features.

Feature	Chronic Bronchitis	Emphysema	α_1-Antitrypsin Deficiency
A. Age at onset	_____	_____	_____
B. Family history	_____	_____	_____
C. Smoking	_____	_____	_____
D. Lung volume	_____	_____	_____
E. D_{LCO}	_____	_____	_____
F. FEV_1/FVC	_____	_____	_____
G. X-ray findings	_____	_____	_____

Management

Egan's lists five general goals of management of COPD. We also need to think about how to avoid complications when the patient has an acute exacerbation of the condition.

Copyright © 2003, 1999 Mosby, Inc. All rights reserved.

14. Why would it be important to differentiate asthma from other forms of COPD?

15. What is the minimum spirometric standard for demonstrating significantly improved airflow after bronchodilator administration?

16. Why is bronchodilator therapy recommended for COPD? What types of drugs are used? What is the effect on decline of lung function and survival?
    A. Why?

    B. What drugs?

C. Outcome

17. Discuss the role of inhaled steroids in COPD.

18. What is the primary effect of theophylline (methylxanthines) on patients with COPD? What serum blood levels are currently recommended to avoid side effects?

19. Name the four important elements of managing an acute exacerbation of COPD due to purulent bronchitis.
    A. _____
    B. _____
    C. _____
    D. _____

20. What is the primary goal of pulmonary rehabilitation?

Copyright © 2003, 1999 Mosby, Inc. All rights reserved.

21. What is the effect of pulmonary rehabilitation programs on survival and pulmonary function?

22. A comprehensive smoking cessation program usually includes what three elements?
   A. _____
   B. _____
   C. _____

23. What is the only therapy for COPD that has been shown to prolong survival?

24. What is the relation between bronchodilator therapy and home oxygen therapy?

25. What two vaccines are recommended for patients with COPD? Which one is given annually?
   A. _____
   B. _____

26. Describe the two surgical options for end-stage COPD. Discuss the outcomes of each of these options.
   A.

   B.

► ASTHMA

"All that wheezes is not asthma."
Anonymous RCPs

Asthma is on the rise, and all of our drugs and technology have not been able to solve the problem. A number of interesting theories exist to explain why industrialized countries are experiencing worse problems than underdeveloped nations. For RCPs, however, the situation is a wonderful opportunity to apply our special expertise to help educate the public and our clients regarding prevention, treatment, and control.

Copyright © 2003, 1999 Mosby, Inc. All rights reserved.

Overview

27. What is the difference between older definitions and the more current view of asthma?

28. What percentage of people in the United States are believed to have asthma?

29. What is the difference between the death rate of asthma and that of other common, treatable conditions?

Etiology and Pathogenesis

30. What are the two primary effects of asthma that result in airflow obstruction?
    A. _____
    B. _____

31. What happens when patients with asthma inhale an allergen to which they are sensitized?

32. Describe the early (EAR) and late (LAR) asthmatic reactions.
    A. EAR

    B. LAR

Clinical Signs

33. What factor plays a key role in suggesting and establishing a diagnosis of asthma?

34. What are the four classic symptoms of asthma?
    A. _____
    B. _____
    C. _____
    D. _____

Copyright © 2003, 1999 Mosby, Inc. All rights reserved.

35. List five conditions that can mimic the wheezing of asthma.

A. _____

B. _____

C. _____

D. _____

E. _____

36. How is reversibility of airflow obstruction demonstrated?

37. Bronchial provocation is the specialized test regimen used to demonstrate obstruction in a patient with suspected asthma who has no symptoms at testing. Name the drug used for this test and what response indicates hyperresponsiveness.

A. Drug

B. Response

38. Describe the role of ABGs in the diagnosis of asthma.

Management

The goal of asthma management is to maintain a high quality of life without symptoms or limitations. The patient should be relatively free of side effects from treatment. To achieve this, the NIH recommends a four-step approach.

39. Complete the chart below to show your understanding of the stepwise approach.

Severity	Symptoms	Long-term Medications
A. 1, Intermittent	_____	_____
B. 2, Mild persistent	_____	_____
C. 3, Moderate persistent	_____	_____
D. 4, Severe persistent	_____	_____

40. Explain control of asthma in terms of the following criteria:

A. Symptoms

Copyright © 2003, 1999 Mosby, Inc. All rights reserved.

B. β$_2$-Agonists

C. Exercise

D. Peak expiratory flow rate (PEFR)

41. Give the criteria and actions for green, yellow, and red peak flow zones.

Zone	PEFR % of Predicted	Treatment/ Action
A. Green	_____	_____
B. Yellow	_____	_____
C. Red	_____	_____

42. Compare the use of inhaled corticosteroids with that of bronchodilators in asthma.

43. Name the two common side effects of inhaled steroids and two ways to control them.
    A. _____
    B. _____
    C. Control/reduce

44. Discuss the use of cromolyn sodium in asthma treatment.
    A. Indications
        1. Adults

        2. Children

    B. Acute attacks

45. When is use of nedocromil indicated?

Copyright © 2003, 1999 Mosby, Inc. All rights reserved.

46. What types of drugs are first-line therapy for all types of acute bronchospasm?

51. Give the criteria for hospital discharge for each of the following:
   A. Pa_{O_2}

47. What is the primary indication for use of salmeterol?

   B. PEFR

   C. Symptoms

48. Describe the use of methylxanthines such as theophylline in the management of asthma.

   D. Discharge medications

49. What is the benefit of using ipratropium in the day-to-day management of asthma?

52. How can you prevent allergic reactions in asthmatic patients?

50. Name three factors you should monitor for a patient hospitalized with acute asthma.
   A. _____
   B. _____
   C. _____

Copyright © 2003, 1999 Mosby, Inc. All rights reserved.

53. Name three common outdoor and indoor allergens.
    A. Outdoor
       1. _____
       2. _____
       3. _____
    B. Indoor
       1. _____
       2. _____
       3. _____

54. What is EIA? List three prophylactic drug treatments.
    A. EIA_____
    B. Prophylaxis
       1. _____
       2. _____
       3. _____

55. Define occupational asthma. What is the most common cause?

56. What is the only way to eliminate occupational asthma once an individual is sensitized?

57. What drug is particularly helpful in the management of cough-variant asthma?

58. List three medications that may be helpful in managing nocturnal asthma.
    A. _____
    B. _____
    C. _____

59. What recommendations would you make to a patient who has aspirin sensitivity?

60. What is the effect of pregnancy on asthmatic women?

61. Discuss the use of asthma medications during pregnancy.

► BRONCHIECTASIS

Bronchiectasis is a condition in which airways are deformed and destroyed by chronic inflammation.

Copyright © 2003, 1999 Mosby, Inc. All rights reserved.

62. What is the clinical hallmark of bronchiectasis?

63. What test is now considered definitive for diagnosing bronchiectasis?

64. List the causes of local and diffuse bronchiectasis.
    A. Local
       1. _____
       2. _____
    B. Diffuse
       1. _____
       2. _____
       3. _____

65. Name the two primary therapies for bronchiectasis.
    A. _____
    B. _____

▶ CASE STUDIES

Case 1

Forest Henry is a 70-year-old man whose chief complaint is dyspnea on exertion. He has a smoking history of 2 packs-per-day for the last 50 years. Mr. Henry has a barrel-shaped chest and very decreased breath sounds. His chest x-ray shows hyperinfla-tion, especially in the apices, flattened diaphragms, and a small heart. He admits to a morning cough but denies significant sputum production.

66. What is the most likely diagnosis?

67. Calculate Mr. Henry's "pack-years."

68. On which factor should you focus to help Mr. Henry control his condition?

Case 2

Billy-Bob Thorn is a 60-year-old man who has smoked a pack of cigarettes per day since he was a teenager. He reports having a chronic productive cough that is producing thick yellow sputum. He is admitted to the medical floor with a fever and shortness of breath. Blood gas analysis reveals pH, 7.35; $Paco_2$, 50 mm Hg; Pao_2, 57 mm Hg. Physical exam shows pedal edema, distended neck veins, and use of accessory muscles of ventilation. The patient has scattered wheezing and rhonchi on auscultation.

Copyright © 2003, 1999 Mosby, Inc. All rights reserved.

69. What type of COPD is most likely in Mr. Thorn's case?

70. What should you do with the sputum the next time the patient coughs productively?

71. What is the immediate respiratory treatment in this case?

72. What other respiratory medications would you recommend?

Case 3

Aaron Defaut is a 44-year-old man with dyspnea on exertion. He is a nonsmoker but drinks wine with his meals. Mr. Defaut has a barrel-shaped chest and very decreased breath sounds. The chest radiograph shows hyperinflation, especially in the bases. History reveals the patient's father and uncle both died of "lung problems."

73. What is the most likely cause of the COPD symptoms? Justify your answer on the basis of the information presented.

74. What treatments are available for this condition?

Case 4

Pierre Poussif is a 15-year-old boy who reports that he cannot catch his breath when he exercises. He states that he coughs a lot, especially in winter. Pierre's breath sounds are clear, and his physical examination findings are unremarkable.

75. What do you suspect is the problem?

Copyright © 2003, 1999 Mosby, Inc. All rights reserved.

76. How could a definitive diagnosis be made?

▶ WHAT DOES THE NBRC SAY?

It will come as no surprise that the board exams place a special emphasis on COPD and asthma. The Clinical Simulation examination matrix states that you will see at least "two problems involving adult patients with COPD." You may also see a pediatric patient with asthma. *All* aspects of treating these patients may be included, from PFT to rehabilitation. Multiple choice exams, such as the Written Registry and Entry Level examinations, do not specifically mention COPD or asthma in the matrices; however, diagnosis and management of these disorders are heavily represented on the tests. Here are some sample questions.

A 20-year-old woman who has a history asthma is brought to the emergency department in respiratory distress. Your assessment of the patient reveals:

pH	7.47
Pa_{CO_2}	33 mm Hg
Pa_{O_2}	72 mm Hg
HCO_3^-	23 mEq/L
Respiratory rate	28 breaths/min
Heart rate	115 beats/min
PEFR	200 L/min

76. Which of the following breath sounds would you expect to hear in this patient?
    A. Inspiratory crackles
    B. Expiratory wheezing
    C. Inspiratory stridor
    D. Expiratory rhonchi

77. The arterial blood gas results indicate the presence of
    A. Acute respiratory alkalosis
    B. Acute metabolic alkalosis
    C. Chronic respiratory acidosis
    D. Acute respiratory acidosis

78. You are asked to initiate oxygen therapy. What would you recommend?
    A. Simple mask at 10 L/min
    B. Nonrebreathing mask at 15 L/min
    C. Nasal cannula at 2 L/min
    D. Air entrainment mask at 50% F_{IO_2}

79. What therapy would you recommend after the oxygen is in place?
    A. Two puffs ipratropium (Atrovent) via MDI
    B. 0.5 mL albuterol (Proventil) via SVN
    C. Intravenous aminophylline (theophylline) administration
    D. Intravenous antibiotics

80. Blood gases are repeated 30 minutes after the oxygen therapy is initiated.

pH	7.42
Pa_{CO_2}	38 mm Hg
Pa_{O_2}	86 mm Hg
HCO_3^-	23 mEq/L
Respiratory rate	24 breaths/min
Heart rate	88 beats/min
PEFR	210 L/min

Which of the following has shown significant improvement according to this information?

Copyright © 2003, 1999 Mosby, Inc. All rights reserved.

A. Compliance
B. Resistance
C. Oxygenation
D. Ventilation

81. Intravenous steroids and repeated doses of bronchodilators have been given. The patient is now receiving 40% oxygen.

pH	7.34
$PaCO_2$	53 mm Hg
PaO_2	74 mm Hg
HCO_3^-	26 mEq/L
Respiratory rate	18 breaths/min
Heart rate	125 beats/min
PEFR	110 L/min

What would you suggest at this point?
A. Increase the FIO_2 to 50%
B. Continuous nebulization of bronchodilators
C. Administration of intravenous bicarbonate
D. Intubation and mechanical ventilation

82. A patient with COPD and CO_2 retention is admitted because of acute exacerbation of disease. The physician requests your suggestion for initiating oxygen therapy. Which of the following would you recommend?
A. Nasal cannula at 6 L/min
B. Air-entrainment mask at 28%
C. Simple mask at 2 L/min
D. Partial rebreathing mask at 8 L/min

83. A PFT performed on a 65-year-old woman indicates airflow obstruction with mild air trapping. The patient is coughing up thick sputum. Which of the following diagnoses is most likely?
A. Cystic fibrosis
B. Pneumonia
C. Pulmonary fibrosis
D. Bronchiectasis

84. A PFT performed on a 56-year-old man with a history of smoking shows increased TLC and RV. The D_{LCO} is reduced. What diagnosis is suggested by these findings?
A. Emphysema
B. Pneumonia
C. Sarcoidosis
D. Pneumoconiosis

85. Spirometry is performed before and after bronchodilator administration. Which of the following indicates a therapeutic response?
   I. FEV_1 increased by 10%
  II. FVC increased by 300 mL
 III. PEFR increased by 50 L/min
A. I only
B. II only
C. I, II only
D. III only

▶ FOOD FOR THOUGHT

Whew, that was a long, hard chapter. You deserve a break. (Nah, just kidding!)

Copyright © 2003, 1999 Mosby, Inc. All rights reserved.

86. Because only 15% of smokers actually show large declines in airflow, why should we encourage all patients to quit smoking?

87. Patients with α_1-antitrypsin deficiency may be eligible for IV augmentation therapy. Discuss the pros and cons of this treatment.

88. Leukotriene inhibitors are now considered useful tools for controlling asthma. How do they work?

▶ INFORMATION AGE

There are hundreds of thousands of references to this topic online.

The ALA is a good place to start.

Chronic bronchitis:
www.lungusa.org/diseases/lungchronic. html
Emphysema:
www.lungusa.org/diseases/lungemphysem. html
Asthma:
www.lungusa.org/asthma/index. html

All of these topics are nicely covered. Lots of clear information, statistics, patient teaching materials, and more. After all, the lung association is the national expert on this subject.

One more thing—asthma. Respiratory care practitioners can hardly know too much about asthma. The National Heart, Lung, and Blood Institute (NHLBI) of the NIH is the definitive reference. You can find the latest version of this cornerstone of asthma therapy at:
www.nhlbi.nih.gov/guidelines/asthma/ asthgdln.htm

Copyright © 2003, 1999 Mosby, Inc. All rights reserved.

Interstitial Lung Disease

> "I do the very best I know how—
> the very best I can; and I mean to keep
> on doing so until the end."
> **Abraham Lincoln**

There are an unbelievable number of interstitial lung diseases (ILDs). Individually they are not very common, but as a group, they represent a significant set of lung disorders. Sooner or later you will encounter some of the members of this broad category of restrictive conditions. Fortunately, there are many common elements in the clinical signs, PFT abnormalities, and management of ILD.

▶ GAME, SET, AND MATCH!

Because there so many new terms related to ILD in Chapter 21, a quick review will help you keep them straight.

1. _____ Asbestosis
2. _____ Corticosteroid
3. _____ Cytotoxic agent
4. _____ Eosinophilic granuloma
5. _____ Hypersensitivity pneumonitis
6. _____ Idiopathic pulmonary fibrosis (IPF)
7. _____ Interstitial lung disease
8. _____ Lupus erythematosus (systemic)
9. _____ Occupational lung disease
10. _____ Pneumoconiosis
11. _____ Rheumatoid arthritis
12. _____ Sarcoidosis
13. _____ Silicosis

A. Formation of scar tissue in the lung without known cause
B. Respiratory disorder characterized by fibrotic infiltrates in the lower lobes
C. Inflammatory reaction provoked by inhalation of organic dusts
D. Chemical lethal to living cells
E. Interstitial lung disease associated with inhalation of small inorganic particles
F. Restrictive disorder associated with pleural abnormalities and lung tumors
G. Disorder of unknown origin that results in formation of epithelioid tubercles
H. Hormones associated with control of body processes
I. Bone growth associated with numerous histiocytes and specific WBCs
J. Serious pulmonary form of inflammatory skin disease
K. Occupational disease that occurs most commonly among coal workers
L. Disorder caused by long-term exposure to sand and stone dust
M. Connective tissue disease associated with inflammation of the joints

Copyright © 2003, 1999 Mosby, Inc. All rights reserved.

► CLINICAL SIGNS AND SYMPTOMS OF INTERSTITIAL LUNG DISEASE

14. Patients with ILD of many different causes usually come to medical attention with which two common problems?
    A. _____
    B. _____

15. Describe the breath sounds usually heard in ILD.

16. What two explanations does *Egan's* give for wheezing heard in patients with ILD?
    A.

    B.

17. Name at least two of the late signs of ILD.
    A. _____
    B. _____

18. Physical signs of underlying connective tissue disease include which four features?
    A. _____
    B. _____
    C. _____
    D. _____

19. Describe the classic radiographic findings in IPF. What are the late-stage findings?

20. Describe the effects of ILD on the following pulmonary function variables.

Variable	Effect of ILD
A. FEV_1	_____
B. FVC	_____
C. FEV_1/FVC	_____
D. D_{LCO}	_____
E. Lung volume	_____
F. PaO_2	_____
G. Compliance	_____

► SPECIFIC TYPES OF INTERSTITIAL LUNG DISEASE

Because there are so many causes of ILD, it will help you to look at the primary groupings and some representative examples of each category.

21. What are the three most common types of occupational ILD?
    A. _____
    B. _____
    C. _____

Copyright © 2003, 1999 Mosby, Inc. All rights reserved.

22. What do these examples have in common?

23. Give at least one specific example of each of the following general categories of drugs associated with the development of ILD.

Category	Example
A. Antibiotic	_____
B. Antiinflammatory	_____
C. Cardiovascular	_____
D. Chemotherapeutic	_____
E. Illegal drugs	_____
F. Miscellaneous agents	_____

24. Why is pulmonary involvement in connective tissue disorders often undetected until late in the course of the disease?

25. Name three common connective disorders associated with lung disease.
    A. _____
    B. _____
    C. _____

26. What is the name for chronic exposure to inhaled organic material that can result in progressive scarring of the lungs?

27. What is the key to identifying the cause of this condition?

28. What is meant by the term *idiopathic*?

29. Let's compare the two idiopathic lung diseases discussed in *Egan's*.

	IPF	Sarcoidosis
A. Patient age	_____	_____
B. Symptoms	_____	_____
C. Treatment	_____	_____
D. Prognosis	_____	_____

Copyright © 2003, 1999 Mosby, Inc. All rights reserved.

► TREATMENT

30. Discuss therapy for hypersensitivity pneumonitis and occupational lung disease.

31. What is the traditional primary medical therapy for ILD?

32. When traditional medicine isn't enough, what type of drugs are used?

33. What condition is managed with colchicine?

34. What is the therapy of last resort for end-stage ILD?

► CASE STUDIES

Case 1

Herb Foin is a 48-year-old man admitted for dyspnea on exertion and a dry cough of unknown origin. The chest radiograph shows bilateral reticulonodular infiltrates. Pulse oximetry shows mild hypoxemia on room air. History reveals that Mr. Foin is a hay farmer.

35. What is the most likely diagnosis?

36. What is the most likely cause of the lung disease? What are some other possible causes?

Case 2

Vincent Kealoha is a retired Pearl Harbor shipyard worker. He states that he has had a cough for some time but recently began expectorating blood. He has bibasilar inspiratory crackles with otherwise clear breath

Copyright © 2003, 1999 Mosby, Inc. All rights reserved.

sounds. A chest radiograph shows reticulonodular infiltrates in both lower lobes. The radiologist notes the presence of a small right-sided pleural effusion, pleural plaques, and pleural fibrosis. Results of PFTs reveal a normal FEV_1, decreased TLC and RV, and decreased D_{LCO}.

37. What is the most likely pulmonary diagnosis?

38. What other information would be helpful in making a determination?

39. What type of disorder is suggested by the PFT results?

► WHAT ABOUT THOSE BOARD EXAMS?

The NBRC thinks you should know your PFT and physical examination findings pretty well! Interstitial lung disease doesn't have a particular category on the boards, but they may be included as side issues to material such as interpreting PFT results.

► FOOD FOR THOUGHT

40. What is the general term for all lung diseases that cause a reduction in lung volume without a reduction in flow rate?

41. *Egan's* lists only three occupations that might cause ILD. I know you can think of at least three other possibilities if you try.
    A. _____
    B. _____
    C. _____

42. What is the therapy of last resort for ILD? When is it likely to be effective?

► INFORMATION AGE

National Jewish Medical & Research Center has a good site at **www.njc.org/a4.html**

The ALA is always a great Internet source for diseases. The site has a section called "Diseases A to Z." Interstitial lung disease is found at **www.lungusa.org/diseases/pulmfibrosis. html**

Copyright © 2003, 1999 Mosby, Inc. All rights reserved.

If you are interested in finding out more about how medications cause lung disease, **pneumotox.com** is an excellent source. For example, antineoplastic agents are well known causes of interstitial disease. I use this site as a handy reference to check on drugs and how they may affect the lungs.

Copyright © 2003, 1999 Mosby, Inc. All rights reserved.

Pleural Diseases

**"Some men dream of doing great things.
Others stay awake and accomplish them"**
Author unknown

Imagine a piece of cake enclosed in plastic wrap. Or if you prefer collapsed lungs, a sandwich covered in that thin, tough clear stuff we use to store food. Thinking about pleura always makes me think of plastic wrap. Like that clingy food protector, a breach in the pleura has important consequences. I hope you get a chance to play with some lungs while you're in training, but if you don't, you can always head for the kitchen.

▶ HEY BUDDY, GOT A MATCH?

Chapter 22 introduces lots of important new terms. Match these pleural puzzlers to their definitions. You're going to need the glossary, but it will be worth it. Many of these words are commonly seen on board exams and in clinical practice.

1. _____ Bronchopleural fistula
2. _____ Chylothorax
3. _____ Empyema
4. _____ Exudative effusion
5. _____ Hemothorax
6. _____ Parietal pleura
7. _____ Pleural effusion
8. _____ Pleurisy
9. _____ Pleurodesis
10. _____ Pneumothorax
11. _____ Primary spontaneous pneumothorax
12. _____ Reexpansion pulmonary edema
13. _____ Secondary spontaneous pneumothorax
14. _____ Tension pneumothorax
15. _____ Thoracentesis
16. _____ Transudative pleural effusion
17. _____ Visceral pleura

A. Pleural effusion high in protein
B. Air leak from the lung to the pleural space
C. Membrane covering the surface of the chest wall
D. Pleural fluid rich with triglycerides from a ruptured thoracic duct
E. Pleural pain
F. Pus-filled pleural effusion
G. Blood in the pleural space
H. Abnormal collection of fluid in the pleural space
I. Pneumothorax without underlying lung disease
J. Air under pressure in the pleural space
K. Procedure that fuses the pleura to prevent pneumothorax
L. Air in the pleural space
M. Condition that occurs when the lung is rapidly inflated after compression by pleural fluid
N. Pneumothorax that occurs with underlying lung disease
O. Low-protein effusion caused by CHF or cirrhosis

Copyright © 2003, 1999 Mosby, Inc. All rights reserved.

P. Chest wall puncture for diagnostic or therapeutic purposes

Q. Membrane that lines the lung surface

▶ THE PLEURAL SPACE

18. How is the pleura of the American buffalo different from that of humans? What is the clinical significance for the buffalo, and when are humans in the same situation?

19. Describe the so-called pleural space.

20. What is normal intrapleural pressure, and what effect does this have on fluid movement?

21. Explain why pleural pressure is different at the apex and the base of the lung.

▶ PLEURAL EFFUSIONS

22. Give a brief explanation of how each of the following conditions can cause transudative pleural effusions.

Condition	Mechanism
A. CHF	_____
	_____
B. Hypoalbu-minemia	_____
C. Liver disease	_____
	_____
D. Lymph obstruction	_____
E. Central venous pressure (CVP) line	_____
	_____

23. What is the most common cause of clinical pleural effusions?

24. What is the general cause of exudative pleural effusions?

Copyright © 2003, 1999 Mosby, Inc. All rights reserved.

25. Give a brief explanation of the cause of the following exudative pleural effusions.

Effusion	*Cause*
A. Parapneumonic	_____ _____
B. Malignant	_____ _____
C. Chylothorax	_____ _____
D. Hemothorax	_____ _____

26. What change in pulmonary function is associated with pleural effusion?

27. In what specific portion of the upright chest radiograph is pleural effusion visualized?

28. Describe the specific type of chest radiograph used to improve visualization of pleural effusions.

29. What type of imaging is the most sensitive for identification of pleural effusions?

30. What are the three major risks of thoracentesis?
    A. _____
    B. _____
    C. _____

31. Identify the purpose of each of the chambers in the three-bottle chest tube drainage system shown on p. 198.
    A. _____
    B. _____
    C. _____

Copyright © 2003, 1999 Mosby, Inc. All rights reserved.

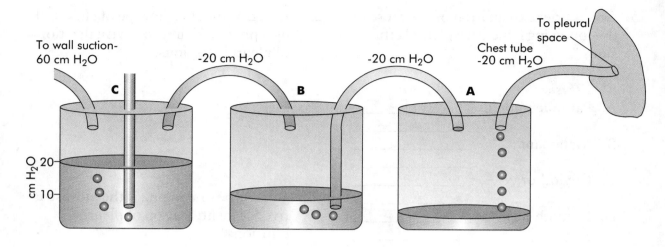

The standard three-bottle system is the basis for all commercial chest tube drainage systems.

▶ PNEUMOTHORAX

32. What two symptoms are common to almost all cases of pneumothorax?
    A. _____
    B. _____

33. What is the most common type of traumatic pneumothorax and how is it treated? Give three examples.

34. Compare blunt and penetrating chest trauma as causes of pneumothorax. How does treatment differ in these two situations?

35. What special technique may be helpful for visualizing pneumothorax in a newborn?

36. Compare the two major types of spontaneous pneumothorax.

37. Tension pneumothorax can be a life-threatening medical emergency.
    A. Definition

Copyright © 2003, 1999 Mosby, Inc. All rights reserved.

B. Radiographic finding

C. Clinical signs

D. Treatment

38. Compare the outcome of early clinical diagnosis and treatment of tension pneumo with that of delayed diagnosis.

39. How does oxygen administration assist in resolution of a pneumothorax?

40. What is BPF? How does mechanical ventilation perpetuate this problem? What special modes of ventilation may be indicated?

► CASE STUDIES

Case 1

Mrs. Ima Dink, a mathematics instructor with a history of CHF, is admitted with pain on inspiration. Her respirations are rapid and shallow. Heart rate is 104 beats/min. The pulse oximeter shows a saturation of 93% on room air. Breath sounds are very decreased on the right side, crackles are present in the left base. Chest wall movement is markedly less on the right. The chest radiograph shows opacification of the right lung with shift of mediastinal structures to the left. Diagnostic percussion reveals a dull note on the right side.

Copyright © 2003, 1999 Mosby, Inc. All rights reserved.

41. What do you think is wrong with Mrs. Dink's right lung? Support your conclusion with at least five pieces of information from the case presentation.
    A. I think Mrs. Dink has
    _____ because
    1.

    2.

    3.

    4.

    5.

42. What would you recommend as the first respiratory intervention?

43. How could this disorder be resolved?

Case 2

Steve Fink, a tall, thin, young male respiratory care instructor, is admitted with pain on inspiration. His respirations are rapid and shallow. Heart rate is 104 beats/min. The pulse oximeter shows a saturation of 93% on room air. Breath sounds are very decreased on the right side, clear in the left base. Chest wall movement is markedly less on the right. The chest radiograph shows a dark area without lung markings on the right side with shift of mediastinal structures to the left. Diagnostic percussion reveals increased resonance on the right side.

Copyright © 2003, 1999 Mosby, Inc. All rights reserved.

44. What do you think is wrong with Fink's right lung? Support your conclusion with at least five pieces of information from the case presentation.
    A. I think Mr. Fink has
    _____ because
    1.

    2.

    3.

    4.

    5.

45. What would you recommend as the first respiratory intervention?

46. How could this disorder be resolved?

▶ WHAT DOES THE NBRC SAY?

Because pneumothorax can be iatrogenic and in mechanically ventilated patients can be life-threatening, you will be expected to know how to recognize and manage this problem. Although there is no special category called *pneumothorax,* you can expect at least three questions related to this topic. In addition, you are expected to understand the causes of pleural effusions and how effusions are diagnosed and managed. Assisting the physician in performing thoracentesis is found in the Certified Respiratory Therapist Entry Level examination and the Written Registry Examination for the Registered Respiratory Therapist credential. Equipment such as chest tubes and drainage systems is found on both exams.

Copyright © 2003, 1999 Mosby, Inc. All rights reserved.

47. Immediately after insertion of a central line through the subclavian vein, an intubated patient becomes dyspneic. The respiratory care practitioner should recommend which of the following diagnostic tests?
   A. 12-Lead ECG
   B. Chest x-ray
   C. ABG
   D. Bedside spirometry

48. The middle bottle of a three-bottle chest drainage system is used as
   A. A water seal
   B. A fluid collection
   C. A means of applying vacuum to the chest
   D. A measurement of improvement of the pneumothorax

49. A chest tube is placed anteriorly between the second and third ribs. The tube is probably intended to manage
   A. Chylothorax
   B. Hemothorax
   C. Transudative pleural effusion
   D. Pneumothorax

50. A patient is believed to have a pleural effusion. Which radiographic position is most appropriate to confirm this diagnosis?
   A. AP chest film
   B. Lateral decubitus chest film
   C. Apical lordotic chest film
   D. PA chest film

51. Thoracentesis is performed, and 1500 mL of fluid is removed from the right side of the chest. Which of the following is likely to occur as a result?
   A. Pulmonary edema in the right lung
   B. Stridor and respiratory distress
   C. Pneumothorax in the right lung
   D. Atelectasis in the right lung

52. All of the following would be useful in differentiating right mainstem intubation from left-sided pneumothorax *except*
   A. Chest x-ray
   B. Diagnostic percussion
   C. Auscultation
   D. Lung compliance measurement

53. After an IPPB treatment, a COPD patient reports sudden severe chest pain. What is the RCP's first priority in this situation?
   A. Notify the physician of the problem
   B. Initiate oxygen therapy
   C. Recommend a chest x-ray
   D. Perform arterial blood gas analysis

54. A patient experiences subcutaneous emphysema after a motor vehicle accident involving multiple rib fractures. What action should the RCP take in this situation?
   A. Perform bedside spirometry
   B. Initiate oxygen therapy
   C. Recommend a chest x-ray
   D. Perform arterial blood gas analysis

Believe me, there are endless variations on these themes. The subject material in Chapter 22 is limited and probably seems pretty straightforward. Be prepared to encounter this topic many times in both the clinical and board examination settings.

Copyright © 2003, 1999 Mosby, Inc. All rights reserved.

► FOOD FOR THOUGHT

55. What is meant by the term *ascites?* Besides causing effusions, how could this condition affect respiratory function?

56. How is thoracentesis modified to prevent reexpansion pulmonary edema?

57. What is subcutaneous emphysema, and what relation does it have to pneumothorax?

► INFORMATION AGE

Let's go back to Virtual Hospital. They have a good section on pleural effusions: **www.vh.org/adult/provider/internalmedicine/PulmonaryCoreCurric/PleuralEffusion/PleuralEffusion.html**

As for the many forms of pneumothorax, you might try **www.vh.org/adult/provider/internalmedicine/PulmonaryCoreCurric/Pneumothorax/Pneumothorax.html,** also at Virtual Hospital.

For something thorough but less glamorous: **www.emedicine.com/EMERG/topic470.htm**

If you just need a simple explanation: **health.yahoo.com/health/encyclopedia/000087/0.html**

Copyright © 2003, 1999 Mosby, Inc. All rights reserved.

Pulmonary Vascular Disease

> "If you ever need a helping hand,
> you'll find one at the end
> of your arm."
>
> **Yiddish Proverb**

The invisible miles of delicate vessels in the lung remain hidden and ignored as they play their vital role in gas exchange and pressure regulation. Then a clot breaks loose and lodges in the pulmonary vascular highway, an accident that frequently has fatal consequences. Rarely recognized, pulmonary embolism (PE) results in thousands of deaths each year in the United States. Chapter 23 reviews the incidence, pathophysiology, and management of pulmonary embolus and pulmonary hypertension, two conditions the RCP will encounter many times in the hospital setting.

▶ WORD POWER

When the pressure inside the lung vessels is elevated, a condition called pulmonary _____ exists. This could be caused by a blood clot that travels to the lung, or pulmonary _____. Other, less common causes include bits of fat or air. If this process results in death of lung tissue, it is called a pulmonary _____. Chronic elevation of pulmonary blood pressure eventually causes a form of right-heart failure known as cor _____.

▶ MEET THE OBJECTIVES

1. Each year in the United States, how many patients are admitted to the hospital for venous thromboembolism?

2. What is the yearly mortality related to thromboembolism?

3. Where do most pulmonary emboli originate?

Copyright © 2003, 1999 Mosby, Inc. All rights reserved.

4. Blood clots to the brain or heart often cause death of the tissue. Why is this uncommon in the lung?

5. Explain how PE increases alveolar dead space.

6. Why does hypoxemia develop in some cases of PE?

7. What is the primary hemodynamic consequence of PE?

8. The combination of what two symptoms should raise the suspicion of PE?
   A. _____
   B. _____

9. What are the three most frequent physical findings associated with PE?
   A. _____
   B. _____
   C. _____

10. What is the incidence of hemoptysis associated with PE?

11. What percentage of patients with PE have a normal ECG?

12. Name the two most common ECG abnormalities associated with PE.
    A. _____
    B. _____

13. How is the chest radiograph helpful in the diagnosis of PE?

14. How helpful are ABGs in ruling out PE? What benefit does ABG analysis provide in these cases?

Copyright © 2003, 1999 Mosby, Inc. All rights reserved.

15. What are the three modalities most widely used for diagnosis of deep venous thrombosis (DVT)?
   A. _____
   B. _____
   C. _____

16. Which test is considered the standard of reference for diagnosis of DVT?

17. What is the test of choice for diagnosis of symptomatic proximal DVT?

18. Because of the high mortality, it is important to make a definitive diagnosis of PE. What two invasive tests are reasonably sensitive and reliable in confirming this diagnosis?
   A. _____
   B. _____

19. What is the relation between the ventilation ($\dot{V}$) and perfusion ($\dot{Q}$) portions of scans in making a high-probability diagnosis of PE?

20. Name two relatively new, noninvasive imaging techniques that show promise in the detection of PE.
   A. _____
   B. _____

21. Prophylaxis for DVT is either pharmacological or mechanical. Give three examples of each.
   A. Pharmacological prophylaxis
      1. _____
      2. _____
      3. _____
   B. Mechanical prophylaxis
      1. _____
      2. _____
      3. _____

22. What is the standard pharmacological therapy for existing thrombosis or embolism? What is the mechanism of action? What are the risks?
   A. Drug

   B. Action

   C. Risks

Copyright © 2003, 1999 Mosby, Inc. All rights reserved.

23. How are thrombolytics different from anticoagulants? Can they be given together?

24. Give three examples of thrombolytic drugs.
    A. _____
    B. _____
    C. _____

25. List the mechanical options available for treatment of management PE.

26. When are vena caval filters indicated?

27. Define PPH.

28. Describe the epidemiology of PPH in terms of age, sex, symptoms, mortality, and genetic factors.
    A. Age

    B. Sex

    C. Genetics

    D. Symptoms

    E. Mortality

29. How is this condition diagnosed?

30. Give three medical therapies for PPH
    A. _____
    B. _____
    C. _____

31. What is the only real cure for PPH?

32. Pulmonary hypertension is a frequent complication of COPD. What percentage of elderly patients with COPD will develop significant pulmonary hypertension?

Copyright © 2003, 1999 Mosby, Inc. All rights reserved.

33. Explain the role of alveolar hypoxia in the development of pulmonary hypertension.

34. What other factors seen in COPD contribute to this condition?

35. What is the only treatment that improves survival in patients with COPD and pulmonary hypertension?

▶ CHAPTER HIGHLIGHTS

36. Venous _____ is an important cause of morbidity and _____ in hospitalized patients.

37. One third of all deaths caused by pulmonary _____ occur within _____ hour(s) of the symptoms.

38. The point of origin of PE is DVT of the _____ extremities or _____ in _____ % of cases.

39. The clinical presentation of PE and DVT is _____.

40. _____ therapy reduces the risk of venous thromboembolism.

41. Management of venous thromboembolism includes anticoagulants such as _____ and _____.

42. Primary pulmonary hypertension is a rare disease that affects _____ patients.

43. Drug treatment of PPH includes _____ and vasodilators such as _____ channel blockers.

▶ CASE STUDIES

Case 1

Mortimer Kent is a 60-year-old man who undergoes total knee replacement. Two days after surgery he reports dyspnea and anxiety. Physical examination reveals a heart rate of 110 beats/min, respiratory rate of 28 breaths/min, blood pressure of 115/80 mm Hg, and SpO_2 of 93% on room air. Breath sounds are clear except for faint inspiratory crackles in both bases.

44. Why is this patient at risk of PE?

Copyright © 2003, 1999 Mosby, Inc. All rights reserved.

45. What additional diagnostic tests would be helpful in ruling out other potential pulmonary problems?

46. What treatment would you provide as an RCP?

47. What medical treatment should be initiated if the diagnosis of PE is confirmed?

► WHAT DOES THE NBRC SAY?

Pulmonary embolism is so nonspecific in clinical presentation that it does not have a separate category in the registry examination matrices. On the other hand, dead space to tidal volume ratio (V_{DS}/V_T) definitely is included. Evaluation of dyspnea, pulmonary hypertension, hypoxemia, and $\dot{V}/\dot{Q}$ scans all are mentioned. Cor pulmonale associated with COPD may be included. Recommending anticoagulants is included in the pharmacology section.

You are expected to be able to make a differential diagnosis between heart attack, pneumothorax, and PE when a patient reports sudden chest pain. I don't see any of this included at the entry level.

48. A patient receiving mechanical ventilation has an increased V_{DS}/V_T ratio. Which of the following disorders could be responsible?
    A. Atelectasis
    B. Pneumonia
    C. Pulmonary embolism
    D. Pleural effusion

49. Which of the following is the most appropriate test for confirming the presence of suspected pulmonary embolism?
    A. Chest x-ray
    B. Pulmonary angiography
    C. Bronchogram
    D. Arterial blood gas

50. A ventilation/perfusion scan reveals a defect in perfusion in the right lower lobe without a corresponding decrease in ventilation. Which of the following is the most probable diagnosis?
    A. Right lower lobe atelectasis
    B. Acute pulmonary embolus
    C. Pneumothorax
    D. Pneumonia

No doubt we'll see more about this subject when we get to hemodynamic monitoring.

Copyright © 2003, 1999 Mosby, Inc. All rights reserved.

► FOOD FOR THOUGHT

51. What is the most common cause of pulmonary hypertension worldwide?

52. Discuss the pros and cons of moving a critically ill ventilator patient to imaging for a $\dot{V}/\dot{Q}$ scan to confirm a suspected diagnosis of PE.

► INFORMATION AGE

The ALA site has some good, basic stuff: **www.lungusa.org/diseases/pphfac.html**

Better you should go to the Pulmonary Hypertension Association site: **www.phassociation.org**

Of special interest to RCPs is information on that site about inhaled prostacyclins for management of pulmonary hypertension.

There are lots of others, of course: **www.phcentral.org** is the site for Pulmonary Hypertension Central, which bills itself as the "definitive Internet resource for pulmonary hypertension."

For information on PE try the NIH site: **www.nlm.nih.gov/medlineplus/ pulmonaryembolism.html**

Copyright © 2003, 1999 Mosby, Inc. All rights reserved.

Acute Lung Injury, Pulmonary Edema, and Multiple System Organ Failure

"To be good is noble, but
to teach others to be good
is nobler—and less trouble."

Mark Twain

1. ALI

Pulmonary edema is one mean clinical problem you will encounter frequently in the emergency department and ICU. Although the symptoms and initial goals of management may be similar, cardiogenic (hydrostatic) and noncardiogenic (nonhydrostatic) pulmonary edema have very different causes and treatments. These are complex syndromes that will challenge you to use every skill and to apply all you've learned. In spite of all we have learned over the years, a fairly high mortality rate still exists, especially for acute respiratory distress syndrome (ARDS).

2. APRV

3. ARDS

▶ ACRONYM SOUP

4. CHF

My favorite acronym is snafu: situation normal, all fouled up. Unfortunately, most medical acronyms aren't all that much fun, but you still need to learn them if you want to be a player. Write out the definitions of Chapter 24's alphabet soup.

Copyright © 2003, 1999 Mosby, Inc. All rights reserved.

5. ECMO

6. ECCO$_2$R

7. GI tract

8. HFV

9. MODS

10. PMNs

11. PEEP

▶ *I always hear people asking me to pass the Ambu (now a brand name) bag: the original AMBU meant air mask bag unit.*

▶ **MEET THE OBJECTIVES**

General Considerations

Let's talk about how to differentiate these two conditions and what causes them.

12. Name two common conditions leading to hydrostatic pulmonary edema for each of the following general categories:

	Category	*Condition*
A.	Cardiac	
	1. _____	_____
	2. _____	_____
B.	Vascular	
	1. _____	_____
	2. _____	_____
C.	Volume overload	
	1. _____	_____
	2. _____	_____

Copyright © 2003, 1999 Mosby, Inc. All rights reserved.

13. List four primary and four secondary risk factors for acute lung injury (ALI)/ARDS.
    A. Primary
        1. _____
        2. _____
        3. _____
        4. _____
    B. Secondary
        1. _____
        2. _____
        3. _____
        4. _____

14. Compare CHF and ARDS in terms of the following criteria for diagnosis.

	CHF	ARDS
A. Chest radiograph		
1. Heart	_____	_____
2. Effusions	_____	_____
3. Infiltrates	_____	_____
B. Pulmonary capillary wedge pressure (PCWP)	_____	_____
C. Broncho-alveolar lavage fluid (BALF)	_____	_____

15. Briefly describe the pathophysiology of hydrostatic pulmonary edema.

16. Briefly describe the pathophysiology of nonhydrostatic pulmonary edema.

17. What five areas must be addressed to avoid *secondary* lung injury in ARDS?
    A. _____
    B. _____
    C. _____
    D. _____
    E. _____

18. What two general approaches are used to maintain adequate tissue oxygen delivery (DO_2) in ARDS?
    A.

    B.

Ventilator Strategies

Most patients with ARDS need artificial ventilatory support. The following questions address the currently accepted methods for providing mechanical ventilation.

19. How does optimal positive end-expiratory pressure (PEEP) differ from PEEP that delivers the best PaO_2? (The NBRC loves this one!)

Copyright © 2003, 1999 Mosby, Inc. All rights reserved.

20. In general, what level of PEEP is considered optimal?

24. What is meant by *permissive hypercapnia*? What is the goal of this ventilator strategy?

21. We can avoid barotrauma by maintaining mean airway pressure at what value?

25. In what two conditions is permissive hypercapnia contraindicated? Why?
A.

22. PEEP should be adjusted to maintain what FIO_2 and PaO_2?

B.

23. Compare tidal volumes delivered in conventional mechanical ventilation versus volumes delivered to ARDS patients (see later, Innovative Strategies).

Innovative Strategies

When the foregoing techniques are not successful, we have to try something different. Each of these methods has had limited success. None is foolproof for every patient. In general, innovative strategies protect patients from lung injury and are especially useful for patients who need high levels of support, such as FIO_2 greater than 0.60.

Copyright © 2003, 1999 Mosby, Inc. All rights reserved.

26. The ARDSNet study showed that mortality is reduced when volume is reduced to what level? (This is so important I've asked you twice!)

27. Describe high-frequency ventilation (HFV).

28. How does inverse-ratio ventilation (IRV) differ from conventional ventilator modes?

29. What is the effect of IRV on survival of ARDS patients?

30. What pharmacologic interventions are needed with IRV?
    A.

B.

31. What are the two ways airway pressure release ventilation (APRV) optimizes ventilation in ARDS patients?
    A.

B.

32. How does APRV compare with IRV in terms of the patient?

33. How can patient positioning be radically altered to improve gas exchange?

34. Both extracorporeal membrane oxygenation (ECMO) and extracorporeal CO_2 removal ($ECCO_2R$) facilitate gas exchange via what type of device?

Copyright © 2003, 1999 Mosby, Inc. All rights reserved.

35. What is the recommendation regarding ECMO and ECCO$_2$R in routine management of ARDS?

36. Exogenous surfactant is helpful in managing infant respiratory distress syndrome and when surfactant is washed out of the adult lung. What is the story on using this agent with ARDS in adults?

37. How is liquid ventilation accomplished?

38. What quality of perfluorocarbon compounds makes them attractive for use in ARDS? What are we waiting for?

39. What type of surfactant is being administered in ARDS clinical trials? How is it being delivered?

40. What is the potential role of nitric oxide (NO) in the management of ARDS?

41. What type of patients would benefit most from NO?

42. What type of abnormal hemoglobinemia is associated with administration of NO?

Pharmacologic Treatments

A variety of drugs have been used to try to turn the tide in ARDS. A few have some limited success.

Copyright © 2003, 1999 Mosby, Inc. All rights reserved.

43. What is the consequence of sudden discontinuation of inhaled NO?

44. What *specific* role do corticosteroids play in the management of ARDS?

► CHAPTER HIGHLIGHTS

45. Congestive heart failure and ARDS are common causes of acute _____ failure that have similar initial _____ presentations.

46. Congestive heart failure–associated pulmonary edema is caused by elevated _____ pressures in the pulmonary _____.

47. Acute respiratory distress syndrome–associated pulmonary edema results from _____ injury to the lungs.

48. It may be necessary to perform _____ or _____ to differentiate CHF from ARDS.

49. Recommendations regarding the management of ARDS have focused on supporting _____ _____ and systemic _____ function until the patient recovers from the underlying illness.

50. Ventilator strategies for patients with ARDS are designed to minimize ventilator _____ lung _____ by using _____, low _____ volumes, and nontoxic levels of inspired _____.

► CASE STUDIES

Case 1

Allen is a 5-foot, 6-inch tall, 143-lb (65 kg) teenager who wouldn't listen when his mom told him not to pop his pimples. Now he is in the ICU with fever of 103° F (39.4° C), blood pressure of 80/50 mm Hg, heart rate of 120 beats/min, and SpO_2 of 88% on 100% oxygen. His PCWP is 14 mm Hg, and cardiac output is 8 L/min. Breath sounds reveal coarse crackles throughout the lungs. Allen is intubated and currently being ventilated with a tidal volume of 800 mL, rate of 14 breaths/min, and PEEP of 0 cm H_2O.

51. What is the most likely diagnosis? Why?

Copyright © 2003, 1999 Mosby, Inc. All rights reserved.

52. With regard to the oxygenation status, what changes would you recommend?

55. What is the most likely diagnosis? What is the underlying cause?

53. With regard to the volume, what changes would you recommend?

56. With regard to oxygenation status, what changes would you recommend?

54. What is the maximum recommended mean airway pressure that should be delivered to this patient to prevent alveolar damage?

▶ WHAT DOES THE NBRC SAY?

You need to be able to differentiate CHF and ARDS on the basis of clinical presentation and diagnostic information. You should be able to maintain oxygenation and determine optimal PEEP. Interpretation of wedge pressure, shunt, and pulmonary edema on radiographs are in the Written Registry matrix. So are IRV, HFV, and APRV. The Clinical Simulation examination matrix specifically mentions CHF as a possible case. ARDS is not specifically mentioned, but it is implied as a possible case.

Case 2

Mabel Frother is a 65-year-old, 143 lb (65 kg) woman who was intubated after arriving in the emergency department with pulmonary edema and severe respiratory distress. Now she is in the ICU with temperature of 97° F (36.1° C), blood pressure of 80/50 mm Hg, heart rate of 120 beats/min, and SpO_2 of 90% on 60% oxygen. Her PCWP is 24 mm Hg, and cardiac output is 3 L/min. Breath sounds reveal coarse crackles throughout the lungs. Mabel is intubated and currently being ventilated with a tidal volume of 700 mL, rate of 14 breaths/min, and PEEP of 10 cm H_2O.

57. Which of the following would be useful in managing elevated shunt in a patient with ARDS who is receiving mechanical ventilation?
   A. Initiating SIMV mode
   B. Initiating PEEP
   C. Increasing the FIO_2
   D. Adding expiratory retard

Copyright © 2003, 1999 Mosby, Inc. All rights reserved.

58. Which of the following indicates the optimal PEEP setting?

PEEP	PaO_2	Cardiac Output
A. 5 cm H_2O	53 mm Hg	4.5 L/min
B. 10 cm H_2O	60 mm Hg	4.3 L/min
C. 15 cm H_2O	74 mm Hg	3.9 L/min
D. 20 cm H_2O	88 mm Hg	3.4 L/min

59. A patient is admitted to the ICU with a diagnosis of pulmonary edema. Which of the following breath sounds is consistent with this diagnosis?
    A. Inspiratory stridor
    B. Inspiratory crackles
    C. Expiratory rhonchi
    D. Pleural friction rub

60. A patient with ARDS being ventilated with the following settings:

Mode	Assist Control
FIO_2	0.80
Rate	10 breaths/min
PEEP	15 cm H_2O
V_T	600 mL
SpO_2	82%

Which of the following would you recommend as possible ways to improve oxygenation?
    I. Change to inverse ratio ventilation
    II. Increase the tidal volume
    III. Attempt prone positioning
    IV. Consider changing to APRV
    A. I, II
    B. I, III, IV
    C. II, III, IV
    D. I, IV

61. Which of the following would provide necessary information regarding fluid management in the care of a critically ill patient with pulmonary edema?
    A. Bedside pulmonary function testing
    B. Intake and output measurements
    C. Daily weights
    D. Pulmonary artery catheter

62. Chest x-ray changes associated with noncardiogenic pulmonary edema include
    I. Pleural effusion
    II. Bilateral infiltrates
    III. Enlarged left ventricle
    A. I, II only
    B. II only
    C. II, III only
    D. I, II, III only

63. Which of the following ventilator techniques have been suggested as useful in managing ARDS that does not respond to conventional therapy?
    I. High-frequency ventilation
    II. Airway pressure release ventilation
    III. Inverse ratio ventilation
    IV. Pressure support ventilation
    A. I, II only
    B. II, III only
    C. I, II, III only
    D. I, II, III, IV

We'll come back to this subject when we get to the chapter on hemodynamic monitoring.

▶ FOOD FOR THOUGHT

Shock lung, Da Nang lung, adult respiratory distress syndrome, wet lung, liver lung, and noncardiogenic pulmonary edema all are names for ARDS. This syndrome has been recognized ever since we began to save trauma victims during modern warfare.

Copyright © 2003, 1999 Mosby, Inc. All rights reserved.

64. What is the recommendation regarding IRV in routine management of ARDS?

65. Is ARDS a homogenous or heterogenous lung condition? Explain.

66. Lower inflection point (LIP or P_{FLEX}) is useful in setting appropriate PEEP and tidal volume levels. What is meant by the term LIP? How is it determined?

▶ INFORMATION AGE

Acute lung injury is a hot topic that requires you to be current in your clinical thinking. The Internet is an ideal tool for staying on top of things. The American Thoracic Society has an important statement available in pdf format at: **www.thoracic.org/adobe/statements/ acute1-5.pdf**

When you are searching for information on this subject use the following terms: Multiple organ dysfunction syndrome ARDS Acute lung injury

You will get lots of results that vary depending on the pathophysiology you want to research.

One really good site on this subject for RCPs is **hedwig.mgh.harvard.edu/ardsnet**

ARDSNet is definitive!

For the patient and family perspective try **www.ards.org**

Finally, the ALA: **www.lungusa.org/diseases/ ards_factsheet.html**

Copyright © 2003, 1999 Mosby, Inc. All rights reserved.

Lung Neoplasms

> "I kissed my first woman and smoked my first cigarette on the same day. I have never had time for tobacco since."
> **Arturo Toscanini**

Respiratory cancer is a popular disease of the rich and famous. John Wayne, Humphrey Bogart, Sigmund Freud—the list goes on and on. Yet there is hardly a more dreaded word in our society than *cancer*. Lung cancer is the most frequently diagnosed cancer in the world. Yet it is relatively easy to avoid.

▶ NEW WORDS

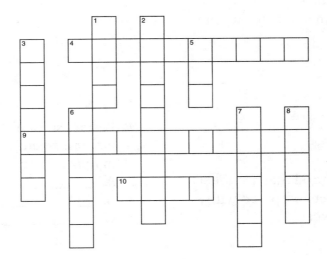

ACROSS

4. process by which tumor cells spread to distant parts of the body
9. Drug treatment to cure cancer; the "N" in the TNM
10. staging system

DOWN

1. small _____ cancer, also called oat _____ cancer
2. treatment of neoplastic growth using gamma rays
3. _____ genic carcinoma—cancer originating in the airway
5. staging system
6. opposite of malignant
7. malignant tissue growth
8. type of nodes where cancer spreads

Copyright © 2003, 1999 Mosby, Inc. All rights reserved.

► MEET THE OBJECTIVES

1. How many cases of bronchogenic carcinoma were newly diagnosed in the United States in 2001? How many cases does the World Health Organization (WHO) estimate worldwide?

   A. _____

   B. _____

2. What percentage of cancer deaths are caused by bronchogenic cancer?

3. Compare the incidence of bronchogenic carcinoma in men with that in women.

4. What is the likelihood that a smoker will get lung cancer compared with that of a nonsmoker?

5. What five smoking factors are related to the risk of development of cancer?

   A. _____

   B. _____

   C. _____

   D. _____

   E. _____

6. How many smokers are there in the United States? What percentage of the total population? Which group of smokers has actually increased? (Which group are you in?)

   A. US smokers

   B. Percentage of population

   C. Increased number of smokers

7. What is another name for passive exposure to smoke?

8. Describe the health risks of passive exposure to smoke.

9. Besides smoking, name the four other major influences linked to an increase in lung cancer.

   A. _____

   B. _____

   C. _____

   D. _____

10. What is meant by a *synergistic relationship* between smoking and the other factors? Give an example.

Copyright © 2003, 1999 Mosby, Inc. All rights reserved.

11. List the four major histopathologic types of bronchogenic carcinoma along with the percentage of cases they represent and a brief description of the cells.

	Type of Cancer	Percentage	Description
A.	_____	_____	_____
	_____	_____	_____
B.	_____	_____	_____
	_____	_____	_____
C.	_____	_____	_____
	_____	_____	_____
D.	_____	_____	_____
	_____	_____	_____

12. What are the two most common sites of metastasis of cancer originating in the lungs?
    A. _____
    B. _____

13. What percentage of patients with bronchogenic lung cancer have no symptoms?

14. Local tumor growth in the central airways can cause many symptoms. Name five that an RCP can easily recognize.
    A. _____
    B. _____
    C. _____
    D. _____
    C. _____

15. Patients with pleural or chest wall involvement typically have which three symptoms?
    A. _____
    B. _____
    C. _____

16. Bronchorrhea may be present with lung cancer. What is bronchorrhea, and what is the presence of this symptom likely to indicate?
    A. _____
    B. _____

17. Explain what is meant by the term *paraneoplastic syndrome.*

18. Give three examples of paraneoplastic syndromes commonly associated with bronchogenic carcinoma.
    A. _____
    B. _____
    C. _____

Diagnosis

19. Name the four common methods for obtaining tissue for lung cancer diagnosis.
    A. _____
    B. _____
    C. _____
    D. _____

Copyright © 2003, 1999 Mosby, Inc. All rights reserved.

20. Why is tumor staging so important?

23. What is the consensus on mass screenings for people at high risk of lung cancer?

21. Explain the meaning of the TNM staging system.
    A. T

Treatment

24. Why is surgical resection the treatment of choice for all non–small cell lung cancers?

    B. N

25. Which patients are not candidates for surgery in terms of staging?

    C. M

26. How are RCPs involved in determining who is a candidate for surgery?

22. How is small cell cancer staged?

Copyright © 2003, 1999 Mosby, Inc. All rights reserved.

27. Which test values suggest a patient may safely (or may not) undergo lobectomy or pneumonectomy?

28. Name two palliative therapeutic modalities.

    A.

    B.

29. What is the choice of therapy for small cell cancer?

30. What is the long-term disease-free survival rate among patients with extensive small cell disease?

► CHAPTER HIGHLIGHTS

31. _____ carcinoma is the leading cause of cancer deaths in the United States.

32. Approximately _____% of all cases of lung cancer are linked to smoking.

33. _____ represents 30% to 35% of all cases of lung cancer and currently is the most common type.

34. The _____ classification groups patients in stages or categories that correlate with _____.

35. _____ cancer is classified in two stages: limited or extensive.

36. The most commonly used modalities of treatment of patients with non–small cell lung cancer are surgical resection, _____, and _____.

37. The most effective way to prevent lung cancer is to prevent _____.

► CASE STUDIES

Chapter 25 has five excellent case studies in the form of Mini-Clinis, so I'm not going to reinvent the wheel. Four of these cases are particularly useful to RCPs.

Copyright © 2003, 1999 Mosby, Inc. All rights reserved.

Pancoast's Tumor

38. Will you be caring for patients with weakness and drooping eyelids? How is this different?

Paraneoplastic Syndrome

39. Confusion and generalized weakness often are signs of what type of serious neurological vascular accident?

Evaluating Surgical Risk

40. Which therapeutic modalities might improve lung function before surgery for lung resection?

No Response to Antibiotics

41. What methods of diagnosis might be useful for patients with copious amounts of clear, frothy sputum?

▶ WHAT DOES THE NBRC SAY?

For once, the NBRC is relatively silent. Hallelujah! Obviously you need to recognize that hemoptysis is an important sign of dysfunction that may relate to cancer or tuberculosis, among other disorders.

▶ FOOD FOR THOUGHT

42. Besides lung cancer, what are the health risks of smoking?

43. With the high incidence and known risk factors for lung cancer, you would expect to see screening techniques. Discuss this issue.

44. What is brachytherapy?

Copyright © 2003, 1999 Mosby, Inc. All rights reserved.

45. What is the DUTY of every respiratory therapist in regard to patients who continue to smoke?

▶ INFORMATION AGE

Here's a good example of how search engines differ. Ask for "lung neoplasms" on Google and you'll get a lot of hits. Try "lung neoplasms" on Teoma and you'll get suggestions for refinement and collections of expert information. I found the following British site useful: **omni.ac.uk/browse/mesh/detail/C002412 1L0024121.html**

Also try Virtual Hospital: **www.vh.org/adult/provider/radiology/Lu ngTumors/TitlePage.html**

And don't forget the ALA: **www.lungusa.org/diseases/lungcanc.html** is only one of many pages on this excellent site.

Copyright © 2003, 1999 Mosby, Inc. All rights reserved.

CHAPTER 26

Other Diseases of the Chest Wall (and Neuromuscular Diseases)

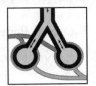

"Expert: Someone who brings confusion to simplicity."
Gregory Nunn

Even if your lungs are normal, diseases that affect the brain, nerves, muscles, and bony thorax can lead to respiratory failure or hypoxemia. There are so many unusual conditions that produce muscular weakness that it can be difficult to keep them all straight. You will do fine if you focus on the general principles that apply to assessment and maintenance of the airway in these complex and often sad cases.

▶ POWER WORDS

I've always wondered whether *neuromuscular* really means you have a strong mind. Let's find out when you try matching these diseases to their definitions.

1. _____ Ankylosing spondylitis
2. _____ Amyotrophic lateral sclerosis
3. _____ Flail chest
4. _____ Guillain-Barré syndrome
5. _____ Lambert-Eaton syndrome
6. _____ Myasthenia gravis
7. _____ Myotonic dystrophy
8. _____ Polymyositis
9. _____ Scoliosis

A. Neuromuscular conduction disorder that particularly affects the face, throat, and respiratory muscles
B. Chronic inflammatory disease that fuses the spine and affected joints
C. Muscle wasting disease characterized by delayed relaxation of contracted groups
D. Degenerative disease of motor neurons characterized by progressive atrophy. Inflammation of muscles caused by a rheumatologic disorder
E. Inflammation of muscles caused by a rheumatological disorder
F. Instability of the chest due to rib fractures exhibiting paradoxic movement on inspiration
G. Idiopathic polyneuritis characterized by ascending weakness
H. Abnormal lateral curvature of the spine that can compromise ventilation
I. Neuromuscular conduction disorder associated with underlying malignant disease

Copyright © 2003, 1999 Mosby, Inc. All rights reserved.

▶ **MEET THE OBJECTIVES**

General Principles

10. Neuromuscular abnormalities affect four major groups of muscles and can result in respiratory problems. Name these four groups.

    A. _____

    B. _____

    C. _____

    D. _____

11. The three best-recognized pulmonary dysfunctions of respiratory muscle weakness are

    A. _____

    B. _____

    C. _____

12. What are the three common complaints of patients with respiratory muscle weakness due to neuromuscular disease?

    A. _____

    B. _____

    C. _____

13. Give two representative diseases that affect each of the following locations in the respiratory system.

Location	*Diseases*
A. Cortex, upper motor	_____
B. Spinal cord	_____
	_____
C. Lower motor neurons	_____
	_____
D. Peripheral nerves	_____
	_____
E. Neuromuscular junction	_____
	_____
F. Muscle tissue	_____
	_____
G. Interstitial lung tissue	_____
	_____

14. Pulmonary function testing of patients with neuromuscular disease and otherwise normal lung tissue demonstrates what type of ventilatory defect?

15. What three specific tests are most useful in monitoring ventilatory function in patients with neuromuscular weakness?

    A. Assess volumes with _____ _____

    B. Assess muscle strength with _____ _____

    C. Assess hypoxemia and hypercapnia with _____

16. How well does PFT assess ability to protect the airway?

17. What signs and symptoms suggest the need for nocturnal oximetry or formal sleep testing?

Copyright © 2003, 1999 Mosby, Inc. All rights reserved.

18. What is the primary therapy for severe respiratory muscle weakness?

19. What problem that may necessitate respiratory therapy is often overlooked?

Specific Neuromuscular Diseases

20. What is myopathic disease? Give two examples of common myopathies.
    A. What is it?

    B. Example 1

    C. Example 2

21. Discuss the role of nocturnal ventilation in the care of patients with myopathic disease.

22. Most cases of myasthenia gravis arise from what abnormality at the cellular level?

23. What general category of drugs is used to manage myasthenia gravis?

24. What surgical treatment may be effective in some cases of myasthenia gravis?

25. List four predisposing factors for Guillain-Barré syndrome (GBS).
    A. _____
    B. _____
    C. _____
    D. _____

26. What percentage of patients with GBS have respiratory muscle compromise?

Copyright © 2003, 1999 Mosby, Inc. All rights reserved.

27. Bilateral interruption of the phrenic nerves that results in diaphragmatic paralysis is seen in what type of injury?

28. Reversible unilateral diaphragmatic paralysis occurs frequently after what commonly performed operation?

29. Describe the chest radiographic presentation of unilateral diaphragmatic paralysis.

30. How is the paralyzed diaphragm visualized during flouroscopy?

31. What is the percentage of new spinal cord injuries in the United States each year, and what percentage of these cases result in quadriplegia?
    A. _____
    B. _____

32. Define the high and middle/low classification of cervical cord lesions.
    A. High

    B. Middle/low

33. Describe the muscle groups affected by each of the following spinal injuries. See the MiniClini.

Level	Muscle Groups
A. C1-2	_____
B. C3-5	_____
C. C4-8	_____
D. T1-12	_____
E. T7-L1	_____

34. What type of breathing is the hallmark sign of significant diaphragmatic weakness?

35. What percentage of patients with C3-5 injury will ultimately become liberated from mechanical ventilation?

Copyright © 2003, 1999 Mosby, Inc. All rights reserved.

36. Both stroke and traumatic brain injury lead to disordered breathing. What is a stroke?

37. What are the two basic types of stroke?
    A. _____
    B. _____

38. Give examples of the effect on the respiratory system of strokes in the following locations in the brain (see Table 26-2 in *Egan's*).

Location	Effect on Respiration
A. Cerebral cortex	_____
	_____
B. Bilateral hemispheric infarct	_____
	_____
	_____
C. Lateral medulla	_____
	_____
D. Midpons	_____
	_____

39. Aside from problems similar to stroke, brain trauma can cause what respiratory "fluid" problems?
    A. _____
    B. _____

Disorders of the Thoracic Cage

40. Describe these two chest wall deformations that often occur together.
    A. Kyphosis

    B. Scoliosis

41. Describe the ventilatory defects and pulmonary function changes associated with severe kyphoscoliosis.
    A. Ventilation

    B. Pulmonary function

42. How is kyphoscoliosis managed in younger patients?

Copyright © 2003, 1999 Mosby, Inc. All rights reserved.

43. Describe the role of nocturnal ventilation in treating patients with kyphoscoliosis.

44. Describe the paradoxic chest motion that is the hallmark of flail chest.

45. Name three other pulmonary injuries frequently associated with flail chest.
    A. _____
    B. _____
    C. _____

46. Regardless of the physiologic mechanisms behind respiratory dysfunction, what are the mainstays of management of flail chest?
    A. _____
    B. _____
    C. _____

▶ CHAPTER HIGHLIGHTS

47. The key components of the respiratory neuromuscular system are the _____, the nerves, the _____ junction, and the _____ of inspiration.

48. Weakness or _____ failure is the most important respiratory dysfunction in many neuromuscular diseases.

49. Neuromuscular diseases can also cause _____ or hypoventilation, sleep _____, aspiration, _____, and pulmonary hypertension.

50. Signs and symptoms of muscle weakness include exertional _____, orthopnea, soft vocalizations, and a weak _____.

51. Pulmonary function tests typically show decreased _____ lung capacity, decreased _____ capacity, and decreased _____ inspiratory pressure.

▶ CASE STUDIES

Case 1

Martha Greene is a 27-year-old woman admitted from her doctor's office after stating she felt fatigue. During her interview, Ms. Greene reports that she becomes weak after any exertion, especially in her arms. She also reports difficulty swallowing. She denies having any recent illness. Vital signs show a normal temperature and slightly increased heart rate and respiration. Inspection reveals that she has drooping eyelids and appears to have little tone in her facial muscles.

52. According to this information, what is the most likely diagnosis?

Copyright © 2003, 1999 Mosby, Inc. All rights reserved.

53. What drug therapy might help to confirm this diagnosis?

54. Why is measurement of inspiratory and expiratory pressures a more sensitive test of muscle function than measurement of vital capacity?

Case 2

Gregory Brown is a 52-year-old man admitted from his doctor's office after reporting fatigue. During his interview, Mr. Brown reports that his feet felt numb yesterday and that his legs were weak when he got up this morning. He went to the doctor because he thought he might be having a stroke. He states that he had the flu about 2 weeks ago. Vital signs show a normal temperature and slightly increased heart rate and respiration.

55. According to this information, what neuromuscular condition is likely?

56. How would analysis of CSF be useful in making a diagnosis?

57. What two treatment strategies have improved outcome in this syndrome?
    A. _____
    B. _____

▶ **WHAT DOES THE NBRC SAY?**

One or two cases on the Clinical Simulation Examination will be devoted to adult patients with neuromuscular or neurologic conditions. Myasthenia gravis, GBS, tetanus, muscular dystrophy, and drug overdose are listed as examples in the matrix. You should be able to recommend or interpret the results of bedside tests such as vital capacity and maximum inspiratory pressure. So while there won't be too many multiple choice questions on neuromuscular diseases, this is a very important part of the testing process. Chest and spinal trauma also are included on your boards. In particular, you should pay attention to the subject of flail chest.

58. A 23-year-old patient with flail chest is transferred to the ICU for observation after a motor vehicle accident. After 2 hours, the patient reports increasing dyspnea, and arterial blood gas analysis is performed with the following results.

    pH   7.27
    $PaCO_2$ 55 mm Hg
    PaO_2 61 mm Hg

Copyright © 2003, 1999 Mosby, Inc. All rights reserved.

What action should the respiratory care practitioner recommend at this time?
A. Place the patient on oxygen therapy
B. Initiate mask CPAP
C. Administer a bronchodilator drug
D. Initiate mechanical ventilation

59. A patient with Guillain-Barré syndrome has had serial vital capacity measurements with the following results.

0900	3.1 L
1100	2.6 L
1300	2.1 L
1500	1.6 L

In regard to these data, what should the respiratory care practitioner recommend?
A. Increase the monitoring to q1h
B. Administer edrophonium chloride (Tensilon)
C. Perform intubation and start mechanical ventilation
D. Continue to evaluate the patient every 2 hours

60. A vital capacity less than what value indicates the need for intubation and ventilation in the care of a patient with acute neuromuscular disease?
A. 30 mL/kg
B. 20 mL/kg
C. 15 mL/kg
D. 10 mL/kg

61. A patient with myasthenia gravis arrives in the emergency department with profound muscle weakness. Administration of which of the following will improve ventilation?
A. Pancuronium
B. Neostigmine
C. Epinephrine
D. Atropine

62. The presence of paradoxic chest motion on inspiration following a motor vehicle accident most likely indicates
A. Flail chest
B. Pulmonary contusion
C. Pneumothorax
D. Hypoxemia

▶ FOOD FOR THOUGHT

63. What is the long-term prognosis for the following conditions?
A. Myasthenia gravis

B. Guillain-Barré syndrome

C. Duchenne's muscular dystrophy

▶ INFORMATION AGE

There are many kinds of neuromuscular and chest wall diseases. The Internet is a fair resource for general information. Dr. Sharma's site has a nice presentation on restrictive lung diseases:

Copyright © 2003, 1999 Mosby, Inc. All rights reserved.

www.ssharma.com/presentations/
restrictive/tsld001.htm

The Internet Handbook of Neurology is interesting:
www.neuropat.dote.hu/nmd.htm

Once you know the specific illness you want to look up, the Internet is an excellent way to get information. For specific diseases such as myasthenia gravis try
www.nlm.nih.gov/medlineplus/
myastheniagravis.html

To students working on a paper or practitioners working with specific patient populations, I highly recommend conducting a web search.

Copyright © 2003, 1999 Mosby, Inc. All rights reserved.

Disorders of Sleep

> "Most people spend their lives going to bed when they're not sleepy and getting up when they are."
> **Cindy Adams**

Does someone you love snore excessively? Whenever I ask that question, hands go up in the audience. Does that mean the snorer has sleep apnea? Have you ever wondered just exactly what you do while you're sleeping? The polysomnography lab is just the place to find out. Many RCPs have found rewarding careers in the sleep or neurodiagnostic lab setting. Another reason RCPs are interested in disorders of sleep are the cardiopulmonary consequences of sleep apnea. Finally, even in the acute care setting, you will be called on to deal with patients who use CPAP or bilevel airway pressure devices to control apnea. Once again, you will find yourself in the position of being the expert on the assessment and equipment involved in managing this not so unusual condition.

▶ ACRONYM-O-PHILIA

These things can be fun if they sound cool, like *scuba*—self-contained underwater breathing apparatus. Too bad most of the medical acronyms are so dull. I think it was all the bad publicity after that pin-index thing. . . . Give the full name of the following acronyms from Chapter 27 (Some of them should be old friends by now!).

1. BiPAP

2. CSA

3. CPAP

4. EDS

5. EEG

6. EPAP

7. IPAP

8. OSA

9. PSG

10. UVPPP

11. UARS

Copyright © 2003, 1999 Mosby, Inc. All rights reserved.

► **MEET THE OBJECTIVES**

12. What is the definition of sleep apnea? What about hypopnea?

13. How does obstructive sleep apnea (OSA) differ from central sleep apnea?

14. What is the estimated incidence of OSA in the adult population?

15. Why does airway closure occur during sleep?

16. Name five cardiopulmonary consequences of uncontrolled OSA.
    A. _____
    B. _____
    C. _____
    D. _____
    E. _____

17. Name four neurobehavioral consequences of uncontrolled OSA.
    A. _____
    B. _____
    C. _____
    D. _____

18. List three factors that predispose a patient to OSA.
    A. _____
    B. _____
    C. _____

19. Describe the five common clinical features seen in many cases of OSA.
    A. _____
    B. _____
    C. _____
    D. _____
    E. _____

20. What is the current standard for making a diagnosis of OSA?

21. An apnea-hypopnea index of what value is consistent with moderate to severe sleep apnea? What is considered normal?

22. What are the three goals of management of OSA?
    A. _____
    B. _____
    C. _____

Copyright © 2003, 1999 Mosby, Inc. All rights reserved.

23. Discuss the behavioral options that should be pursued in the care of all patients with sleep-disordered breathing.

24. Why do you think nocturnal CPAP has become the first-line medical therapy for OSA?

25. How does CPAP work to relieve OSA?

26. Discuss the issue of patient compliance with nasal CPAP therapy.

27. Explain how the titration of BiPAP therapy differs from that of CPAP.

28. Describe five of the common minor side effects of positive pressure therapy. Identify what you can do to help the patient solve these annoying problems.

    A. _____
       _____
    B. _____
       _____
    C. _____
       _____
    D. _____
       _____
    E. _____
       _____

29. What is the role of tracheostomy in the management of sleep apnea?

30. What is the success rate of uvulopalatopharyngoplasty (UPPP), and what is the current recommendation regarding this procedure as therapy for OSA?

▶ CHAPTER HIGHLIGHTS

31. The three types of sleep apnea are obstructive, _____, and _____.

Copyright © 2003, 1999 Mosby, Inc. All rights reserved.

32. The predominant risk factor for airway narrowing or closure during sleep is a _____ or _____ upper airway.

33. The long-term adverse consequences of OSA include poor _____ functioning as well as increased risk of _____ morbidity and mortality.

34. Risk factors for OSA include _____ sex, age greater than _____ years, upper body _____, and habitual _____.

35. The first-line medical therapy for OSA is _____.

36. _____ positive airway pressure therapy may be useful salvage treatment of patients who have difficulty with conventional positive pressure treatments.

37. _____ therapy may be an option for a select group of patients who have undergone extensive upper airway analysis and comply with medical therapy.

► CASE STUDIES

KISS is another one of my favorite acronyms. Keep it simple . . . , and this is simple. No way could I improve on the excellent cases in your textbook.

► WHAT DOES THE NBRC SAY?

The NBRC usually considers CPAP to be a ventilator or freestanding strategy for improving oxygenation, but that is changing.

Nasal CPAP and BiPAP, which is a trademark of a particular company, not a generic term, are included on the Written Registry Examination. Remember that these techniques for increasing airway pressure also are used to help prevent intubation and mechanical ventilation in the acute care setting. The Clinical Simulation matrix does mention obesity-hypoventilation as a potential case. So although this is not a large area of the boards and it is relatively new, some of the information from Chapter 27 is included.

38. A respiratory care practitioner notes in the medical record that a patient is receiving BiPAP therapy with a machine brought from home. Which of the following is the most likely diagnosis?
    A. Pulmonary emphysema
    B. Congestive heart failure
    C. Obstructive sleep apnea
    D. Atrial fibrillation

39. A sleep study shows simultaneous cessation of airflow and respiratory muscle effort. These findings are consistent with
    A. Pulmonary hypertension
    B. Obstructive sleep apnea
    C. Congestive heart failure
    D. Central sleep apnea

40. Which of the following is true regarding BiPAP therapy?
    I. Expiratory pressure is always set above inspiratory pressure
    II. BiPAP units are pneumatically powered
    III. IPAP should be increased until snoring ceases
    A. I, III
    B. II only
    C. II, III
    D. III only

Copyright © 2003, 1999 Mosby, Inc. All rights reserved.

► FOOD FOR THOUGHT

41. What do tennis balls have to do with OSA?

If you want to gain more expertise on this subject, look no further than the April and May 1998 issues of the journal *Respiratory Care*, which are completely devoted to sleep-disordered breathing! Or you can surf on into the . . .

► INFORMATION AGE

The trick here is to get the info you want. Searching for "sleep apnea" will give you a headache, believe me. "Obstructive sleep apnea" will yield better results and so will "sleep disordered breathing" and "polysomnography." Some keywords work better than others.

The American Sleep Apnea Association is a nonprofit organization that maintains a good site:
www.sleepapnea.org

The British site **www.sleepstudy.org/ Index. htm** has lots of useful information including an excellent historical section.

I found lots more, including a good PowerPoint presentation you can download at
www.aasmnet.org/MEDSleep/psgslides. htm

TTFN (ta ta for now)!

Copyright © 2003, 1999 Mosby, Inc. All rights reserved.

Neonatal and Pediatric Disorders

"Any man who hates dogs and babies can't be all bad."

Leo Rosten

There's hardly a more joyous event than bringing new life into the world. Unless you look at it from the perspective of the respiratory therapist. We don't see the healthy babies—only the sick ones. And it's difficult enough rearing children these days without having to deal with health problems. Sometimes I'm surprised that respiratory therapists even have children of their own.

▶ WORDS

Try this matching exercise to test your ability to understand the new terms and acronyms found in Chapter 28.

1. _____ RDS
2. _____ Croup
3. _____ Apnea of prematurity
4. _____ PPHN
5. _____ MAS
6. _____ TTN
7. _____ SIDS
8. _____ Epiglottitis
9. _____ BPD
10. _____ Bronchiolitis

A. Poor clearance of lung fluids (type II RDS)
B. Aspiration of fetal poop
C. Chronic problem from alveolar trauma and oxygen toxicity
D. Life-threatening upper airway infection
E. Virus-induced subglottic swelling
F. Acute infection of the lower airways
G. Leading cause of death among infants younger than 1 year
H. Complex syndrome of newborn hypertension
I. Immature respiratory drive to breathe
J. Surfactant deficiency in preemies

▶ BABY BLUES

11. How many babies in the United States have respiratory distress syndrome (RDS)?

12. What is the primary pathophysiology in infants with RDS?

Copyright © 2003, 1999 Mosby, Inc. All rights reserved.

13. State four clinical signs of RDS.
    A. Respiratory rate
    B. Breathing pattern
    C. Auscultation
    D. Audible sounds

14. How is the definitive diagnosis usually made?

15. What are the three main therapies for RDS?
    A. _____
    B. _____
    C. _____

16. How does the chest radiograph of a baby with transient tachypnea of the newborn (TTN) (type II RDS) differ from that of primary RDS?

17. List two typical respiratory treatments for TTN.
    A. _____
    B. _____

18. Meconium aspiration syndrome (MAS) is usually associated with what fetal event?

19. What age baby usually has MAS?

20. Name the three primary problems in MAS.
    A. _____
    B. _____
    C. _____

21. Immediate treatment of MAS babies is vital. What should you do?
    A. As the head presents

    B. Immediately on delivery

    C. If the condition worsens

Copyright © 2003, 1999 Mosby, Inc. All rights reserved.

22. In some ways, bronchopulmonary dysplasia (BPD) is a result of our efforts to save preterm infants. What are the four events implicated in causing BPD?
    A. _____
    B. _____
    C. _____
    D. _____

23. What is the "best management" of BPD?

24. What is periodic respiration?

25. Describe the two types of drug therapy for apnea of prematurity.

26. Persistent fetal circulation may result in hypertension in the newborn. Name the three types of persistent pulmonary hypertension of the newborn (PPHN) and at least one factor that might have caused the problem.

Type	Factors
A. _____	_____
B. _____	_____
C. _____	_____

27. What is the basic idea behind initial management of PPHN?

28. An infant with profound cyanosis at birth most likely has one of two conditions. Name them.
    A. _____
    B. _____

29. What are the four defects seen in tetralogy of Fallot?
    A. _____
    B. _____
    C. _____
    D. _____

30. Acyanotic heart diseases are also seen in newborns. Patent ductus arteriosus (PDA) is of special interest to RCPs. Describe PDA (not the electronic gadget!). Name two treatments.
    A. Description

    B. Treatment

Copyright © 2003, 1999 Mosby, Inc. All rights reserved.

C. Treatment

► PEDI PROBLEMS

Kids get sick a lot, and they have small airways. The combination of infection and airway problems such as reactive airways and cystic fibrosis makes for many visits to the emergency department.

► SUDDEN INFANT DEATH SYNDROME

Sudden infant death syndrome (SIDS) is the leading cause of death among infants younger than 1 year in the United States, with approximately 7000 deaths each year. The diagnosis is not made until a previously healthy baby dies unexpectedly.

31. What is the cause of SIDS?

32. Describe the typical profile of a baby who dies of SIDS.

33. What sleeping position is strongly linked with SIDS?

34. Identify the four infant characteristics often seen near the time of death.
    A. _____
    B. _____
    C. _____
    D. _____

35. Once an at-risk infant is identified, what can be done to try to prevent SIDS?

► GASTROESOPHAGEAL REFLUX DISEASE

36. What is gastroesophageal reflux disease (GERD)? Name a few of the many respiratory problems this condition can cause.

Copyright © 2003, 1999 Mosby, Inc. All rights reserved.

37. What group of kids usually gets bronchiolitis?

38. One particularly nasty virus is the culprit in many cases of bronchiolitis. What is it?

39. Dyspnea, tachypnea, wheezing, and cough are common in these kids. If the children have to be hospitalized, what respiratory treatments are indicated? Name at least four.
    A. _____
    B. _____
    C. _____
    D. _____

with albuterol in the emergency department has no effect. Vital signs are essentially normal, except for a slight elevation in respiratory rate. The chest radiograph shows mild hyperinflation with no signs of consolidation. Pulse oximetry shows a saturation of 94%.

40. What diagnosis is most likely?

41. How can a diagnosis of respiratory syncytial virus (RSV) infection be ruled out?

42. The physician decides to send mom and baby home. What treatment would you recommend?

▶ CASE STUDIES

Bronchiolitis, croup, epiglottitis, and cystic fibrosis all are serious and relatively common pediatric respiratory disorders that you should be able to recognize and differentiate from each other.

Case 1

A mother brings her previously healthy 1-year-old to the emergency department. She states that her baby had a cold 2 days ago, but he still has a slight fever and has been coughing. Mom became concerned when she heard audible wheezing. A treatment

Case 2

A 3-year-old is brought to the emergency department with respiratory distress and a barking cough. The child has been sick for several days with a low-grade fever and stuffy nose. Examination reveals moderate inspiratory stridor and retractions. The pulse oximeter shows a saturation of 88% on room air. A lateral neck radiograph shows subglottic narrowing with a steeple sign.

Copyright © 2003, 1999 Mosby, Inc. All rights reserved.

43. What is the most likely diagnosis?

47. What is the most likely diagnosis?

44. What aerosolized medication is traditionally delivered?

48. What organism usually is responsible for this condition? How could you confirm?

45. When should you add nebulized budesonide?

49. What is the immediate therapy for this condition? Who should perform the intervention and where?

46. How would you deliver oxygen to this child?

50. What shouldn't be done?

Case 3

A 5-year-old is brought to the emergency department with labored breathing and a high fever. Examination reveals marked inspiratory stridor. The child is listless, and dad says the child has had a sore throat. When you talk to the boy, he responds very quietly with short answers. A lateral neck radiograph shows a thumb sign.

Case 4

Grandma brings her son's 2-year-old in to the clinic because "his breathing just isn't right." She states, "This boy is coughing all the time. Besides, he isn't growing very well, and when I kiss him his skin tastes salty!" (Have I given it away yet?)

Copyright © 2003, 1999 Mosby, Inc. All rights reserved.

51. How would your diagnosis be confirmed?

52. What dietary modifications are needed in cystic fibrosis?

53. Name four respiratory treatments aimed at decreasing airway obstruction.
    A. _____
    B. _____
    C. _____
    D. _____

54. What new drug can be aerosolized to thin the secretions?

Collect perinatal data:

- Maternal history
- Perinatal history
- Apgar score
- Gestational age
- Lecithin/sphingomyelin (L/S) ratio

Recommend procedures:

- Umbilical line
- Transcutaneous monitoring

Inspect the patient:

- Apgar score
- Gestational age
- Retractions
- Nasal flaring

Inspect lateral neck radiograph:

- Epiglottitis
- Subglottic edema
- Foreign bodies

Use equipment:

- Oxygen hoods and tents
- Specialized ventilators-oscillators, high frequency

The Clinical Simulation examination matrix makes it clear that you will have one pediatric and one neonatal problem. They list these cases as examples:

Neonatal
Delivery room management, resuscitation, infant apnea, meconium aspiration, RSD, congenital heart defect

Pediatric
Epiglottitis, croup, bronchiolitis, asthma, cystic fibrosis, foreign body aspiration, toxic substance ingestion, bronchopulmonary dysplasia

▶ WHAT DOES THE NBRC SAY?

The Entry Level examination may ask you a couple of questions related to pediatrics, usually recall questions, but this not the primary proving ground for this area of knowledge. The Registry tests make detailed references to the material in Chapter 28. The examination matrices (all of them) contain these items (just a partial list!):

Copyright © 2003, 1999 Mosby, Inc. All rights reserved.

Try these multiple choice questions on for size.

55. A premature infant is experiencing episodes of apnea and cyanosis. The respiratory therapist should recommend which of the following?
    A. Albuterol
    B. Naloxone hydrochloride (Narcan)
    C. Colfosceril palmitate (Exosurf)
    D. Aminophylline

56. A 5-year-old child arrives in the emergency department with a severe sore throat. The child has inspiratory stridor and muffled phonation. He has a fever of 40° C. His mother states he will not drink anything, so she brought him in. The most likely diagnosis is
    A. Croup
    B. Bronchiolitis
    C. Foreign body aspiration
    D. Epiglottitis

57. Which of the following tests is helpful in establishing a diagnosis of cystic fibrosis?
    A. Sweat chloride
    B. L/S ratio
    C. Apgar score
    D. Pneumogram

58. Which of the following is the most appropriate imaging technique to help confirm a diagnosis of croup?
    A. Computed tomography
    B. PA chest film
    C. Lateral neck radiograph
    D. Bronchogram

59. A 4-year-old child with LTB arrives in the emergency department with moderate stridor and harsh breath sounds. The respiratory therapist should recommend which of the following?
    A. Albuterol
    B. Racemic epinephrine
    C. Immediate intubation
    D. Aminophylline

▶ FOOD FOR THOUGHT

By now you must be thinking about having your tubes tied, or at least using birth control. My students were just asking me, "What's the difference between an infant, baby, child . . . ?" Here are some definitions that aren't in *Egan's*:

Fetus: The unborn offspring from the end of the eighth week after conception (when the major structures have formed) until birth. Up until the eighth week, the developing offspring is called an embryo.

Premature baby: A baby born before 37 weeks of gestation have passed. Historically, the definition of prematurity was 2500 g (about 5½ pounds) or less at birth. The current WHO definition of prematurity is a baby born before 37 weeks of gestation.

Neonate: A newborn baby. A baby who leaves the newborn nursery, goes home, and comes back to the hospital may be put into the pediatric unit.

Postterm baby: A baby born 2 weeks (14 days) or more after the usual 9 months (280 days) of gestation.

Copyright © 2003, 1999 Mosby, Inc. All rights reserved.

Child: A person 6 to 12 years of age. A person 2 to 5 years of age is a preschool-aged child. Sometimes 1 to 8 years is the criterion for a child. Size is important when you're talking about endotracheal tubes and drug dosages, because some children are quite large.

▶ INFORMATION AGE

It's easy enough to look up information about any of these specific conditions on the Internet. Virtual Children's Hospital is a great place to start:
www.vh.org/pediatric

If you need to look up words, you might try the following site. I know I do.
www.medterms.com

Copyright © 2003, 1999 Mosby, Inc. All rights reserved.

CHAPTER 29

Airway Pharmacology

> "All things are poison and nothing is without poison. It is the dose only that makes a thing not a poison."
>
> **Paracelsus**

When the first edition of *Egan's* came out in 1969, only a limited number of drugs were available by inhalation. Most of those medications are no longer used because of the advent of newer, more specific agents with longer action and fewer side effects. New categories of inhaled medicines require the respiratory practitioner to have a strong grasp of pharmacologic principles and the specific indications and actions for these newer tools for managing the airway. You will need to be able to advise physicians, nurses, and patients on methods and options for producing bronchodilation, reducing the inflammatory response, clearing secretions, and managing infection.

▶ BETTER LIVING THROUGH CHEMISTRY

Try this matching exercise to test your ability to understand the new terms found in Chapter 29. (You may have to really dig for some of these—use the chapter, the glossary, and a medical dictionary if necessary.)

1. _____ Indicationu
2. _____ Tolerance
3. _____ Adrenergic
4. _____ Vasopressor
5. _____ Pharmaceutical
6. _____ Muscarinic
7. _____ Pharmacodynamic
8. _____ Side effect
9. _____ Absolute contraindication
10. _____ Leukotriene
11. _____ Mydriasis
12. _____ Agonist
13. _____ Pharmacokinetic
14. _____ Cholinergic
15. _____ Antagonist
16. _____ Tachyphylaxis
17. _____ Onset
18. _____ Peak effect
19. _____ Duration
20. _____ Half-life

A. Length of time to metabolize one-half the drug dosage
B. Drug may not be given for any reason
C. Effect of acetylcholine on smooth muscle
D. Reason for giving a drug to a patient
E. Undesired effect of a drug
F. Drugs that mimic the effect of epinephrine
G. Has receptor affinity and exerts an effect
H. Mimics the effect of acetylcholine
I. Drug that exerts a constricting effect on blood vessels
J. Phase related to route of administration
K. Dilation of the pupil of the eye
L. Phase related to mechanism of action
M. Maximum effect from a drug dosage

Copyright © 2003, 1999 Mosby, Inc. All rights reserved.

N. How long it takes a drug to start working
O. How long a drug effect lasts
P. Increasing dose needed for effect
Q. Has receptor affinity but produces no effect
R. Rapidly developing tolerance
S. Compounds that produce allergic or inflammatory responses
T. Phase related to metabolism of a drug

▶ JUST SAY YES

21. What is the most common route of administration used by RCPs?

22. Name four advantages of this route.
    A. _____
    B. _____
    C. _____
    D. _____

23. Name two disadvantages.
    A. _____
    B. _____

24. How do medications delivered by this route usually end up in the systemic circulation?

25. Describe the two primary divisions of the autonomic nervous system in terms of name, neurotransmitter, and effect on bronchial smooth muscle.

Division
A. Sympathetic
   1. Other name _____
   2. Neurotransmitter _____
   3. Airway muscle effect _____

B. Parasympathetic
   1. Other name _____
   2. Neurotransmitter _____
   3. Airway muscle effect _____

▶ ADRENERGIC BRONCHODILATORS

26. State the three receptors of the sympathetic nervous system and their basic effects.

	Receptor	*Primary Effect*
A.	α	_____
B.	β_1	_____
C.	β_2	_____

27. Give the generic name, brand name, strength, and dose for the following commonly used β-adrenergic bronchodilators.
A. Racemic epinephrine_____
   Brand name _____
   Strength _____
   Dose _____
B. Terbutaline (SC)_____
   Brand name _____
   Strength _____
   Dose _____
   Terbutaline (MDI)_____
   Brand name _____
   Strength _____
   Dose _____

Copyright © 2003, 1999 Mosby, Inc. All rights reserved.

C. Formoterol (DPI)_____
   Brand name _____
   Strength _____
   Dose _____
D. Albuterol (SVN)_____
   Brand name _____
   Strength _____
   Dose _____
   Albuterol (MDI) _____
   Brand name _____
   Strength _____
   Dose _____
E. Bitolterol (SVN)_____
   Brand name _____
   Strength _____
   Dose _____
   Bitolterol (MDI)_____
   Brand name _____
   Strength _____
   Dose _____
F. Pirbuterol (MDI)_____
   Brand name _____
   Strength _____
   Dose _____
G. Salmeterol (MDI)_____
   Brand name _____
   Strength _____
   Dose _____
   Salmeterol (DPI) _____
   Brand name _____
   Strength _____
   Dose _____
H. Epinephrine (SVN) _____
   Brand name _____
   Strength _____
   Dose _____
I. Levalbuterol (SVN)_____
   Brand name _____
   Strength _____
   Dose _____

28. Epinephrine and racemic epinephrine
    are bronchodilators, but these drugs
    are usually administered to achieve
    what effects? Give examples of clinical
    conditions.

	Effect	*Clinical Uses*
A.	_____	_____
B.	_____	_____

29. Discuss the use of salmeterol
    (Serevent) in the management of
    asthma. When should it be used?
    When should it be avoided? What
    patient teaching would be important
    with this drug?

30. It is especially important that you
    know how long it takes for a drug to
    start working, reach its maximum
    effect, and last. Fill in the information
    for the drugs listed below.

Drug	*Onset*	*Peak Effect*	*Duration*
A. Levalbuterol (Xopenex)	_____	_____	_____
B. Epinephrine (microNefrin)	_____	_____	_____
C. Albuterol (Proventil)	_____	_____	_____
D. Salmeterol (Serevent)	_____	_____	_____

31. List the most common side effects of
    bronchodilator drugs.
    A. _____
    B. _____
    C. _____
    D. _____

Copyright © 2003, 1999 Mosby, Inc. All rights reserved.

32. Adverse reactions are more serious but are less frequently seen. List six potential adverse effects you must watch for in patients receiving adrenergic bronchodilators.

   A. _____
   B. _____
   C. _____
   D. _____
   E. _____
   F. _____

33. What should you monitor when administering any drugs by the aerosol route?

34. What specific tests or data can be obtained for monitoring the effects of bronchodilator therapy?

► ANTICHOLINERGIC BRONCHODILATORS

35. Generally, ipratropium is indicated for use in what types of patients?

36. Fill in the blanks to complete your knowledge of ipratropium.

Name	Brand Name	Strength	Dose
Ipratropium bromide			
MDI	_____	_____	_____
SVN	_____	_____	_____

37. Now try this one.

Drug	Onset	Peak Effect	Duration
Ipratropium	_____	_____	_____
Tiotropium	_____	_____	_____

38. What medication is available by MDI with both ipratropium and albuterol? What are the possible advantages and disadvantages of this medication?

39. Describe the side effects and adverse reactions to watch for when administering this drug.

40. Why does *Egan's* recommend that atropine no longer be used by inhalation?

Copyright © 2003, 1999 Mosby, Inc. All rights reserved.

► MUCUS-CONTROLLING AGENTS

41. Describe the two drugs approved for inhalational management of secretion problems in the United States.

Drug	Brand Name	Dose	Indication
A. _____	_____	_____	_____
B. _____	_____	_____	_____

42. Bronchospasm is a common side effect of the administration of mucolytic agents. How would you recommend modifying the therapy to prevent or manage this problem?

43. What types of short- and long-term assessments should you make to monitor the effectiveness of these drugs?

44. How long will it take for inhaled steroids to have a noticeable effect on the symptoms of asthma?

45. What significance does this have in terms of patient education?

46. The most common side effects of inhaled steroids are local ones (as opposed to systemic). Name the four most common problems.
    A. _____
    B. _____
    C. _____
    D. _____

47. Why should reservoir devices always be used with the administration of aerosolized steroids via MDI?

► INHALED CORTICOSTEROIDS

Like bronchodilators, there are a lot of inhaled steroids out on the market. You can expect many of your patients to be receiving these medications. Physicians, patients, and family members have many misconceptions about steroids, including "steroid phobia." Again, it's up to you to be the expert and be able to clearly explain the use of these very important tools in the fight against asthma.

48. Describe the short- and long-term methods used to assess the effectiveness of inhaled steroids.

Copyright © 2003, 1999 Mosby, Inc. All rights reserved.

The NIH 1997 Asthma Education and Prevention Program (NAEPP) guidelines contain definitive information on the use of drug therapy for asthma. You can get a copy of these guidelines from the ALA or your instructors, or download the information from the NIH website (see later, "Information Age" for access to the NAEPP guidelines and the most current update.)

▶ NONSTEROIDAL ANTIASTHMA DRUGS

Drugs that prevent the release of histamine or block the release or effects of other mediators of inflammation are hot items right now. These drugs, whether oral or inhaled, hold tremendous promise for managing asthma and preventing the long-term pulmonary consequences of this increasingly serious condition. The drugs fall into the category of "controllers" rather than "quick relief" drugs such as albuterol.

49. What is believed to be the mode of action of cromolyn sodium?

50. Which two mediator anatagonists are recommended for use in young children? *(Hint:* Look at Table 29-6 in *Egan's)*

51. Which of these mediator anatagonists is available by inhalation?

52. List the chief side effect of each of the following
    A. Cromolyn sodium (Intal)

    B. Nedocromil (Tilade)

    C. Zafirlukast (Accolate)

    D. Zileuton (Zyflo)

    E. Montelukast (Singulair)

▶ MANAGING INFECTION BY THE AEROSOL ROUTE

It should make sense to you that lung infections can be managed with aerosolizing medications. This technique for delivery is limited to very specific situations.

53. What agent may be nebulized to manage *Pneumocystic carinii* pneumonia (PCP) seen in severely immunocompromised patients?

Copyright © 2003, 1999 Mosby, Inc. All rights reserved.

54. Discuss how to determine whether to give this drug by the inhalational route.

55. What special precautions must be taken when administering this medication by aerosol?

56. What are the common undesired respiratory side effects of administration? What modification of therapy would you recommend if side effects were to occur?

57. Although PCP is not a hazard to healthy persons (like you), patients with AIDS often have what other disease that is transmitted by the airborne route?

58. Describe the use of ribavirin in terms of indication, patient population, and special equipment needed for administration.
    A. Indication

    B. Type of patient

    C. Special equipment

59. What other antiinfective agent is approved for aerosol administration? What type of organism is it used against? What special nebulizer is recommended?
    A. Drug

Copyright © 2003, 1999 Mosby, Inc. All rights reserved.

B. Organism

C. Nebulizer

60. Influenza can be fatal to the elderly and those with heart or lung problems. Although vaccination is still the best protection, a new inhaled drug can shorten the course and alleviate symptoms. What is the drug? What is the problem with giving it to asthma and COPD patients?
    A. Drug

    B. Problem

61. Invasive pulmonary fungal infections such as aspergillosis love the lungs of the immunocompromised. Intravenous amphotericin B is the drug of choice. But when poor blood flow limits IV delivery to the lungs, you may consider aerosolizing amphotericin B. Describe a dosing and treatment plan for a patient with this problem.

► CASE STUDIES

Case 1

Wendy Wheezer has asthma. She is admitted to the hospital for the second time in 2 months. She has not been able to get relief and is using her albuterol inhaler frequently.

62. In addition to inhaled β-agonists, steroids are commonly administered to *reduce* inflammation associated with asthma. Name one inhaled steroid and recommend a dose.

Copyright © 2003, 1999 Mosby, Inc. All rights reserved.

63. What device is important to use along with an MDI to prevent deposition of these drugs in the mouth?

64. Why should Wendy rinse her mouth after use of her inhaled steroid?

65. Recommend another drug that can be delivered by MDI as a long-term controller to *prevent release* of inflammatory mediators.

66. What long-acting bronchodilator may help Wendy sleep through the night without being awakened by dyspnea and wheezing?

Case 2

Cystic fibrosis is diagnosed in a 7-year-old white boy. This patient has extremely thick mucus (like glue!). Auscultation reveals scattered wheezing and rhonchi.

67. What drug would you recommend aerosolizing for control of the thick mucus?

68. What other drug should be given to control the wheezing?

Case 3

Bob Bloater is a 67-year-old man with long-standing COPD characterized by chronic bronchitis. He is coughing up copius amounts of very thick white sputum. Bob says his chest feels tight, and he cannot catch his breath. His albuterol inhaler is not providing relief.

69. What bronchodilator is appropriate to add to the therapeutic regimen?

Copyright © 2003, 1999 Mosby, Inc. All rights reserved.

70. What mucolytic can be considered if other means of sputum clearance are ineffective? Why might this drug be counterproductive?

▶ **WHAT ABOUT THOSE BOARD EXAMS?**

Sure enough, those scholastic scoundrels at the NBRC have scattered a number of drug questions strategically throughout the tests. Pharmacology appears in at least six parts of the matrix.

71. A patient with *Pnueumocystis carinii* pneumonia is unable to tolerate oral antibiotics because of gastrointestinal side effects. Which of the following would you recommend?
    A. Aerosolized acetylcysteine (Mucomyst)
    B. Aerosolized albuterol (Proventil)
    C. Aerosolized Dornase alfa (Pulmozyme)
    D. Aerosolized pentamidine iethion-ate (NebuPent)

72. An asthmatic patient presents in the emergency department with dyspnea, hypoxemia, and wheezing. All of the following are appropriate at this time *except*
    A. Administration of oxygen
    B. Nebulized cromolyn sodium (Intal)
    C. Nebulized albuterol (Ventolin)
    D. Measurement of peak expiratory flow rates

73. After extubation, a patient has mild stridor. Which of the following would you recommend at this time?
    A. Administration of oxygen
    B. Aerosolized albuterol (Proventil)
    C. Aerosolized ribavirin (Virazole)
    D. Aerosolized racemic epinephrine (Vaponefrin)

74. After administering a corticosteroid via MDI, the respiratory care practitioner should ask the patient to perform which of the following actions?
    A. Rinse and gargle with water
    B. Deep breathe and cough
    C. Inhale an adrenergic bronchodilator
    D. Inhale via a spacer device

75. The heart rate of a patient receiving an adrenergic bronchodilator rises from 80 to 94 beats/min during the treatment. Which of the following actions is most appropriate?
    A. The respiratory care practitioner should discontinue the therapy
    B. Let the patient rest for 5 minutes and continue therapy
    C. Continue the treatment
    D. Reduce the dosage of the bronchodilator in future treatments

76. A physician calls in an order for bronchodilator therapy for a patient with COPD. The order states ".05 mL of albuterol in 3 mL of normal saline via SVN four times per day." The respiratory care practitioner should
    A. Deliver the treatment as ordered
    B. Recommend substituting ipratropium (Atrovent)
    C. Carefully monitor heart rate during the treatment
    D. Call the doctor to verify the order

Copyright © 2003, 1999 Mosby, Inc. All rights reserved.

▶ FOOD FOR THOUGHT

You might be wondering how you can retain all this drug information. It's not easy! Especially when you might not use many of these medications on a regular basis. One suggestion is a time honored technique. Make drug cards. All you need is some 3 × 5 or 4 × 6 index cards. Write out the following on each card (or type on the computer and glue or tape to the card):

- Generic and brand names of the drug
- Route, such as MDI, oral, small-volume nebulizer (SVN)
- Dose
- Strength
- Adverse reactions and side effects
- Contraindications
- Patient teaching points

77. Besides management of excessively thick mucus, what can acetylcysteine (Mucomyst) be used for?

78. Primatene Mist is a commonly used asthma inhaler that is available without a prescription. What drug is found in this MDI? What are potential problems of patients taking this drug?

▶ INFORMATION AGE

Naturally you can look up any particular drug on the Internet, so that's easy enough. There are other things you can do with the Web. For example, the FDA site is a great place to find out what's happening now. Is tiotropium approved? Is fluticasone plus salmeterol (Advair) safe? Go to **www.fda.gov**

Or maybe you want the 2002 asthma guidelines from the NIH: **www.nhlbi.nih.gov/guidelines/asthma/index.htm**

Pharmacology is always changing, always new. No textbook can keep up to date with the latest information, so your journals and the Internet are the best source. I really appreciate this site: **pneumotox.com**

Pneumtotox.com tells you all about the effects of drugs on the lung. For example, amiodarone is used to manage various cardiac arrythmias. What are the long-term pulmonary problems with this medication?

Copyright © 2003, 1999 Mosby, Inc. All rights reserved.

Airway Management

"When you can't breathe,
nothing else matters."
American Lung Association Motto

Airway management is one of my favorite subjects. It is very satisfying to help patients breathe better in such a dramatic fashion. Although there is no substitute for experience, Chapter 30 helps you learn how to use equipment, tubes, and techniques to deal with airway emergencies. You will want to become an expert in every aspect of this subject so that you can become a skilled, knowledgeable provider and a resource for other healthcare professionals. The chapter is divided into three parts:

• Airway clearance techniques
• Insertion and maintenance of airways
• Special airway management procedures

▶ "THE HALLS ARE ALIVE WITH THE SOUND OF MUCUS . . ."

Patients who can't clear their own secretions are at risk of all kinds of problems, such as increased work of breathing, atelectasis, and lung infections. It's our job to get in there and clean out those airways.

Respiratory care practitioners suction both the upper and lower airways.

1. Oral suctioning alone usually is accomplished with a rigid plastic tube called a tonsil tip. What is the other common name for this device?

2. Why do you need to be careful when you're putting a device in someone's mouth? (*Hint:* Did you ever stick your toothbrush too far into the back of your mouth?)

Endotracheal (ET) suctioning is a vital, but potentially risky procedure. Closely following the rules will greatly reduce your chances of causing an adverse reaction. The AARC Clinical Practice Guideline in *Egan's* gives a good overview of this slimy subject.

Copyright © 2003, 1999 Mosby, Inc. All rights reserved.

Ten Commandments of Endotracheal Suctioning

I. Thou shalt assess thy patient.

II. Thou shalt use the correct vacuum setting.

III. Thou shalt use the correct catheter size.

IV. Thou shalt preoxygenate and hyperinflate thy patient.

V. Thou shalt withdraw 1 to 2 cm before suctioning.

VI. Thou shalt suction on withdrawal only.

VII. Thou shalt limit the duration to 10 to 15 seconds

VIII. Thou shalt reoxygenate and hyperinflate after each attempt.

IX. Thou shalt irrigate only when indicated.

X. Thou shalt monitor thy patient.

3. Describe the cause and how to prevent each of the following complications.

Complication	Cause	Prevention
A. Hypoxemia	_____	_____
B. Cardiac arrhythmia	_____	_____
C. Hypotension	_____	_____
D. Atelectasis	_____	_____
E. Mucosal trauma	_____	_____
F. Increased ICP	_____	_____

4. Discuss the advantages and disadvantages of closed-system multiuse catheters.

A. Advantages

B. Disadvantages

5. What special catheter is used to facilitate entry into the left main bronchus?

6. How should you position a patient for nasotracheal suctioning?

7. What additional supply is needed to prevent trauma during this procedure?

8. What specialized airway is used to facilitate repeated nasal suctioning?

Copyright © 2003, 1999 Mosby, Inc. All rights reserved.

9. What device do you need to include when you want to collect a sputum specimen during suctioning?

► ESTABLISHING THE ARTIFICIAL AIRWAY

Start by learning the parts of the two most important artificial airways used to maintain adequate ventilation.

► TUBE TERMS

_____ tubes are long, semirigid tubes, usually made of _____ chloride or some other type of plastic. A typical ET tube has nine basic parts. The proximal end (sticking out of the mouth) has a standard _____ -mm adaptor. The body of the tube has _____ markings in centimeters. The tube ends in a _____ tip. A port, or slot, cut in the side of the tip is called a _____ eye. This slot helps ensure gas flow if the tip is obstructed. Just above the tip, a _____ is bonded to the tube and can be inflated to seal the airway to prevent aspiration or provide for _____ pressure ventilation. A small filling tube leads to a _____ balloon. This small balloon has a spring-loaded _____ with a connector where a syringe can be attached to allow inflation or deflation. A _____ indicator is embedded in the wall of the tube body to make it easier to see the tube position on a chest radiograph.

Another commonly used tube, inserted through a surgical opening in the trachea, is called a _____ tube. These tubes are also made of plastic, or occasionally metal such as _____. The _____ cannula forms the primary structural unit of the tube. As on an ET tube, a _____ may be attached near the end to seal the airway. A _____ is attached to the proximal end to prevent slippage and provide a means to secure the tube to the neck. Many tubes have a removable _____ cannula with a standard _____-mm adaptor. This cannula can be removed for cleaning. A special device called an _____ has a rounded blunt end and is used to facilitate insertion.

► YOU'RE SO SPECIAL

There are two specialized ET tubes you should know about: double lumen and jet ventilation.

10. What type of lung disease requires the use of a double-lumen ET tube?

These are also called *Carlen's* or *endobronchial tubes*.

11. High-frequency jet ventilation tubes look like conventional tubes with two additional lines:
    A. _____
    B. _____

Copyright © 2003, 1999 Mosby, Inc. All rights reserved.

▶ INTUBATION PROCEDURES

12. What is the preferred route for establishing an emergency tracheal airway?

13. Name the four practitioners who most commonly perform ET intubation.
    A. _____
    B. _____
    C. _____
    D. _____

14. Why is suction equipment needed for intubation?

15. Describe two common troubleshooting procedures used when the laryngoscope doesn't light up properly.

16. How are tube sizes selected for babies?

17. What about adults? How does size differ for men and women?

18. Before insertion, how should the RCP test the tube?

19. How is the head positioned to align the mouth, pharynx, and larynx?

20. What other actions *must be taken* before making any attempt to intubate?

21. How long may you attempt intubation? Why?

Copyright © 2003, 1999 Mosby, Inc. All rights reserved.

22. Name at least two anatomic land-
marks to be visualized before
intubation.

C.

D.

23. Compare the use of the Miller and
Macintosh laryngoscope blades during
the intubation procedure.

25. What is the disadvantage of using
capnographic or colorimetric analysis
of CO_2 to assess intubation in a
cardiac arrest victim?

24. Your textbook describes eight methods
for bedside assessment of correct tube
position. Although none absolutely
confirms position, these methods are
essential assessments to make immediately after the tube is placed. Name at
least four of these methods.
A.

26. What are the two methods used to
absolutely confirm tube placement?
A.

B.

B.

Copyright © 2003, 1999 Mosby, Inc. All rights reserved.

27. Give two examples of clinical situations in which nasotracheal intubation might be preferred over oral intubation.
    A. _____
    B. _____

28. Describe the two techniques of nasal intubation.
    A.

    B.

29. Let's compare oral and nasal intubation. Each has advantages and disadvantages. Place a letter "O" by items that match oral intubation and a letter "N" by items that go with nasal intubation. Refer to Table 30-1 for help.
    A. Avoids epistaxis
       and sinusitis   _____
    B. Greater comfort
       for long-term use   _____
    C. Easier to suction   _____
    D. Larger tube   _____
    E. Greater risk of extubation   _____
    F. Improved oral hygiene   _____
    G. Bronchoscopy more difficult   _____
    H. Increased salivation   _____
    I. Reduced risk of kinking   _____
    J. Decreased laryngeal
       ulceration   _____
    K. Increased risk of sinusitis   _____

► **TRACHEOTOMY**

30. What is the primary indication for tracheotomy?

31. When is tracheotomy the preferred primary route of airway management?

32. Describe the sequence for removing an ET tube during the tracheotomy procedure.

33. Compare percutaneous and traditional surgical tracheostomy in terms of placement.

Copyright © 2003, 1999 Mosby, Inc. All rights reserved.

34. Name at least three advantages of the percutaneous technique over traditional surgical tracheotomy.

A.

B.

C.

► AIRWAY TRAUMA

35. Compare the following laryngeal injuries associated with intubation in terms of symptoms and treatment.
    A. Glottic edema
       Symptoms _____
       Treatment _____
    B. Vocal cord inflammation
       Symptoms _____
       Treatment _____
    C. Laryngeal ulceration
       Symptoms _____
       Treatment _____
    D. Polyp/granuloma
       Symptoms _____
       Treatment _____

E. Vocal cord paralysis
   Symptoms _____
   Treatment _____
F. Laryngeal stenosis
   Symptoms _____
   Treatment _____

36. Name the three most common tracheal lesions.
    A. _____
    B. _____
    C. _____

37. Compare tracheal malacia and tracheal stenosis in terms of cause, pathology, and treatment.
    A. Malacia
       Cause _____
       Pathology _____
       Treatment _____
    B. Stenosis
       Cause _____
       Pathology _____
       Treatment _____

38. Describe tracheoesophageal (TE) fistula in terms of cause, complications, and treatment.

39. Tracheoinnominate fistula is a rare but serious complication. What are the clues and what are the immediate and corrective actions taken? What is the survival rate?

Copyright © 2003, 1999 Mosby, Inc. All rights reserved.

▶ CARE AND FEEDING OF YOUR NEW AIRWAY

Once placement of an artificial airway is successfully completed, the real fun begins. As an RCP you will be expected to secure the airway, maintain adequate humidification, manage secretions, care for the cuff, and troubleshoot problems that arise—some of which are life-threatening.

40. What is the most common material used to secure ET tubes? Tracheostomy tubes?

41. How do flexion and extension of the neck affect tube motion? What is the average distance the tube will move (in centimeters)?

Talk to Me, Baby

42. People with ET tubes can't talk, and they shouldn't try. What device is used to help with communication?

43. What is a "talking" trach? What are some of the problems with these gadgets?

44. A trach can be temporarily closed with a finger (the patient's finger or yours, with a glove of course). A more elegant solution is the Passy Muir valve. What do you need to do with the cuff? How about the ventilator?

Humidity Anyone?

45. What is the worst problem that results from inadequate humidification of the artificial airway?

46. What temperature range must be maintained in a heated humidification system to provide adequate inspired moisture?

Copyright © 2003, 1999 Mosby, Inc. All rights reserved.

47. What device can be used as an alternative to heated humidifiers for short-term humidification of the intubated patient?

Look into Chapter 32 for more details on this soggy subject.

48. State at least four reasons why tracheal airways always increase the risk of infection.
    A. _____
    B. _____
    C. _____
    D. _____

49. Describe three techniques that can be used to decrease the risk of infection.
    A.

    B.

    C.

50. What is the most common cause of airway obstruction in critically ill patients?

▶ CUFF CARE

51. Describe the shape of a modern tube cuff.

52. What is the recommended safe cuff pressure? What is the consequence of elevated cuff pressure?

25 cm H_2O is considered the top number for the board exams!

53. Describe the two alternative cuff inflation techniques.
    A. Minimal occlusive volume (MOV)

Copyright © 2003, 1999 Mosby, Inc. All rights reserved.

B. Minimal leak technique (MLT)

54. What happens to cuff pressures when the tube is too small for the patient's trachea?

55. How is the methylene blue test performed?

▶ TRACH CARE

Respiratory therapists and nursing personnel may share tracheostomy care duties. The tubes require daily care to keep the wound clean and the tube functioning properly.

56. What protective gear do you need when performing trach care?

57. Briefly describe the eight basic steps of tracheostomy care.
A.

B.

C.

D.

E.

Copyright © 2003, 1999 Mosby, Inc. All rights reserved.

F.

G.

H.

Your textbook makes changing a trach tube sound so simple. It can be, or it can be a harrowing experience. The first change often is performed by the surgeon. Be especially careful when

• The neck is thick
• The site is inflamed or infected
• The trach is fresh

▶ AIRWAY EMERGENCIES

58. State the three airway emergencies.
    A. _____
    B. _____
    C. _____

59. Give four reasons why a tube may become obstructed.
    A.

    B.

    C.

    D.

60. What simple technique is used to assess tube obstruction not relieved by repositioning the head or deflating the cuff?

Copyright © 2003, 1999 Mosby, Inc. All rights reserved.

61. If you cannot clear the obstruction, what action should you be prepared to take?

62. What additional troubleshooting step often can be performed on patients with tracheostomies?

63. What effects will occur with a cuff leak when a patient is being mechanically ventilated?

64. What action should you be prepared to take if the cuff is blown?

▶ **EXTUBATION AND DECANNULATION**

Extubation is a procedure commonly performed by the RCP. You will need to be familiar with the indications for extubation and techniques used to minimize risk during this procedure.

65. The decision to remove the airway is *not the same* as the decision to remove the ventilator! What kind of patients might need to remain intubated even after the ventilator is removed?

66. Describe two methods for performing a "cuff-leak test."
A.

B.

67. List five types of equipment you will want to assemble *before* extubation.
A. _____
B. _____
C. _____
D. _____
E. _____

Copyright © 2003, 1999 Mosby, Inc. All rights reserved.

68. You will need to suction what two places before extubating? Name them and describe the correct sequencing for this important step.

69. Describe the two different strategies for removing the tube itself.
    A.

    B.

70. What therapeutic modality usually is applied immediately after extubation?

71. List two or three of the most common problems that occur after extubation.

72. The worst complication of extubation is laryngospasm. What can you do if laryngospasm persists more than a few seconds?

73. A common complication of extubation is glottic edema. How will you recognize *and* manage this problem?

74. Oral feeding should be withheld for how long after extubation? Why?

75. State the three methods for weaning from a tracheostomy tube. Give one advantage and one disadvantage for each technique.

    A. Technique_____
       Advantage _____
       Disadvantage_____
    B. Technique_____
       Advantage _____
       Disadvantage_____
    C. Technique_____
       Advantage _____
       Disadvantage_____

Copyright © 2003, 1999 Mosby, Inc. All rights reserved.

▶ ALTERNATIVE AIRWAY

You might need to have a few more airway tricks up your sleeve. Laryngeal mask airways (LMAs) are increasingly popular devices, especially in the OR and in emergency medical services (EMS) settings. Combitube devices also are used in the prehospital setting. Both of these tubes are now a part of Advanced Cardiac Life Support (ACLS) training. Emergency cricothyroidotomy may be needed if the upper airway is obstructed. Paramedics may insert the devices, but therapists usually do not.

76. Give three advantages of the LMA.
    A. _____
    B. _____
    C. _____

77. What about disadvantages?
    A. _____
    B. _____

78. Why is the Combitube device so useful in the field?

▶ BRONCHOSCOPY

Although rigid scopes usually are used in the OR, flexible bronchoscopy often is performed at the bedside with the RCP playing a key role in patient preparation and monitoring during the procedure.

79. State one advantage and three disadvantages of use of a rigid bronchoscope.

80. Give an example of a specific drug and the general goal for each of the following classes of premedication used in bronchoscopy.

Drug Class	Example	Goal
A. Tranquilizer	_____	_____
B. Drying agent	_____	_____
C. Narcotic analgesic	_____	_____
D. Anesthetic	_____	_____

Copyright © 2003, 1999 Mosby, Inc. All rights reserved.

81. What drugs would respiratory thera-
    pists nebulize before the procedure on
    a nonintubated patient? What about
    after the procedure?
    A. Before
    B. After

82. What three types of cardiopulmonary
    monitoring devices are considered
    essential for this procedure?
    A. _____
    B. _____
    C. _____

83. What are some of the activities we
    might perform while assisting with the
    procedure?
    A. _____
    B. _____
    C. _____

▶ CASE STUDIES

Case 1

During your first day of clinical training in
the ICU, a patient suffers a cardiac arrest.
Your clinical instructor asks you to assist in
preparing the equipment needed for ET
intubation. The patient is a small 56-year-
old woman.

84. What size ET tube should you select?

85. How should you test the tube before
    insertion?

86. How will you test the laryngoscope
    and blade for proper function?

87. Once the tube is inserted, how can you
    quickly assess placement?

88. A colorimetric CO_2 detector is
    attached to the ET tube. The end-tidal
    CO_2 is 2% on exhalation and 0% on
    inhalation as the chest rises with bag-
    ging. What does this suggest regarding
    the effectiveness of the chest
    compressions?

Case 2

After your heart-pounding initiation into
resuscitation, it is time to check the other
ventilator patients in the unit. Mrs. Barbara
Doll, a 19-year-old with a head injury, is

Copyright © 2003, 1999 Mosby, Inc. All rights reserved.

receiving mechanical ventilation through a cuffed No. 8 tracheostomy tube with an inner cannula. As you enter the room, the high pressure alarm is sounding.

89. How will you determine the need for suctioning in this situation?

90. What vacuum pressure should be set before suctioning?

91. What size suction catheter is suggested according to the rule of thumb in *Egan's*?

92. How long, and with what FIO_2, should you preoxygenate this patient?

93. After suctioning, you will need to check the cuff pressure. What is a safe cuff pressure?

▶ WHAT ABOUT THOSE BOARD EXAMS?

Chapter 30 is the longest one we've had so far! That must mean this is extremely important material. The NBRC agrees! The examination matrix says you must perform procedures to achieve maintenance of the airway, including artificial airway care, adequate humidification, cuff monitoring, positioning, and removal of secretions. It goes on to include modification of the management of artificial airways, including changing the type of humidification, inflating or deflating the cuff, and initiating suctioning. You should be able to assemble and check the function of the airways and the intubation equipment. Finally, you need to assist the physician in performing bronchoscopy, tracheostomy, and, of course, intubation. The actual number of airway questions varies from exam to exam, but you should be prepared for at least 8 to 10 questions on any given test.

94. Which of the following will decrease the risk of damage to the trachea from the endotracheal tube cuff?
   I. Minimal leak technique
   II. Maintaining cuff pressure of 30 to 35 cm H_2O
   III. Minimum occluding volume technique

Copyright © 2003, 1999 Mosby, Inc. All rights reserved.

A. I only
B. I, II only
C. I, III only
D. I, II, III

95. The diameter of the suction catheter should be no larger than
A. One-tenth the inner diameter of the ET tube
B. One-third the inner diameter of the ET tube
C. One-half the inner diameter of the ET tube
D. Three-fourths the inner diameter of the ET tube

96. A patient with a tracheostomy tube no longer needs mechanical ventilation. All of the following would facilitate weaning from the tracheostomy *except*
A. A fenestrated tracheostomy tube
B. A cuffed tracheostomy tube
C. A tracheostomy button
D. An uncuffed tracheostomy tube

97. Extubation is performed on a patient with an endotracheal tube. The presence of which of the following suggests the presence of upper airway edema?
A. Rhonchi
B. Crackles
C. Wheezes
D. Stridor

98. All of the following are useful in nasotracheal intubation *except*
A. Laryngoscope handle
B. Stylette
C. Miller blade
D. Magill forceps

99. While performing endotracheal suctioning, a respiratory care practitioner notes that flow through is minimal and secretion clearance is sluggish. Which of the following can cause this problem?
I. The vacuum setting is greater than 120 mm Hg
II. The suction canister is full of secretions
III. There is a leak in the system
A. I only
B. I, II only
C. II only
D. II, III only

100. Rapid, initial determination of endotracheal tube placement can be achieved by
I. Auscultation
II. Arterial blood gas analysis
III. Measurement of end-tidal CO_2
IV. Measurement of SpO_2
A. I, II only
B. I, III only
C. II, III, IV
D. I, III, IV

101. A patient with a tracheostomy tube shows signs of severe airway obstruction. A suction catheter passes only a short distance into the tube. The respiratory care practitioner should
A. Remove the tracheostomy tube
B. Deflate the cuff of the tube
C. Ventilate the tube with positive pressure
D. Remove the inner cannula

102. Which of the following can be used to measure the adequacy of pulmonary circulation during closed-chest cardiac compressions?
A. Capnometry
B. Arterial blood gas analysis
C. Pulse oximetry
D. Blood pressure monitoring

Copyright © 2003, 1999 Mosby, Inc. All rights reserved.

103. Before performing bronchoscopy, a respiratory care practitioner is asked to administer a nebulized anesthetic to the patient. What medication is most appropriate to place in the nebulizer?
    A. Midazolam (Versed)
    B. Atropine
    C. Morphine
    D. Lidocaine

► FOOD FOR THOUGHT

104. What are the advantages and disadvantages of commercial tube holders or harnesses compared with tape or cloth ties for securing ET or trach tubes?

105. Hi-Lo Evac tubes have been approved for use in the United States to prevent ventilator-associated pneumonia. Try the Internet for more on these terrific tubes. I am sure you'll be seeing them in your ICU!

► INFORMATION AGE

When I searched Google for "endotracheal tube PowerPoint presentations" I got 149 hits! The Internet journal of airway management **www.ijam.at** has good stuff and a cool virtual airway museum.

Emedicine has a good area on tracheostomy at **www.emedicine.com/ent/topic356.htm**

There is an astonishing amount of material on airway management on the Internet, so you need to have a pretty good idea of what you are looking for when you start to search.

Copyright © 2003, 1999 Mosby, Inc. All rights reserved.

Emergency Life Support

"We're in the resuscitation
business, not the
resurrection business."
Anonymous RCP

Nothing is more satisfying than being a part of the team that helps save someone's life! A successful resuscitation is an exciting event that you will remember forever. Of course, a poorly managed effort is completely frustrating, and attempting to save someone who should never receive CPR in the first place is about as depressing as it gets. Because RCPs play an integral role in hospital resuscitations, you need know both basic and advanced life support techniques. *There is no substitute for formal training and certification in basic and advanced life support!* Chapter 31 summarizes the important concepts of these two activities and helps you to gain knowledge and skills you will be expected to demonstrate on your boards.

► ACRES OF ACRONYMS

You must have noticed by now that medicine loves acronyms. I found 15 in Chapter 31 that will enable you to talk the talk. (Walking the walk is another story altogether!)

Write out the full definition of each acronym below.

1. ABCD

2. ACLS

3. AED

4. AHA

Copyright © 2003, 1999 Mosby, Inc. All rights reserved.

5. ARC

10. CPR

6. BLS

11. SVT

7. BVM

12. EMS

8. CDC

13. OSHA

9. CNS

14. PALS

Copyright © 2003, 1999 Mosby, Inc. All rights reserved.

15. PVC

I'm sure I left some out, but you get the idea.

▶ CAUSES AND PREVENTION OF SUDDEN DEATH

16. What is the primary cause of sudden death among adults in the United States?

17. Give an estimate of how many lives could be saved each year by a comprehensive community-wide system of life support implemented throughout the country.

18. Identify five types of accidental death among persons younger than 40 years in the United States.
    A. _____
    B. _____
    C. _____
    D. _____
    E. _____

19. Discuss death by foreign body obstruction of the airway in children.

▶ BASIC LIFE SUPPORT

20. Use Box 31-1 on p. 707 to help you describe the following steps of *adult* basic life support.

Action	Description
A. First step	_____
B. Act	_____
C. Airway	_____
D. Breathing	_____
E. Circulation	_____
F. Defibrillation	_____
G. Obstructed airway	_____

Copyright © 2003, 1999 Mosby, Inc. All rights reserved.

21. Compare adult, child, and infant resuscitation for the following categories (Table 31-1).

Category	Adult	Child	Infant
A. Obstructed			
1. Conscious	_____	_____	_____
2. Unconscious	_____	_____	_____
B. Breathing	_____	_____	_____
C. Compress			
1. Hands	_____	_____	_____
2. Ratio	_____	_____	_____
3. Cycles	_____	_____	_____
4. Depth	_____	_____	_____
5. Rate	_____	_____	_____
6. Pulse	_____	_____	_____

22. When is the jaw-thrust maneuver indicated?

23. How can you determine whether a victim is breathing?

24. Describe the technique for mouth-to-mouth breaths for adults and children. What is this the hazard to the victim in this procedure?
A. Adults

B. Children

Copyright © 2003, 1999 Mosby, Inc. All rights reserved.

C. Infants

28. How is hand positioning for chest compression different in adults, children, and infants?
    A. Adult

D. Hazard

    B. Children

25. When is mouth-to-nose indicated in adults?

    C. Infant

26. Mouth-to-tube or stoma? Seriously folks, you might be able to bring yourself to do this on a loved one, but in the hospital, you will want to modify this technique. What would you do?

29. Describe the modifications to CPR that you need to consider under these special circumstances:
    A. Near drowning

27. How is assessment of pulselessness different in adults and infants?

    B. Electrocution

Copyright © 2003, 1999 Mosby, Inc. All rights reserved.

C. Pacemaker (Don't shock the pacemaker site!)

D. Artificial heart valve

30. Once CPR is begun, it is normally stopped only for what three reasons?
    A. _____
    B. _____
    C. _____

31. A person with sudden cardiac arrest is probably in what rhythm?

32. What is the management of this rhythm?

33. The American Heart Association (AHA) has added the letter "D" to the ABCs. Explain what this means. What's the easiest way to do this? Why is it so important in terms of sudden cardiac arrest? Are there any patients on whom we don't usually use an automated external defibrillator (AED)?

34. How can you easily and quickly determine the effectiveness of ventilations and compressions delivered during CPR?
    A. Ventilation

    B. Compression

35. State the three major common complications of CPR.
    A. _____
    B. _____
    C. _____

36. CPR is contraindicated under what two circumstances?
    A. _____
    B. _____

Copyright © 2003, 1999 Mosby, Inc. All rights reserved.

37. What is the universal distress signal for foreign body obstruction of the airway?

38. When should back blows be used on an adult victim?

39. Give another name for the abdominal thrust maneuver. When should you avoid this maneuver in an adult?
A.

B.

40. What should you do if you cannot or should not perform the abdominal thrust on a choking victim?

41. Describe four ways you can tell that you have effectively removed a foreign body from the airway.
A. _____
B. _____
C. _____
D. _____

▶ ADVANCED CARDIAC LIFE SUPPORT

Respiratory care practitioners often are called on to perform oxygenation, assessment, and airway management techniques during resuscitation. In addition, I recommend that you take the AHA course in ACLS. Besides making you a smarter member of the code team, it will enhance your marketability to employers.

42. What concentration of oxygen should be administered during a life-threatening emergency?

43. Compare mouth-to-mask and bag-valve-mask methods of ventilation in terms of oxygen delivery and ease of performance.

Copyright © 2003, 1999 Mosby, Inc. All rights reserved.

44. List five characteristics of the ideal mask.
    A. _____
    B. _____
    C. _____
    D. _____
    E. _____

45. What is the technique for selecting the best-sized oropharyngeal airway (OPA)?

46. Name and describe the two basic types of oral airways.
    A. _____
    B. _____

47. What could go wrong if you insert an oral airway in a conscious victim?

48. What airway would you choose for a patient who cannot tolerate an oral airway?

49. Describe two ways to insert an oral airway without pushing back the tongue.
    A.

    B.

50. How would you lubricate the following airways before insertion?
    A. Oral

    B. Nasal

51. Why is an ET tube the preferred method for securing the airway during CPR?

Copyright © 2003, 1999 Mosby, Inc. All rights reserved.

52. What is the recommended maximum duration of an intubation attempt?

53. Describe the four ways of achieving a high FIO_2 with a self-inflating resuscitation bag.
    A.

    B.

    C.

    D.

54. When should the ET route of drug administration be used?

55. What is the primary management of pulseless ventricular tachycardia and ventricular fibrillation?

56. Give three examples of drugs that can be delivered by the ET route.
    A. _____
    B. _____
    C. _____

57. What modification of dosage and technique must be made for ET instillation of emergency drugs?

58. What initial energy level is recommended for electrical countershock during ventricular fibrillation? How about the second and third shocks?

Copyright © 2003, 1999 Mosby, Inc. All rights reserved.

59. Explain the difference between cardioversion and defibrillation.

60. When is electrical pacing indicated?

61. What are the two primary types of pacing?
    A. _____
    B. _____

▶ THE RETURN OF JUST SAY YES

62. Identify the drug indicated to manage each of the following (see Table 31-2).

Event	Drug Therapy
A. Ventricular tachycardia	_____
B. Pulseless electrical activity	_____
C. Asystole	_____
D. Poor cardiac contractility	_____
E. Hypotension	_____
F. Hypertension	_____
G. Ventricular fibrillation	_____
H. Supraventricular tachycardia (SVT)	_____
I. Coronary arterial occlusion	_____
J. CHF/pulmonary edema (fluid overload)	_____

▶ CASE IN POINT

We're going to skip the cases and get straight to the board exam questions for once.

▶ NBRC HIGHLIGHTS

The Entry Level examination matrix no longer makes it clear what you need to know in regard to resuscitation. Isn't that nice? You are told there will be six questions on the subject. The answers are mostly simple recall and application of facts. The matrix also mentions laryngoscopes, all the tubes, and CO_2 detectors. If you pay attention to this one chapter, you'll get those six questions right! You must

A. Recognize when to perform CPR
B. Call for help (Help! Help!)
C. Establish an effective airway
D. Ventilate with the three methods described in Chapter 31 (and watch the chest)
E. Perform chest compressions
F. Remember to check for a pulse
G. Provide oxygen
H. Ask for blood gases

The Registry examinations cover much, much more (12 questions). They won't specify what you need to know, but they do add the issue of cardiac drugs. The questions are more difficult as well. You can expect

A. Endotracheal instillation of drugs
B. Cardioversion and defibrillation
C. Use of capnometry to determine tube placement and adequacy of perfusion
D. Intubation
E. Cardiac and vasoactive drugs
F. Initiation and interpretation of ECG monitoring
G. Check on the pupils (of the eye)

Copyright © 2003, 1999 Mosby, Inc. All rights reserved.

Admittedly, there is a lot to know. I don't think there is any substitute for an ACLS course to complete your knowledge in preparation for work in the ICU or the examinations. In fact, the examination matrices are clear that you must know ACLS, Basic Life Support (BLS), Pediatric Advanced Life Support (PALS), and Neonatal Resuscitation Program (NRP) information even if you are not certified in these techniques! Chapter 31, along with the previous material (such as Chapter 30), will give you most of what you need.

63. When is the jaw-thrust technique indicated to help maintain an open airway?
    A. When foreign body obstruction is suspected
    B. After trauma to the head
    C. In cases of suspected neck injury
    D. During most CPR efforts

64. While attempting mask-to-mouth ventilation, a respiratory care practitioner notes that the chest does not rise with each breath. The most appropriate action to take at this time is to
    A. Intubate the patient
    B. Switch to bag-mask ventilation
    C. Use an oxygen-powered breathing device
    D. Give another breath after repositioning the head

65. Where should you check the pulse of an unresponsive infant?
    A. Brachial artery
    B. Carotid artery
    C. Femoral artery
    D. Radial artery

66. Upon entering a hospital room you see a physical therapist administering CPR to a patient who is lying on the floor. Your first action would be to
    A. Move the patient onto the bed
    B. Call for help
    C. Take over chest compressions
    D. Deliver two slow breaths to the airway

67. What is the correct number of rescue breaths to deliver during mouth-to-mouth ventilation of an adult victim?
    A. 10 breaths per minute
    B. 12 breaths per minute
    C. 16 breaths per minute
    D. 20 breaths per minute

68. An unconscious patient begins gagging during your attempt to insert an oropharyngeal airway. The correct action to take at this time would be to
    A. Insert a smaller oral airway
    B. Intubate the patient
    C. Perform the jaw-thrust maneuver
    D. Insert a nasal airway

69. The correct ratio of ventilations to compressions during two-rescuer CPR is
    A. 5:1
    B. 1:15
    C. 1:5
    D. 2:15

70. The ideal airway to use during a resuscitation effort is
    A. An oropharyngeal airway
    B. A nasopharyngeal airway
    C. A fenestrated tracheostomy tube
    D. An oral endotracheal tube

Copyright © 2003, 1999 Mosby, Inc. All rights reserved.

71. A patient is coughing and wheezing after accidentally aspirating a piece of meat. At this time, the respiratory care practitioner should
    A. Do nothing but reassure the patient
    B. Perform the Heimlich maneuver
    C. Deliver five back blows
    D. Call for help

72. Upon entering an ICU room, a respiratory care practitioner observes ventricular fibrillation on the cardiac monitor. The most appropriate management of this rhythm is
    A. CPR
    B. Administration of lidocaine
    C. Administration of epinephrine
    D. Electrical countershock

73. During a resuscitation effort, no IV line can be established. The respiratory care practitioner should recommend
    A. Intraosseus infusion of the medications
    B. Endotracheal instillation of the medications
    C. Insertion of a central line
    D. Aerosol administration of the medications

74. The effectiveness of chest compressions in producing circulation can be measured by
     I. Pulse oximetry
    II. Capnography
    III. Transcutaneous monitoring
    IV. Arterial blood gas analysis
    A. I, II only
    B. II, III only
    C. II, IV only
    D. I, II, III, IV

75. A patient has atrial fibrillation with serious signs and symptoms that do not respond to medications. The treatment of choice would be
    A. Vagal stimulation
    B. Defibrillation
    C. Oxygen administration
    D. Cardioversion

Get the picture? Any question on the subject of resuscitation is fair game. Start by learning the basic rates, depths, and management techniques. Then move on to the advanced material.

▶ FOOD FOR THOUGHT

76. Why doesn't anyone want to do mouth to mouth in the hospital? What are the alternatives?

77. How do you "activate EMS" in a hospital?

78. Who provides emotional support to the family of a resuscitation victim? The healthcare providers?

Copyright © 2003, 1999 Mosby, Inc. All rights reserved.

▶ INFORMATION AGE

You can get plenty of help on-line. One good place to look is:
www.acls.net

My students tell me this site is a lot of help when you are learning ACLS.

For kid stuff try this:
www.cs.nsw.gov.au/rpa/neonatal/html/ newprot/resuscit.htm

Of course there's more, but this subject is pretty easy to search.

Copyright © 2003, 1999 Mosby, Inc. All rights reserved.

Humidity and Bland Aerosol Therapy

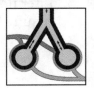

> **"Water, taken in moderation, cannot hurt anyone."**
> **Mark Twain**

I recently traveled to Las Vegas to attend a conference. After the first night in the hotel room I woke up with a dry, sore nose. (It even bled a little when I blew it!) Have you ever traveled to a low-humidity environment and experienced a humidity deficit? Imagine what happens to patients when we give them dry gases to breathe. Or worse, when we bypass the natural humidification system of the upper airway. Humidification is a simple thing, really, but then it's often the simple things in life that matter most.

▶ WET WORDS

The amount of relative humidity in gas can be measured with a device called a _____. When air does not have enough moisture to meet the normal _____ humidity of 44 mg/L, a humidity deficit is present. This problem can occur when the normal upper airway is bypassed by an ET tube. Secretions can become very thick or _____ and cause airway obstruction. A _____ is a device that adds gaseous water to inspired air. With heat, a humidifier can deliver more water to the lungs. An artificial nose, or _____ and _____ exchanger, is a simple device that does not require a water-filled chamber. _____, or devices that produce particles of water, also are useful for adding moisture to inspired air. An electrically powered device called an _____ nebulizer, works with _____ crystal and produces a large output of small particles of water for deposition in the lung.

▶ MEET THE OBJECTIVES

1. How are heat and moisture normally exchanged in your body?

2. List at least four consequences of prolonged inspiration of improperly conditioned gases.
   A. _____
   B. _____
   C. _____
   D. _____

Copyright © 2003, 1999 Mosby, Inc. All rights reserved.

301

3. Liter flows exceeding what value require humidification?

4. Give one other situation in which you would *always* provide humidification.

5. List the two primary and two secondary indications for humidification (Box 32-1).

   Primary   *Secondary*
   A. _____   A. _____
   B. _____   B. _____

6. What are the three variables that determine how well a humidifier works?
   A. _____
   B. _____
   C. _____

Which is most important?

7. Bubble humidifiers are added to what type of oxygen delivery system?

8. What is the typical range for absolute humidity delivered by a bubble humidifier? What does this amount convert to in terms of relative body humidity?
   A. _____
   B. _____

9. What safety device is incorporated into the design of a bubble humidifier?

10. Discuss the three primary advantages of passover humidifiers over bubble humidifiers.
    A.

    B.

    C.

Copyright © 2003, 1999 Mosby, Inc. All rights reserved.

11. Describe the principle of operation of each of the following artificial noses.
A. Condenser humidifier

B. Hygroscopic condenser humidifier

C. Hydrophobic condenser humidifier

12. What are the five contraindications to using heat and moisture exchangers (HMEs), according to the AARC CPG on humidification with mechanical ventilation?
A. _____
B. _____
C. _____
D. _____
E. _____

13. Identify three possible risks of using heated humidifiers. (*Hint:* See Box 32-2 and the CPG.)
A. _____
B. _____
C. _____

14. Identify three hazards associated with water that "rains out," or condenses in humidified breathing circuits.
A. _____
B. _____
C. _____

15. What specialized breathing circuit circumvents (usually) the condensation problem?

16. The AARC recommends what range of alarm settings for electronically controlled heated humidifiers?

17. What is the most reliable and scientific method used to determine the effectiveness of a humidification system? What do secretions tell you about effectiveness of humidification?
A. Scientific method

B. Secretions

Copyright © 2003, 1999 Mosby, Inc. All rights reserved.

18. *Egan's* describes what simple way to estimate the performance of an HME or heated-wire circuit without using a hygrometer? (So simple I wish I'd thought of it.)

19. List the seven indications in the AARC CPG for bland aerosol administration.

A. _____

B. _____

C. _____

D. _____

E. _____

F. _____

G. _____

20. Give three examples of solutions used to make bland aerosols.

A. _____

B. _____

C. _____

21. Identify the parts of the ultrasonic nebulizer (USN) shown below.

A. _____

B. _____

C. _____

D. _____

E. _____

F. _____

G. _____

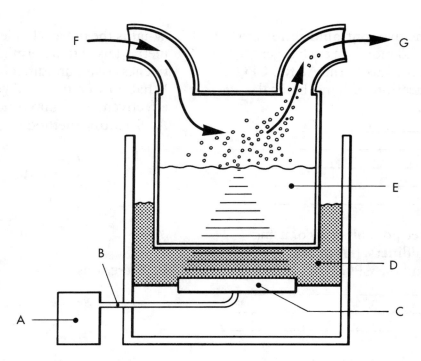

Functional schematic of a typical large-volume ultrasonic nebulizer. (From Barnes TA: *Core textbook for respiratory care practice,* ed 2, Chicago, 1994, Mosby.)

Copyright © 2003, 1999 Mosby, Inc. All rights reserved.

22. What preset variable determines the size of the aerosol particles generated by a USN?

23. What adjustable control determines the actual amount of aerosol produced?

24. Ultrasonic nebs are used primarily to accomplish what specific clinical goal or procedure?

25. When performing this procedure, what type of water is placed in the nebulizer cup?

26. Identify the two primary clinical problems associated with tents and body enclosures.
    A. _____
    B. _____

27. Your text identifies six important problems associated with bland aerosol therapy. For each of these problems, give a possible solution or means of prevention.
    A. Cross-contamination, infection
       Solution _____
    B. Environmental safety
       Solution _____
    C. Inadequate mist
       Solution _____
    D. Overhydration
       Solution _____
    E. Bronchospasm
       Solution _____
    F. Noise
       Solution _____

► **CHAPTER HIGHLIGHTS**

Let's review some basic concepts from Chapter 32. Fill in the blanks.

28. Heat and _____ exchange is done primarily by the _____.

29. Gases delivered to the trachea should be warmed to _____ ° C to _____ ° C.

30. A _____ is a device that adds invisible molecular water to a gas.

31. A _____ generates and disperses particles into the gas stream.

32. _____ is the most important factor affecting humidifier output.

33. At high flows some bubble humidifiers may produce _____, which can carry infectious bacteria.

34. Breathing circuit _____ must always be treated as _____ waste.

Copyright © 2003, 1999 Mosby, Inc. All rights reserved.

35. Bland aerosol therapy with sterile _____ often is used to manage airway _____, overcome humidity _____ in patients with tracheal airways, and help obtain _____ specimens.

► CASE STUDIES

Use the algorithm in Figure 32-17 to choose the correct humidity or bland aerosol system.

Case 1

Gunther Snorkelson has fallen into a lake while ice-fishing. He is brought to the emergency department with a core temperature of 30° C. Gunther is intubated with a No. 8 ET. He is unconscious and needs mechanical ventilation.

36. Give two reasons why you can't use an HME in the care of this patient.
    A.

    B.

37. What humidification system would you recommend?

Case 2

Anthony Marcus is a 32-year-old man admitted to the medical floor with a diagnosis of *Mycoplasma* pneumonia. He is receiving oxygen via nasal cannula at 5 L/min. He reports having a stuffy, dry nose a few hours after admission.

38. What humidification system would you recommend for this patient?

39. Why is Anthony unable to benefit from an HME?

Case 3

Billy Butter is a 57-year-old man who has undergone coronary artery bypass graft (CABG) surgery. He is receiving mechanical ventilation pending recovery from the procedure. Billy has no secretion problems.

Copyright © 2003, 1999 Mosby, Inc. All rights reserved.

40. What humidification system would you recommend?

▶ WHAT ABOUT THOSE BOARD EXAMS?

Sure enough, you should be able to recommend and administer bland aerosol and humidity therapy. You should know when to change to another system. Selecting, assembling, cleaning, and troubleshooting are in there too. Expect three to five questions; especially expect something on HMEs and USNs.

41. A respiratory care practitioner hears a loud whistling sound as she enters the room of a patient receiving oxygen via cannula at 6 L/min. In reference to the humidifier, what is the most likely cause of the problem?
    A. The top of the humidifier is cross-threaded
    B. The humidifier has run out of water
    C. The flow rate is set at less than the ordered amount
    D. There is a kink in the oxygen supply tubing

42. An ultrasonic nebulizer is ordered for sputum induction. Which of the following solutions should be placed in the medication cup to accomplish this goal?
    A. Sterile distilled water
    B. 0.45% NaCl solution
    C. 0.9 % NaCl solution
    D. 3% NaCl solution

43. A large-volume all-purpose nebulizer is set at an FIO_2 of 40% and a flow rate of 10 L/min to deliver humidified oxygen to an patient with a tracheostomy. The nebulizer is producing very little mist. Which of the following could be done to improve the aerosol output?
    I. Check the water level in the nebulizer
    II. Increase the flow rate to the nebulizer
    III. Drain condensate from the supply tubing
    IV. Turn off the nebulizer heating system
    A. I only
    B. I, II only
    C. I, III only
    D. I, III, IV only

44. While performing a ventilator check, the respiratory care practitioner observes a large amount of thin, white mucus in the tubing connected to the HME. Which of the following actions should be taken at this time?
    A. Rinse out the HME with sterile water
    B. Suction the mucus from the tubing
    C. Use a heated humidification system
    D. Replace the HME

45. Sputum induction via USN is ordered. The nebulizer will produce 5 mL of water per minute on the maximum amplitude setting. The treatment is to last 15 minutes. How much solution should the respiratory care practitioner place in the nebulizer?
    A. 5 mL
    B. 15 mL
    C. 50 mL
    D. 75 mL

Copyright © 2003, 1999 Mosby, Inc. All rights reserved.

These questions are only samples! There are many more possibilities in the area of humidification.

▶ FOOD FOR THOUGHT

46. The industry standard for adding simple humidification to an oxygen delivery system is a flow rate of greater than 4 L/min. Can you think of any situations in which you might add humidification when the flow rate is less than 4 L/min?

Just for fun (respiratory fun), place yourself on a nasal cannula at 6 L/min (be sure to use a clean one) or use a simple mask at 10L/min in the laboratory. Breathe through your nose for 10 or 15 minutes. How does it feel?

47. What is an "active HME"?

▶ INFORMATION AGE

I don't usually recommend corporate websites, but Portex has a good one: **www.frca.co.uk/portex/physiology_humid.htm**

The respiratory care program at the University of Medicine and Dentistry of New Jersey (UMDNJ) has a great page that has lots of good resources and information: **www.umdnj.edu/rspthweb/rstn2100/unit3.htm**

If you want more info on the subject of humidification, just do a search using the device you are interested in as the keyword. For example, "active HME" or "bubble humidifiers."

Copyright © 2003, 1999 Mosby, Inc. All rights reserved.

Aerosol Drug Administration

> **"The pen is mightier than the sword! The case for prescriptions rather than surgery."**
> **Marvin Kitman**

Now that you have the drugs, what do you do with them? When I was a student (we walked through the snow for 5 miles to get to clinical . . .) we gave almost all our medications via intermittent positive pressure breathing (IPPV). It was expensive, complicated, time and labor intensive, and most certainly was not customized to the customer! The good news was that we didn't have to know about so many delivery systems. You, of course, are expected to learn a wide variety of ways to deliver aerosolized drugs and to find the most cost-effective and therapeutic method of delivery.

Chapter 33 gets you off to a good start on this quest. This chapter is newly revised and expanded, so it really gets the job done.

▶ TERMINOLOGY TORTURE

By now you must have noticed that respiratory care has a language all its own. You won't go far without the passwords. Drug administration is no different, so you need to start by matching the following terms to their definitions.

1. _____ Aerosol
2. _____ Atomizer
3. _____ Baffle
4. _____ Deposition
5. _____ Hygroscopic
6. _____ Inertial impaction
7. _____ MMAD
8. _____ Nebulizer
9. _____ Propellant
10. _____ Therapeutic index
11. _____ Residual volume

A. Suspension of solid or liquid particles in a gas
B. Difference between therapeutic and toxic drug concentrations
C. Device that produces uniformly sized aerosol particles
D. Device that removes large particles
E. Device that produces nonuniformly sized aerosol particles
F. Deposition of particles by collision
G. Testimony of a witness (or, particles being retained in the respiratory tract)
H. Absorbs moisture from the air
I. Measurement of average particle size
J. Amount of drug left in the SVN
K. Something that provides thrust

▶ CHARACTERISTICS OF THERAPEUTIC AEROSOLS

12. Why is particle size so important in aerosol therapy?

Copyright © 2003, 1999 Mosby, Inc. All rights reserved.

13. What is the primary method of deposition for large, high-mass particles?

14. Particles of 10 μm or larger tend to deposit in what part of the respiratory tract? What about particles between 5 and 10 μm?

15. In what part of the lung would you like to deposit β-adrenergic bronchodilator drugs? What particle size is needed to reach this goal?

16. Because it is extremely difficult to predict exactly what happens to particles once they enter the lung, what is the most practical way to determine how well you are delivering a drug?

▶ HAZARDS OF AEROSOL THERAPY

What is the main hazard of aerosol drug therapy? Why, the drugs themselves, of course! (But you knew that.)

17. Nebulizers are a great source of nosocomial infection. Describe three of the CDC recommendations for preventing this serious problem.
A.

B.

C.

18. List five aerosolized substances associated with increased airway resistance.
A. _____
B. _____
C. _____
D. _____
E. _____

Copyright © 2003, 1999 Mosby, Inc. All rights reserved.

19. What can you do to prevent bronchospasm?

21. What group of patients is most prone to harm from bland aerosols?

20. Aerosolizing drugs *always* carries the risk of inducing bronchospasm. Describe at least four ways you can monitor this potential problem.
A.

22. What is meant by the term "drug reconcentration"? When is this most likely to occur?

B.

C.

D.

▶ AEROSOL DRUG DELIVERY SYSTEMS

I mentioned earlier that many delivery options are available. Naturally, every company claims its system is the best. Let's see if we can figure it out using the information in *Egan's*.

Metered-Dose Inhalers

Metered-dose inhalers are the most widely prescribed aerosol drug delivery system, even though they are not completely socially accepted. It's okay to pop your antacids in the boardroom, but most executives will hide their inhalers!

Copyright © 2003, 1999 Mosby, Inc. All rights reserved.

23. What percentage of patients and healthcare professionals is believed to use MDIs incorrectly?

24. What propellant is used in most MDIs, and why is this a problem? What new propellant is safer for patients and the environment?

25. What other substances are found in MDIs that may produce clinical problems?

26. What percentage of the drug in an MDI is actually deposited in the lung? Why is there so much variability?

27. What MDI-delivered drugs should always be used with a spacer? Why?

28. Put the following steps of optimal MDI delivery in order.
    A. Hold your breath _____
    B. Breathe out normally _____
    C. Wait 1 minute _____
    D. Shake the canister _____
    E. Hold the MDI two fingerbreadths from mouth _____
    F. Slowly inhale as deeply as you can _____
    G. Warm the canister _____
    H. Fire the canister _____

29. What is the difference between a spacer and a holding chamber? Does it matter?

30. How does the recommended breathing pattern with a holding chamber differ from that of a spacer or unassisted MDI?

Copyright © 2003, 1999 Mosby, Inc. All rights reserved.

31. What is a DPI? What's the big deal?

32. How does DPI breathing technique differ from that recommended with an MDI?

33. What patients cannot use DPIs? What warning should patients receive about using their DPIs during an acute episode of bronchospasm?

34. List three potential power sources for driving a small medication nebulizer.
    A. _____
    B. _____
    C. _____

35. How does an atomizer differ from an SVN? When would you want to use an atomizer?

36. What is the optimal flow rate and amount of solution to put in an SVN?
    A. _____
    B. _____

37. What potential problem exists when you deliver an SVN treatment via mask? How can you deal with this problem?

Small-Volume Nebulizers

Small-volume nebulizers have been around a long time and are still widely used. They have an amazing number of aliases: minineb, acorn neb, handheld neb, updraft neb, microneb, med neb—the list seems to go on forever. These devices are indicated when a patient is unable to physically use an MDI or cannot generate sufficient inspiratory flow rates for an MDI or dry powder inhaler (DPI). Some drugs are available only for nebulization.

38. Why is it so important to match nebulizer and compressor systems for home use?

Copyright © 2003, 1999 Mosby, Inc. All rights reserved.

39. Several nebulizers on the market are designed to reduce the amount of drug expelled into the atmosphere and wasted. Name two of these nebs.

    A. _____

    B. _____

40. What is meant by nebulizer "sputter" and why is it important to RCPs?

41. Explain what is meant by the blow-by technique used with babies, and discuss the effectiveness of this technique.

Large-Volume Nebulizers

Large-volume nebulizers are usually used to deliver bland aerosols (see Chapter 32). Special large-volume nebulizers, such as HEART and HOPE nebulizers, are used to deliver continuous bronchodilator therapy. You may want to try one to deliver drugs when a severely obstructed patient does not respond to SVN treatments and needs a repeated series over time.

42. What potential clinical problem may exist with continuous bronchodilator therapy?

43. Why is the small-particle aerosol generator (SPAG) generator unique? When is it indicated?

Small Ultrasonic Nebulizers

Small USNs have a lot of advantages: small uniform particles, high output, and capability of use with ventilators.

44. List three advantages and three disadvantages of USNs for delivering meds (Table 33-2).

	Advantages	Disadvantages
A.	_____	_____
B.	_____	_____
C.	_____	_____

▶ CASE STUDIES

Use the algorithms (Figures 33-24 and 33-26) in *Egan's* to answer the following questions about selection of aerosol drug delivery devices and doses.

Case 1

Big Bob Bloater is an alert, cooperative 52-year-old man who has recently been

Copyright © 2003, 1999 Mosby, Inc. All rights reserved.

given the diagnosis of chronic bronchitis. He quit smoking (60 pack-year history) 6 months ago but still has respiratory symptoms. He is in your pulmonary clinic today to receive his PFT results and medications. The physician has ordered ipratropium bromide (Atrovent) and beclomethasone (Vanceril) for Bob.

45. What method of delivery would you recommend for this patient?

46. What other equipment is indicated?

47. What general considerations for patient education would you emphasize for Mr. Bloater?

48. How will you know that the patient is able to perform the therapy correctly?

Case 2

Randy Andrews arrives in the emergency department with acute respiratory distress. His condition is diagnosed as status asthmaticus. This 27-year-old man has high-pitched diffuse wheezes, a respiratory rate of 24 breaths/min, heart rate of 106 beats/min, and an SpO_2 of 92%. The PEFR is 150 L/min after 4 puffs of albuterol via MDI.

49. What are the possible options for treating Mr. Andrews at this point?

50. What method of bronchodilator delivery would you recommend for Mr. Andrews?

51. What is meant by dose-response assessment?

Case 3

You are asked to deliver a bronchodilator to a patient in the neuro unit. When you arrive to assess the patient, you notice that she is obtunded. Breath sounds reveal scattered rhonchi and wheezing in the upper lobes.

Copyright © 2003, 1999 Mosby, Inc. All rights reserved.

52. What method of bronchodilator delivery would you recommend in this situation?

53. What modification will you need to make?

54. Because peak flow measurement is unlikely to be performed, how will you assess the effectiveness of therapy?

▶ WHAT ABOUT INTUBATED PATIENTS?

Delivering bronchodilators to intubated patients has always been difficult. Much of the drug ends up in the circuit or the endotracheal tube. Assessment of effectiveness can be difficult as well. Both SVN and MDI can be used to achieve good results if you follow some guidelines and use the right equipment.

55. Small-volume nebulizer dosages should be adjusted by what amount when delivered to an intubated patient?

56. What standard starting dosage is recommended for albuterol by MDI to a ventilator patient?

57. Where should you place the SVN in the ventilator circuit?

58. When should an MDI be activated for a ventilator patient?

Copyright © 2003, 1999 Mosby, Inc. All rights reserved.

59. What adjustments to dilution need to be made with the SVN for ventilator delivery?

▶ WHAT ABOUT THOSE BOARD EXAMS?

It will come as no surprise that this information is on your boards. What is unusual is how little of this material is on the test considering the importance and frequency of aerosol drug administration in the clinical setting. One reason is that only recently have good studies been done to provide more scientific conclusions about how best to deliver medications. The matrix specifically mentions MDIs, spacers, and pneumatic-powered nebulizers. Of course peak flows and assessment are included. I could not find continuous nebulization in the matrix. Perhaps it will appear on the new exams that are coming soon.

Asthma has been recently diagnosed in a 16-year-old patient. The respiratory care practitioner is asked to teach the patient how to self-administer beclomethasone (Vanceril) via metered-dose inhaler.

60. In addition to the inhaler, what other equipment would be indicated?
    I. A spacer device
    II. A pulse oximeter
    III. A peak flow meter
    A. I only
    B. I, II only
    C. I, III only
    D. II, III only

61. After performing the inhalation, the respiratory care practitioner instructs the patient to perform a breath-hold maneuver. The purpose of this maneuver is to
    A. Promote a strong cough
    B. Improve venous return
    C. Improve inertial impaction
    D. Increase medication delivery

62. While attempting to administer albuterol via SVN to a patient who has had a recent cerebrovascular accident, the respiratory care practitioner notices that the patient is unable to hold the nebulizer or keep her lips sealed on the mouthpiece. The respiratory care practitioner should recommend
    A. Switching to a metered-dose inhaler
    B. Using an aerosol mask for delivery
    C. Discontinuing the medication
    D. Administering the medication subcutaneously

63. A metered-dose inhaler is ordered for a patient who is intubated and being mechanically ventilated and humidified with a heat and moisture exchanger. Which of the following is the most appropriate way to administer the bronchodilator?
    A. Place the MDI in the expiratory limb of the ventilator circuit
    B. Place the MDI between the HME and the endotracheal tube
    C. Recommend changing the delivery method to a small-volume nebulizer
    D. Remove the HME during delivery of the drug

Copyright © 2003, 1999 Mosby, Inc. All rights reserved.

64. An alert adult patient with asthma is receiving bronchodilator therapy via small-volume nebulizer during a hospitalization. What recommendations should the respiratory care practitioner make in regard to this therapy when the patient is ready for discharge?
    A. Recommend MDI instruction
    B. Recommend oral administration of the medication
    C. Recommend training in home use of the SVN
    D. Recommend administration of the drug via IPPB

65. Which of the following devices is most suitable for delivery of virazole (Ribavirin)?
    A. Continuous large-volume nebulizer
    B. Small-particle aerosol generator
    C. Ultrasonic nebulizer
    D. Atomizer

▶ **FOOD FOR THOUGHT**

Hey, what about me? The guy giving all these treatments? Chapter 33 ends with some important material on the subject of protecting the practitioner from continuous exposure to a wide variety of inhaled agents.

66. What two inhalational drugs have the greatest occupational risk for RCPs?
    A. _____
    B. _____

67. Describe some of the physical ways to control environmental contamination when delivering medications that have potential side effects for the provider.

68. What do the terms HEPA and PAPR refer to?

▶ **INFORMATION AGE**

A good place to start is the AARC website **www.aarc.org** where you will find the CPGs for selection of an aerosol delivery device. The on-line journal **www. rcjournal.co** is another good place to look. For more on Pari and Circulaire nebs try **www.pari.com** and **www.westmedinc.com**

If you are interested in continuous bronchodilator therapy, all you need to do is type this subject into one of the search engines and you'll get an eyeful.

Copyright © 2003, 1999 Mosby, Inc. All rights reserved.

Storage and Delivery of Medical Gases

**"O Lord, help me to be
pure, but not yet."**

St. Augustine

One thing is for certain, every generation of respiratory care students since the dawn of time has had a good laugh at the engineers who thought up the name pin-index safety system. And what's up with that American standard safety system? Another thing I'm sure of is that we all have to learn more about medical gases than any other mortals on this planet! I have to admit this information has come in handy many times in the clinical setting, and it is good to be an expert when the delivery systems malfunction and no one but the RCP knows quite what to do.

▶ GAS POWERED

There's a little puzzle on p. 320 to help you learn the new terms found in Chapter 34.

▶ CHARACTERISTICS OF MEDICAL GASES

1. Nonflammable gases simply will not burn. Name three gases categorized as nonflammable.
   A. _____
   B. _____
   C. _____

2. Most therapeutic gases support combustion. Name three gases in this category.
   A. _____
   B. _____
   C. _____

3. Describe the four basic steps of the fractional distillation process.
   A.

   B.

   C.

   D.

Copyright © 2003, 1999 Mosby, Inc. All rights reserved.

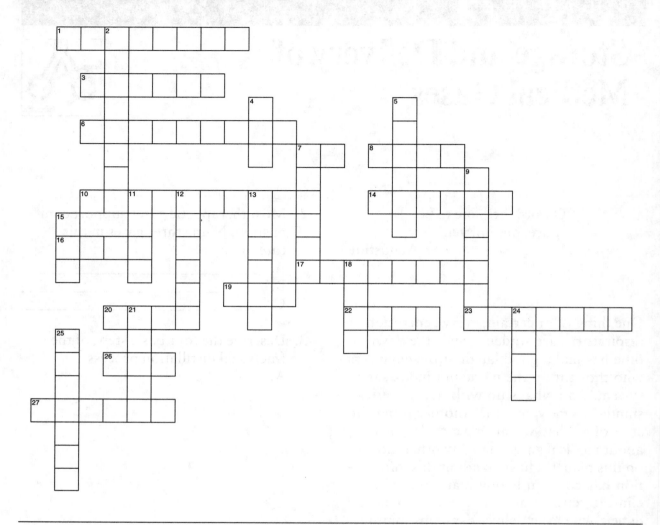

4. What purity level is required for medical-grade O_2?

5. Describe the two methods used to separate O_2 from air. What concentration is produced by each method?

A.

Copyright © 2003, 1999 Mosby, Inc. All rights reserved.

ACROSS

1. Valve that lowers gas pressure
3. _____ dioxide, used to treat hiccups
6. A device that controls both pressure and flow
7. Chemical named for this light gas
8. This meter controls the volume of gas per unit of volume
10. Type of "distillation" that produces oxygen
14. Gas used in treatment of severe asthma
16. Low pressure safety system
17. Pipe with many connections used to link gas cylinders together
19. Gas delivered in a yellow cylinder
20. _____ valves shut off the gas in case of a fire
22. Your mom told you not to say this, but it really is a safety system!
23. Gas delivered in a blue cylinder
26. The "P" in PISS
27. Gas that makes up 20.95% of air

DOWN

2. The "D" in DISS
4. Agency that classifies cylinders
5. Needle _____ adjust the flow in a Thorpe tube
7. Low density gas
9. Fixed orifice, variable pressure measuring or metering device
11. Rear end: also a safety system
12. Variable orifice, constant pressure flow metering device
13. Just say "NO"
15. Agency that sets standards for gas purity
18. Sets standards for design, construction, placement, and use of bulk oxygen systems
21. Gas with only one oxygen molecule
24. Slang term for cylinder
25. Second half of gas made by heating limestone in contact with water

B.

B. Home

6. Describe the devices used to produce medical-grade air for hospital systems and for home use.
   A. Hospital

7. Most medical-grade CO_2 is used for what purpose?

Copyright © 2003, 1999 Mosby, Inc. All rights reserved.

8. What is heliox? What is it used for?

9. What is the primary medical use of nitrous oxide? What are some of the hazards of nitrous oxide administration?

10. How is nitric oxide being used in the neonatal setting?

11. Describe two possible hazards of using nitric oxide.
   A. _____
   B. _____

12. Give the chemical symbol for each of the following medical gases.

Gas	Symbol
A. Oxygen	_____
B. Air	_____
C. Carbon dioxide	_____
D. Helium	_____
E. Nitrous oxide	_____
F. Nitric oxide	_____

▶ STORING MEDICAL GASES

High-pressure medical gas cylinders have been around for more than 100 years. The modern cylinder is the subject of numerous regulations and rules that control manufacture, storage, and transportation of these potentially dangerous steel bottles. Naturally, you will be expected to have considerable knowledge on this subject even if you don't use it on a daily basis!

13. Identify the cylinder markings on the diagram shown on p. 323.
   A. _____
   B. _____
   C. _____
   D. _____
   E. _____

Copyright © 2003, 1999 Mosby, Inc. All rights reserved.

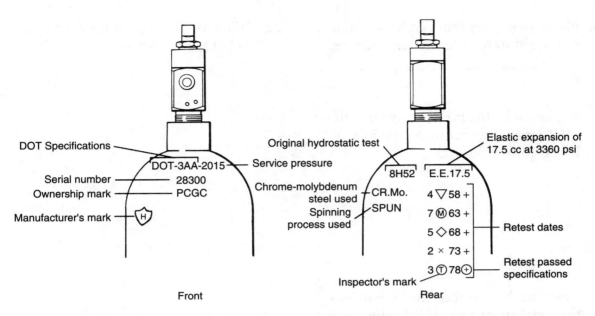

Typical markings of cylinders containing medical gases. Front and back views are for illustration purposes only. Exact location and order of markings vary.

14. What do the symbols * and + mean when stamped on a cylinder?

A. *

B. +

15. Identify the proper color for these gas cylinders (in the United States).
    A. Oxygen_____
    B. Carbon dioxide_____
    C. Nitrous oxide_____
    D. Helium_____
    E. Nitrogen_____
    F. Air_____

16. Because cylinder color is only a guideline, how do you actually determine what gas is in a tank?

17. What is the best way to determine the actual O_2 concentration in a cylinder?

► FILL 'ER UP

Cylinders are filled with either gas or liquid. The liquid is either at room temperature or in a cryogenic state.

Copyright © 2003, 1999 Mosby, Inc. All rights reserved.

18. Name two gases that can be stored in the liquid state at room temperature.
    A. _____
    B. _____

19. Explain why the pressure in a gas-filled cylinder is different from that in a liquid-filled cylinder.

20. Describe the methods for measuring the contents of a gas-filled cylinder and a liquid-filled cylinder.
    A.

    B.

21. Write the formula for calculating the cylinder factor for a gas-filled cylinder.

22. What are the factors for the "E" and "H" O_2 cylinders?
    A.

    B.

23. Now write the formula for calculating duration of flow in minutes.

I promise we'll come back to this and practice these calculations. They are important for clinical practice and for your board exams!

▶ BULK OXYGEN

Try to imagine how much O_2 a large hospital needs every day. If you had 100 patients wearing O_2 at 6 L/min, you would need more than 800,000 L for 1 day! Ventilators draw much more gas! You could provide this O_2 with individual cylinders in each room, but think how much work that would involve. A bulk system, by definition, has at least 20,000 cubic feet of gas.

Copyright © 2003, 1999 Mosby, Inc. All rights reserved.

24. Describe a gaseous bulk system. Be sure to discuss the manifold, the primary, and reserve banks.

25. Why do most hospitals use a liquid bulk O_2 system?

26. Where are small liquid O_2 cylinders usually used?

27. What is the critical temperature of O_2? How is bulk liquid O_2 maintained at this temperature?

28. What is the normal working pressure for a hospital O_2 piping system?

29. What are zone valves? Give two reasons you might need to use these valves.

▶ SAFETY SYSTEMS

Ah, the fabled safety systems. They come in two general types: those built into the cylinder valve stem to prevent rupture from high pressures and indexed systems designed to keep you from giving the wrong gas to a patient.

30. Remember the gas laws? If a cylinder overheats the pressure will rise. Describe the type of pressure release valve usually found in these cylinder stems.
    A. Small cylinder

    B. Large cylinder

Copyright © 2003, 1999 Mosby, Inc. All rights reserved.

31. Name the three basic indexed safety systems for medical gases. Both names!

Abbreviated Name	*Full Name*
A. _____	_____
B. _____	_____
C. _____	_____

32. A large cylinder of O_2 is described as follows: CGA-540 0.903-14NGO-RH-Ext. Explain what this means.

33. What type of cylinder has pins and holes in the safety connection system?

34. What system was established to prevent accidental interchange of low-pressure medical gas connectors? What is meant by "low-pressure"?

35. What is the purpose of the quick-connect system?

► **REGULATING PRESSURE AND FLOW**

Because a large cylinder of O_2 can have a pressure as high as 2400 psi, we need to have a way to lower this pressure and control it, or our equipment (or the patient) could be harmed.

36. Describe the action of the following devices.
    A. Reducing valve

    B. Flowmeter

    C. Regulator

37. Describe the normal way each of the following is used in respiratory care.
    A. Preset reducing valve

Copyright © 2003, 1999 Mosby, Inc. All rights reserved.

B. Adjustable reducing valve

C. Multiple-stage reducing valve

38. What two hazards can occur when you open a cylinder attached to a high-pressure reducing valve?

Three categories of flowmeters are used in respiratory care. The next set of questions tests your knowledge of these commonly used devices.

39. What are two advantages and two disadvantages of flow restrictors?

Advantages	Disadvantages
A. _____	_____
B. _____	_____

40. Describe the Bourdon flowmeter.

41. What is the chief advantage of the Bourdon-type flowmeter?

42. How will indicated flow compare with actual flow when a Bourdon flowmeter meets up with downstream resistance?

43. What do Bourdon gauges actually measure? Thorpe tubes?
A. Bourdon

B. Thorpe

Copyright © 2003, 1999 Mosby, Inc. All rights reserved.

44. Compare indicated flow and actual flow in a compensated Thorpe flowmeter when downstream resistance occurs.

45. What happens to the float in a compensated Thorpe tube when you connect it to a 50-psi gas source?

► CASE STUDY

Case 1

A patient is to be transported from the ICU to the imaging department for a CT scan. The patient needs continuous supplemental O_2 at 10 L/min by mask. You will need to provide portable O_2 for the transport. An E cylinder is available.

46. What type of regulator is most appropriate for transport?

47. How long will the cylinder last at the given flow rate if the pressure is 1000 psi?

Formula: _____

Calculation: _____

48. When you turn on the cylinder valve, a hissing noise is heard from the regulator. The flowmeter is off, so there must be a leak. What should you check to try to correct the leak?
A. _____
B. _____

► MATHEMAGIC

I told you we'd come back to the problem of cylinder duration calculations. This is important—not just because it is on tests! Let's say you have to transport a patient by plane, send someone home with O_2, or just go from the emergency department to the ICU. Will you have enough gas? Running out in the elevator is not acceptable. There are two ways to do the calculations—the board exam, precise way and the rule-of-thumb quick and dirty way. Precise first.

The two most common cylinders you will be using are the small E type, and the larger H or K type. Factors are 0.28 and 3.14.

Example: You are sending a patient home by car. The E cylinder is full (2200 psi), and the patient is wearing a cannula at 2 L/min. How long will the O_2 last?

Start by writing out the formula. (You have to know this one.)

$$\text{Duration} = \text{psi} \times \text{Factor}/\text{Flow}$$

Now plug in the numbers.

Copyright © 2003, 1999 Mosby, Inc. All rights reserved.

Calculation: $2200 \times 0.28/2 = 616/2 = 308$ minutes

OK, how many hours is that?

$$308/60 = 5.1 \text{ hours}$$

Now for the quick and dirty way:

0.28 is roughly 1/3. One third of 2200 is 700. 700 divided by 2 = 350 minutes, divided by 60 minutes in the hour = 5+ hours

Can you see how you could get into trouble with this? Of course, if the patient is taking a 30-minute trip home, it would hardly matter. Be sensible when you take short cuts!

(By the way, everyone knows about short cuts. If you use this on the boards you could get burned.)

▶ WHAT ABOUT THOSE BOARD EXAMS?

You won't see too many questions on the material in Chapter 34. Cylinder duration is one common question and usually involves duration of an E or H cylinder. Here are some typical questions for you to try.

49. An H cylinder of oxygen is being used to deliver oxygen to a patient in a sub-acute care facility where no piped in oxygen is available. The cylinder gauge shows a pressure of 1000 psi. The patient is receiving oxygen at 5 L/min by cannula. Approximately how long will the cylinder gas last at this flow rate?
    A. 1 hour
    B. 8 hours
    C. 10 hours
    D. 628 hours

50. A respiratory care practitioner notices that a flowmeter plugged into the wall outlet continues to read 1 L/min even though it is not turned on. What is the most appropriate action at this time?
    A. Replace the flowmeter
    B. Include the extra liter in any calculations
    C. Disassemble the flowmeter and replace the O-rings
    D. Do nothing; this is not an unusual situation

51. A respiratory care practitioner has to transport a patient via air from the island of Maui to Honolulu. The patient is being manually ventilated with an oxygen flow set at 10 L/min. The cylinder gauge reads 2000 psi. How long will the cylinder last?
    A. 42 minutes
    B. 56 minutes
    C. 60 minutes
    D. 10 hours

52. When a respiratory care practitioner unplugs a Thorpe-type flowmeter, a huge leak occurs from the wall outlet. What action should the respiratory care practitioner take at this time?
    A. Shut off the gas to the room with the zone valve
    B. Shut off the bulk oxygen system
    C. Plug the flowmeter back into the outlet
    D. Call maintenance to fix the outlet

Copyright © 2003, 1999 Mosby, Inc. All rights reserved.

▶ FOOD FOR THOUGHT

53. What would happen if nitrous oxide were to leak in the emergency department or OR?

54. What would you do if the bulk system at your hospital were to fail?

55. What protective gear is appropriate when opening a valve on a high-pressure cylinder?

▶ INFORMATION AGE

Just for your amusement try the site for the Compressed Gas Association: **www.cganet. com**

Now go to **www.osha-slc.gov/SLTC/ compressedgasequipment**

This is the OSHA compressed gas site. For an even better Internet resource try **www.pp.okstate.edu/ehs/links/gas.htm**

This one is devoted to cylinder safety and has lots of useful information. Tons of it!

Copyright © 2003, 1999 Mosby, Inc. All rights reserved.

CHAPTER 35

Medical Gas Therapy

> "I like the dreams of the future
> better than the history
> of the past."
> **Thomas Jefferson**

My first job in respiratory therapy was that of oxygen technician. I was excited by the thought of being responsible for all those cannulas, masks, and humidifiers. We've come a long way since then, but medical gas therapy is still a cornerstone of respiratory care. Of course we think of oxygen as a drug now, and things have changed a lot in our understanding of administering this powerful medication. The modern respiratory therapist must have a much firmer grasp of the goals and objectives of medical gas therapy than I did when I made my patient rounds 25 years ago.

▶ TANK JOCKEY

Let's try something different in the war of the words. My students always have a hard time with the spelling of medical terms. Check your ability by circling the correct spelling for this gas jargon.

1. canulla   cannula
2. reservore   reservoir
3. lasitude   lassitude
4. diaphramatic   diaphragmatic
5. retanopathy   retinopathy

6. hypoxemia   hypoxemea
7. toxicity   toxisity
8. infarction   infraction
9. displasia   dysplasia
10. pendent   pendant
11. concentration   concintration
12. entranement   entrainment
13. wye   why

▶ PLEASE PASS THE GAS

We're not just going to slap the mask on their faces, OK? Any old knob twirler could figure out how to do that part of the procedure. Let's start by reviewing the reasons for giving O_2 and how to clinically recognize those needs.

14. What is acute hypoxemia?

15. What are the threshold criteria for defining hypoxemia in adults and newborns according to the AARC CPG? Give two laboratory values.
    A. Adults (and children)
       1. Pa_{O_2}
       2. Sa_{O_2}
    B. Newborns
       1. Pa_{O_2}
       2. Sa_{O_2}

Copyright © 2003, 1999 Mosby, Inc. All rights reserved.

16. Specifically, what beneficial effect does O_2 have on the symptoms of patients with COPD and chronic hypoxemia (besides relieving hypoxemia)?
    A. COPD (and interstitial disease)

    B. Chronic hypoxemia

17. Describe the two compensatory mechanisms of the cardiopulmonary system in the face of hypoxemia.
    A. Lungs

    B. Heart

18. In what acute cardiac condition is O_2 therapy especially important?

19. What effect does hypoxemia have on the pulmonary blood vessels? What are the long-term consequences of this effect?

20. State the three basic ways to determine whether a patient needs O_2.
    A. _____
    B. _____
    C. _____

21. List six common acute clinical situations in which hypoxemia is so common that O_2 therapy usually is provided.
    A. _____
    B. _____
    C. _____
    D. _____
    E. _____
    F. _____

Copyright © 2003, 1999 Mosby, Inc. All rights reserved.

22. Give two signs of mild and severe hypoxia for each of the following systems.
    A. Respiratory
       Mild _____
       Severe _____
    B. Cardiovascular
       Mild _____
       Severe _____
    C. Neurological
       Mild _____
       Severe _____

▶ WHAT COULD GO WRONG?

There are four great big problems associated with O_2 therapy (besides burning down the hospital). Naturally, you gotta know 'em.

Toxic Talk

23. Oxygen toxicity affects what two organ systems?
    A. _____
    B. _____

24. The harm caused by O_2 is influenced by what two factors?
    A. _____
    B. _____

25. Describe the effects on lung tissue caused by breathing excessive O_2.

26. What is meant by a vicious circle in reference to O_2 toxicity?

27. Although every patient is unique, what general rule of thumb can be applied to prevent O_2 toxicity?

28. When should O_2 be withheld from a hypoxic patient to avoid the consequences of toxicity?

I Feel Depressed

29. What specific type of COPD patient is likely to experience depression of ventilatory drive while breathing O_2?

Copyright © 2003, 1999 Mosby, Inc. All rights reserved.

30. Give two explanations for this effect.

    A.

    B.

31. When should O_2 be withheld from a hypoxic COPD patient to avoid depressing ventilation?

RLF or ROP, It's All the Same to Me!

32. Describe the pathophysiology of how excessive blood O_2 causes blindness in premature newborns.

33. During what time period after birth is retinopathy of prematurity (ROP) likely to develop?

34. How can you reduce the risk of ROP?

Absorbing Information

35. Describe how O_2 can cause atelectasis.

36. What group of patients is at increased risk of absorption atelectasis?

37. How can you reduce the risk of absorption atelectasis?

Copyright © 2003, 1999 Mosby, Inc. All rights reserved.

▶ OXYGEN DELIVERY SYSTEMS

Now that you know why to give a patient O_2 and some of the hazards of administration, it's time to learn how to make tasty selections from the complex choices offered on the medical gas menu.

38. The three basic categories are low flow, high flow, and reservoir. Match the category to the description below.

Category		Description
A. Low flow _____		1. Always exceeds patient's inspiratory needs
B. Reservoir _____		2. Provides some of patient's inspiratory needs
C. High flow_____		3. May meet needs if no leaks occur

▶ LOW FLOW

39. Why do you think the nasal cannula is the most commonly used low-flow system?

40. When should you attach the cannula to a bubble humidifier?

41. What maximum flow does the text suggest for newborns?

Experiment

If you have access to a cannula, humidifier, and some medical O_2, I think you should find out what it feels like to be a patient. First, attach the cannula to a flowmeter with the nipple adaptor (or "Christmas tree" if you like that term better). Insert the prongs in your nose and set the flow to 1 L/min. Try that for 1 minute. Increase the flow by 1 L/min. Continue this until you get to the 8-L/min maximum suggested in the text. Try again with a humidifier.

Questions

How well could you feel the gas at 1 L? What implication does this have for patient care? When did the flow start to become noticeable? Uncomfortable? What happened to the humidifier as the flow rate exceeded 5 L/min?

42. What is the primary advantage of using a transtracheal O_2 catheter?

Copyright © 2003, 1999 Mosby, Inc. All rights reserved.

43. Why does the range of F_{IO_2} delivered by nasal cannulas vary so much?

44. Because you can't tell exactly how much O_2 a patient is receiving at any given moment from a cannula, how can you assess the effects of administering the drug?

45. What are the advantages and disadvantages of reservoir cannulas?
    A. Advantages

    B. Disadvantages

46. In what setting are reservoir cannulas usually used?

▶ RESERVOIR

47. Use Table 35-3 to help you find the information about O_2 masks.

Mask	F_{IO_2} Range	Advantage	Disadvantage
A. Simple	_____	_____	_____
B. Partial	_____	_____	_____
C. Non	_____	_____	_____

48. What is the primary difference between the partial rebreathing and nonrebreathing masks?

49. How can you tell if a nonrebreathing mask has an adequate flow rate?

50. Give a solution for each of these common problems with reservoir masks.

Problem	Solution
A. Confused patient removes mask	_____
B. Humidifier pop-off activated	_____
C. Mask causes claustrophobia	_____
D. Bag collapses on inspiration	_____
E. Bag fully inflated on inspiration	_____

Copyright © 2003, 1999 Mosby, Inc. All rights reserved.

Experiment

Get a nonrebreather (NRB), a simple mask, a bubble humidifier, a nipple adaptor, and a flowmeter. Try to use an NRB with two valves on the mask if you can find one.

First try the simple mask without a humidifier. Set the flowmeter at 2 L/min and breathe from the simple mask for a few breaths. Now take deep breaths. Set the flowmeter at 10 L/min and try again. Next, set up the NRB. Repeat the experiment. Breathe as deeply as you can and adjust the flowmeter until the bag doesn't collapse. Try the mask with one expiratory flap valve in place and with two (if possible). Finally, attach the bubble humidifier, set the flow at 10 L/min, and put on the mask. Increase the flow rate to 15 L/min, then flush.

Questions

- How did it feel to breathe on the simple mask at a low flow rate?
- What happened when you tried the NRB at a low flow?
- How did mask performance vary when you used two valves?
- What difference did the humidifier make?
- What happened to the humidifier when you increased the flow?

▶ HIGH-FLOW

Air-entrainment systems are commonly used to provide high-flow O_2 because they are simple and inexpensive to operate. Oxygen is directed through a small tube, or jet, which creates a very high forward velocity. Air is entrained into the system, which dilutes the O_2 and increases the total flow rate.

51. Describe the effects on F_{IO_2} and total flow rate caused by varying jet size or the entrainment port opening.

Factor	Increased Size	Decreased Size
A. Jet		
1. F_{IO_2}	_____	_____
2. Flow	_____	_____
B. Port		
1. F_{IO_2}	_____	_____
2. Flow	_____	_____

52. Fill in the air-to-O_2 ratios for the following O_2 concentrations (Table 35-7).
    A. 100% _____
    B. 60% _____
    C. 40% _____
    D. 35% _____
    E. 30% _____
    F. 24% _____

53. What is the common name for an air-entrainment mask (AEM)?

54. Why does the AEM have larger openings on the side of the mask than does a simple O_2 mask?

Copyright © 2003, 1999 Mosby, Inc. All rights reserved.

55. What is the effect on the F_{IO_2} delivered by an AEM caused by raising the delivered flow from the flowmeter?

56. Air-entrainment devices are classified as high flow. For what F_{IO_2} settings is this usually true?

57. How do you boost the total flow when using an AEM?

58. Why is this not possible with an air-entrainment nebulizer?

59. Four devices are used to deliver gas from an air-entrainment nebulizer to the patient. Choose the device(s) that fits each of the following patients (see Figure 35-16).

Patient	Aerosol Appliance
A. Tracheostomy tube	_____
B. Endotracheal tube	_____
C. Intact upper airway	_____

60. Describe an easy way to tell if an air-entrainment nebulizer is providing sufficient gas to meet the patient's needs.

61. Give one example of a specialized flow generator that produces an aerosol and one example that produces dry gas. These devices produce high flow and high F_{IO_2}, thus solving the problem created with nebulizers and AEMs. See Figures 35-18 and 35-19.
    A. Aerosol_____
    B. Dry _____

62. What is the effect of downstream resistance to flow on F_{IO_2} and total flow delivered by a typical AEM or nebulizer entrainment system?

Copyright © 2003, 1999 Mosby, Inc. All rights reserved.

Experiment

You will need an AEM, O_2 analyzer, and air-entrainment jet nebulizer with a length of corrugated tubing. First set the AEM at 40% with a flow of 5 L/min of O_2. Analyze the FIO_2 (detach the mask and put the analyzer tee on). Increase the flow to 8 L/min. Analyze again. Set up the nebulizer. Use 40% and a flow of 10 L/min. Analyze the output. Increase the flow to 12 L/min and analyze again. Pour enough water into the tube to *partially* occlude it. Analyze. Add enough water to completely occlude the tubing. Analyze. Finally, drain out the water. Try to increase the flowmeter setting past 15 L/min.

Questions

- What effect does altering flow rate have on the AEM?
- What is the effect of water (resistance) in the tubing of a jet neb?
- What happened when you tried to increase the flow with the neb? Why?

▶ MATHEMAGIC

Oxygen–to–air entrainment ratios and total flow from air-entrainment devices are universal clinical and board exam expectations that have driven countless students to the brink of insanity. Take a slow, deep breath. Exhale. Straighten shoulders. Engage. The way I see it, you have three choices. Memorize the ratios for each FIO_2. Learn the algebraic formula. Learn the magic box. You must learn and master this information!

If you like the first method, you must memorize every detail in Table 35-7.

Read the fine print.

Or

Look at the Mini Clini "Computing the Total Flow Output of an Air-Entrainment Device." A three-step method is provided for calculating the ratio and the subsequent total flow. Let's try one.

A patient is receiving O_2 at 40% via a ventimask with the flowmeter set at 8 L/min. What is the ratio of O_2 to air? What is the total flow?

Step 1: Compute the ratio

$$\frac{\text{Liters of air}}{\text{Liters of } O_2} = \frac{100 - 40}{40 - 21}$$

$$\frac{\text{Liters of air}}{\text{Liters of } O_2} = \frac{60}{19}$$

$$\frac{\text{Liters of air}}{\text{Liters of } O_2} = \frac{3}{1}$$

Step 2: Add the ratio parts

$3 + 1 = 4$

Step 3: Multiply the sum of the parts by the O_2 flow rate

$4 \times 8 = 32$ L/min total flow

Now you try.

63. What are the O_2-to-air entrainment ratio and total flow for a patient who is receiving 60% O_2 via an entrainment nebulizer with the flowmeter set at 10 L/min?
    A. Step 1: Compute the ratio
       Formula _____
       Calculation_____
       Reduce answer
       to get ratio _____
    B. Step 2: Add the parts _____
    C. Step 3: Multiply the sum of the parts by the O_2 flow rate _____

Copyright © 2003, 1999 Mosby, Inc. All rights reserved.

The "magic box" is my favorite (see Figure 35-14). Retry the sample problem above for a patient on 40%. Pretty nifty. The only problem with this method, is that you substitute 20 (instead of 21) to make the math easy. At percentages below 40, your answers will start to vary from the algebraic method. You can solve this by using 21 for low percentages and 20 for 40% or more.

Practice with your chosen method until you can solve for every FIO_2. There is no way out of this!

▶ BLENDERS

Oxygen blenders are another kind of magic box. The blender requires a 50 psi input of air and O_2. When you twirl the knob to set the FIO_2, you are actually adjusting a proportioning valve. Turning toward a high percentage of O_2 makes the opening for O_2 larger and the opening for air smaller; 100% closes the air side and only lets O_2 out. Vice versa for turning the knob toward 21%. Very handy device, the blender. It gives you high flow rates or 50 psi to power equipment at any FIO_2 you desire.

64. Describe the three-step process for confirming the proper operation of a blender (see Box 35-3).
    A.

    B.

    C.

▶ PUT THAT CHILD IN A BOX!

The opening scene of the venerable *Marcus Welby, MD* television show depicts a man in an O_2 tent. You may see this being done on soap operas as well. Today, enclosures are a simple way to deliver O_2 to infants and children.

65. What is the major problem with O_2 tents?

66. What is the highest FIO_2 you can expect to deliver with a tent?

Copyright © 2003, 1999 Mosby, Inc. All rights reserved.

67. Why is a hood the best method for delivering O_2 to an infant?

68. What minimum flow must be set for a hood? Why?

69. What harmful consequence occurs when the flow rate into the hood is too high?

70. What effect will cold air flowing into the hood have on a premature infant?

71. What is the best way to control O_2 delivery to an infant inside an incubator?

72. What is the primary benefit of the infant incubator?

► HBO

Life under pressure: that's hyperbaric O_2, or HBO. We can administer O_2 to the patient at 2 or 3 atmospheres (atmospheric pressure absolute [ATA]) to manage several acute and chronic problems. Originally designed for decompression sickness in divers, HBO operates according to Boyle's law. Respiratory care practitioners often work with patients who need this mode of O_2 administration. It also is common for respiratory therapists to work in hyperbaric units. So pick up your pencils and let's get on with the show!

73. Compare the monoplace and multiplace hyperbaric chambers.

Chamber	O_2 Delivery	Patient	Staff
A. Monoplace	_____	_____	_____
B. Multiplace	_____	_____	_____

74. List three acute and three chronic conditions in which hyperbaric O_2 is indicated (see Box 35-6).

Acute	Chronic
A. _____	_____
B. _____	_____
C. _____	_____

Copyright © 2003, 1999 Mosby, Inc. All rights reserved.

75. Under what circumstances is HBO indicated in cases of carbon monoxide poisoning (see Box 35-7)?

79. Helium is so diffusible that special balloons are used to hold it. What type of gas delivery device is used to administer helium to patients who are not intubated?

▶ WHAT ELSE COULD THERE BE?

76. Two other therapeutic gases are administered by respiratory therapists. Give indications for each.

Gas	Indications
A. NO	_____
	_____
B. Helium	_____
	_____

▶ CASE STUDIES

Case 1

Abraham Dink, a 58-year-old college professor, is admitted for chest pain and possible MI. ECG monitoring reveals sinus tachycardia. The chest pain has been decreased by administration of nitroglycerin. Respirations are 20 per minute, and SpO_2 on room air is 94%.

77. What other gas is always mixed with helium? What is the most common combination?

80. What is your assessment of this patient's oxygenation status?

78. What physical property of helium results in decreased WOB?

81. What is your recommendation in regard to administration of supplemental O_2?

Copyright © 2003, 1999 Mosby, Inc. All rights reserved.

Case 2

Rolly Clemens has been admitted for exacerbation of COPD. He is wearing O_2 at 2 L/min via nasal cannula. The pulse oximeter shows a saturation of 94% while Mr. Clemens is at rest. The nurse calls you to ask for your assistance in evaluation of Rolly's dyspnea during ambulation.

82. What changes occur in breathing pattern during exercise?

83. How are low-flow O_2 devices affected by changes in breathing pattern?

84. How would you assess dyspnea on ambulation for a patient wearing O_2?

Case 3

Linda Loo is recovering from surgery after a head injury. She is trached and needs supplemental O_2 at 60% via T piece. The flowmeter is set at 12 L/min. Each time Linda inhales, the mist exiting the T piece disappears.

85. Air-entrainment nebulizers are considered high-flow delivery systems. Discuss this in terms of the disappearing mist.

86. What should be added to the T piece to help deal with this problem?

87. Describe a common method of increasing the delivered flow when administering high FIO_2 via air-entrainment nebulizers.

88. What is the O_2-to-air entrainment ratio for 60%?

Copyright © 2003, 1999 Mosby, Inc. All rights reserved.

89. What is the total flow in the system described in this case?

▶ BOARD EXAM BROADSIDE

There must be some reason this chapter has gone on forever. The NBRC will expect you to know about all types of delivery systems and when to use them. You should know when O_2 is indicated and recognize and minimize potential hazards and complications. The Entry Level exam will have at least 10 questions based on the topic of "conducting therapeutic procedures to achieve adequate arterial and tissue oxygenation." Heliox administration is covered on the Registry Examination. Nitric oxide and HBO are not currently on the tests, but I would not be surprised to see these therapies in the near future. Pour yourself another cup of java and answer the following questions.

90. During a suctioning procedure, a patient experiences tachycardia with PVCs. Which of the following could be responsible for this response?
    A. Inadequate vacuum pressure
    B. Lack of sterile technique during the procedure
    C. Fear of the suctioning procedure
    D. Inadequate preoxygenation

91. A patient with a history of carbon dioxide retention is receiving oxygen at 6 L/min via nasal cannula. He is becoming lethargic and difficult to arouse. In regard to oxygen delivery, what change would you recommend?
    A. Change to a 40% Venturi mask
    B. Maintain the present therapy
    C. Change to a partial rebreathing mask
    D. Reduce the flow to 2 L/min and obtain an ABG

92. A newborn needs oxygen therapy. Which of the following methods of delivery would you select?
    A. Partial rebreathing mask
    B. Oxygen hood
    C. Venturi mask
    D. Oxygen tent

93. A patient is receiving oxygen therapy from a nonrebreathing mask with a flow rate of 10 L/min. The respiratory care practitioner observes the bag deflating with each inspiration. What action is indicated in this situation?
    A. Replace the mask with a cannula
    B. Immediately perform pulse oximetry
    C. Increase the flow to the mask
    D. Change to a Venturi mask

94. A patient is to receive a mixture of helium and oxygen. Which of the following delivery devices would be appropriate?
    A. Nasal cannula
    B. Oxygen tent
    C. Venturi mask
    D. Nonrebreathing mask

Copyright © 2003, 1999 Mosby, Inc. All rights reserved.

95. An 80/20 mixture of helium and oxygen is administered. The oxygen flowmeter is set at 10 L/min. What is the actual flow delivered to the patient?
    A. 10 L
    B. 14 L
    C. 16 L
    D. 18 L

96. A patient is receiving 40% oxygen via an air-entrainment mask with the flowmeter set at 8 L/min. What is the total flow delivered to the patient?
    A. 24 L/min
    B. 32 L/min
    C. 40 L/min
    D. 48 L/min

97. Water has accumulated in the delivery tubing of an aerosol system. This will result in all of the following *except*
    A. Increased F_{IO_2}
    B. Decreased aerosol output
    C. Increased total flow
    D. Increased backpressure in the system

98. A patient requires a flow rate of 40 L/min to meet his inspiratory demand for gas. He is to receive oxygen via a Venturi mask set at 24%. What is the minimum setting on the flowmeter to produce the appropriate flow?
    A. 1 L/min
    B. 2 L/min
    C. 3 L/min
    D. 4 L/min

► **FOOD FOR THOUGHT**

99. Why does common use of the term "100% nonrebreather" create a clinical problem?

100. Why would an AEM be preferred over an air-entrainment nebulizer for a patient who has asthma or COPD?

► **INFORMATION AGE**

A good place to start is the UMDNJ Respiratory Program site: **www.umdnj. edu/rspthweb/rstn2100/unit2.htm**

The KUMC respiratory care program has a good page on NO therapy: **classes.kumc. edu/cahe/respcared/cybercas/nitricoxide/ nother.html**

or

The nitric oxide home page: **darwin.apnet. com/no**

You could put a term such as "heliox therapy for asthma" or "nonrebreathing mask" into the search engine and get good sites.

One more idea for you that's cool. A hot item in home care is the O_2 conserving regulator. These devices work by sensing

Copyright © 2003, 1999 Mosby, Inc. All rights reserved.

inspiration and pulsing a dose of O_2 to the patient. No flow occurs during exhalation, so a lot of gas is saved. Sure beats a reservoir cannula! You can see one of these at the Salter website: **www.salterlabs.com/ products_con.htm**

Although Salter is a commercial site, if you click on Medical Professionals, you can get a lot of neat resources and links.

I really could go on and on, but you look like you need a break.

Copyright © 2003, 1999 Mosby, Inc. All rights reserved.

CHAPTER 36

Lung Expansion Therapy

> **"Whenever I feel like exercise,
> I lie down until the
> feeling passes."**
> **Robert Maynard Hutchins**

Postoperative complications are dreaded by everyone involved: surgeons, nurses, third-party payers, and yes, even patients. Postop pulmonary complications have been recognized as a problem for as long as surgery has been around, and we respiratory therapists have been at the forefront of the battle against atelectasis and retained secretions for many years. Anesthesia, pain, medications, and preexisting lung disease are the enemy. Fortunately, we have a powerful arsenal of lung expansion devices and treatments on our side.

▶ WORD POWER

One of the problems associated with lung expansion therapy is to explain the goals, procedures, and equipment so the patient can understand. For each of the following terms or treatments, give a simple, short explanation in terms that even your kid brother could understand. (I'll help you get started, but you don't have to use my words if you don't need to.)

1. Atelectasis
   "When you don't take deep breaths . . ."

2. Incentive spirometer (IS)
   A. "The purpose of this treatment is to . . ."

   B. "This device will . . ."

3. Sustained maximal inspiration
   "I want you to take . . ."

Copyright © 2003, 1999 Mosby, Inc. All rights reserved.

4. Intermittent positive pressure breathing (IPPB)
   A. "Your doctor has ordered a breathing treatment that will . . ."

   B. "This machine will . . ."

5. Continuous positive airway pressure (CPAP)
   A. "This treatment will . . ."

   B. "I am going to put a mask on your face . . ."

Maybe you should try out your explanations on friends or family members to see if you make sense.

▶ MEET THE OBJECTIVES

6. What is the definition of *atelectasis*?

7. What is resorption atelectasis, and when is it likely to occur?

8. What causes passive atelectasis?

9. Why are postoperative patients at highest risk of development of atelectasis?

10. Explain why hypoxemia can occur when FRC decreases in the first 48 hours after surgery.

Copyright © 2003, 1999 Mosby, Inc. All rights reserved.

11. What specific group of postop patients is at highest risk?

B. Breaths sounds

C. Respiratory rate

12. Name two other types of patients who have increased likelihood of development of atelectasis. Explain why.
A.

D. Heart rate

B.

E. Chest radiograph

13. Explain how each of the following signs can help provide clues that atelectasis is present. (Can you use the same signs to tell if atelectasis is resolving after lung expansion therapy?)
A. History

14. All modes of lung expansion therapy increase lung volume by increasing the transpulmonary pressure gradient. What are the two methods for increasing the gradient?
A.

B.

Copyright © 2003, 1999 Mosby, Inc. All rights reserved.

15. List three indications for, two contraindications to, and two hazards of IS (see Boxes 36-1, 36-2, and 36-3).
    A. Indications
        1. _____
        2. _____
        3. _____
    B. Contraindications
        1. _____
        2. _____
    C. Hazards
        1. _____
        2. _____

16. By whom and in what year was IPPB first introduced? (Oops! Sorry, I went into Sputum Bowl mode for a minute.)

17. Like IS, IPPB is used to manage atelectasis. Specifically, when would IPPB be indicated rather than IS?

18. What is the one absolute contraindication to IPPB?

19. List at least five additional partial contraindications.
    A. _____
    B. _____
    C. _____
    D. _____
    E. _____

20. Name two common complications of IPPB administration.
    A. _____
    B. _____

21. What outcomes will tell you that your IPPB therapy has been effective? Name at least four.
    A. _____
    B. _____
    C. _____
    D. _____

22. Name the three current positive airway pressure (PAP) therapies. Which one is the best?
    A. _____
    B. _____
    C. _____
    D. The best one is _____

23. Physiologic effects of CPAP are poorly understood but probably include
    A. _____
    B. _____
    C. _____
    D. _____

24. Name two contraindications to CPAP therapy.
    A. _____
    B. _____

Copyright © 2003, 1999 Mosby, Inc. All rights reserved.

25. The text suggests three major complications of this therapy. Discuss each of the following problems.
    A. Hypoventilation

    B. Barotrauma

    C. Gastric distention

26. What alarm system is essential for monitoring patients receiving CPAP?

27. Adequate flow is important to maintain CPAP levels. How can you determine the intitial setting?

► CHAPTER HIGHLIGHTS

28. Atelectasis is caused by persistent _____ with _____ tidal volume.

29. Patients who have undergone upper _____ or _____ surgery are at the greatest risk of atelectasis.

30. A history of _____ disease or _____ is an additional risk factor.

31. _____ is not associated with atelectasis unless the patient also has pneumonia.

32. Patients with atelectasis usually demonstrate _____ _____ breathing.

33. The most common problem associated with lung expansion therapy is the onset of respiratory _____, which occurs when the patient breathes _____.

► CASE STUDIES

Use the protocol found in Figure 36-8 to help answer the following questions.

Case 1

John Babbit is an alert, 34-year-old man admitted for cholecystectomy. John smokes 2 packs of cigarettes per day. After the operation, the surgeon asks for your recommendation for therapy to prevent lung complications.

Copyright © 2003, 1999 Mosby, Inc. All rights reserved.

34. Discuss potential risk factors for atelectasis in this case.

35. What therapy would you recommend for prevention of atelectasis for Mr. Babbit?

Case 2

Maria Contraire is immobilized after hip replacement. Mrs. Contraire is a 70-year-old, 5'2" tall woman. Her predicted inspiratory capacity is 1.8 L. She is performing IS at 600 mL per breath. Breath sounds reveal bilateral basilar crackles, and the patient is coughing up lots of thick mucus.

36. What is the minimum acceptable volume for IS?

37. What treatment would you recommend adding to the therapeutic regimen at this time?

Case 3

Marcy Strongarm is an obese, confused 54-year-old woman. She is recovering from CABG (open-heart surgery). Marcy has persistent atelectasis with mild hypoxemia. A radiograph shows an elevated left hemidiaphragm with air bronchograms in the left base. Vital capacity is 10 mL/kg.

38. What is the significance of the elevated diaphragm and air bronchograms seen on the chest radiograph?

39. What treatment would you recommend? Why? What's the minimum goal for this therapy?

▶ WHAT ABOUT THOSE BOARD EXAMS?

Lung expansion techniques such as IS, IPPB, and CPAP are important parts of your board examinations. Positive expiratory pressure (PEP) usually is discussed under secretion management. The main difference between the CRT and RRT exams is the difficulty level of the questions. For example, the CRT is more likely to ask you to recall facts or to apply them. The RRT asks more difficult questions that require you to analyze information.

Copyright © 2003, 1999 Mosby, Inc. All rights reserved.

40. A patient reports a "tingling" feeling in her lips during an IS treatment. The respiratory therapist should instruct the patient to
    A. Breathe more slowly
    B. Take smaller breaths
    C. Continue with the treatment as ordered
    D. Exhale through pursed lips after each breath

41. Which of the following alarms is a vital part of the system when CPAP therapy is set up for management of atelectasis?
    A. Exhaled volume
    B. High respiratory rate
    C. Pulse oximetry
    D. Low pressure

42. During administration of IPPB therapy, the practitioner observes the system pressure rise above the pressure set to end the inspiration. The respiratory therapist should instruct the patient to
    A. "Help the machine give you a deep breath"
    B. "Inhale slowly along with the machine"
    C. "Exhale gently and normally"
    D. "Exhale through pursed lips after each breath"

43. A patient is having difficulty initiating each breath with an IPPB machine. The practitioner should adjust the
    A. Pressure limit
    B. Peak flow
    C. FIO_2
    D. Sensitivity

44. Which control is used to increase the volume delivered by an IPPB machine?
    A. Pressure limit
    B. Peak flow
    C. FIO_2
    D. Sensitivity

45. Continuous positive airway pressure is used to increase which of the following?
    A. Functional residual capacity
    B. Peak expiratory flow rate
    C. FEV_1
    D. Arterial carbon dioxide levels

46. An IPPB machine cycles on with the patient effort but does not shut off. The most likely cause of this problem is
    A. The pressure is set too low
    B. The sensitivity is set incorrectly
    C. There is a leak in the system
    D. The patient is not blowing out hard enough

47. How should you instruct a patient to breathe during incentive spirometry?
    A. "Exhale gently, then inhale rapidly through the spirometer"
    B. "Inhale deeply and rapidly through the spirometer"
    C. "Exhale until your lungs are empty, then inhale and hold your breath"
    D. "Exhale normally, then inhale slowly and deeply and hold your breath"

48. How often should a patient be instructed to use an incentive spirometer after being taught to perform the procedure correctly?
    A. 10 breaths, 4 times per day
    B. 6 to 10 breaths every hour
    C. 10 to 20 breaths every 2 hours
    D. 6 to 8 breaths tid

Copyright © 2003, 1999 Mosby, Inc. All rights reserved.

49. A patient who has undergone an operation for abdominal aortic aneurysm experiences postoperative arrhythmias and hypotension. The physician asks for your recommendation for lung expansion therapy. The best choice in this situation would be
    A. IS
    B. IPPB
    C. PEP
    D. CPAP

50. When adjusting the flow rate control on an IPPB machine, the respiratory therapist would be altering the
    A. Maximum pressure delivered by the device
    B. The effort required to initiate a breath
    C. The volume delivered by the machine
    D. The inspiratory time for a given breath

I'll stop torturing you now, but I could go on and on. To get good at lung expansion therapy you will need to get out the equipment and practice in the lab. All of these treatments can be delivered to classmates in practice sessions until you are skilled with the devices, the coaching, and the breathing circuits. My students say the hardest part is learning to explain and coach therapy, not the equipment.

▶ FOOD FOR THOUGHT

51. Your textbook refers to using vital capacity or inspiratory capacity as important indicators in lung expansion therapy, especially IS. How can you determine the predicted inspiratory capacity?

▶ INFORMATION AGE

For an interesting treatise on trends in lung inflation therapy try **www.wws.princeton. edu/cgi-bin/byteserv.prl/~ota/disk3/ 1981/8102/810206.PDF**

Your best bet on the subject of LI is the AARC Clinical Practice Guidelines: **www.rcjournal.com/online_resources/ cpgs/cpg_index.asp**

Copyright © 2003, 1999 Mosby, Inc. All rights reserved.

Bronchial Hygiene Therapy

**"Sputum is our
bread and butter."
Anonymous respiratory therapist**

Bronchial hygiene. Well, it sounds better than "pulmonary toilet," which was the catch phrase when I was a student. After medical gas administration, playing with sputum is what makes our profession famous (or infamous). I distinctly remember my early clinical experience of asking a man to "cough it up" while I turned my head away to gag. That was before I got used to that lovely rattling sound. Join me now, for the halls are alive with the sound of mucus, and we've got work to do.

▶ ACRONYMS AGAIN?

After you've read Chapter 37 (you have read it, right?), you will have noticed an awful lot of acronyms. Let's get those out of the way before we dive into bronchial hygiene. Write the definition for each of these mystic medical markings.

1. ACB

2. ARDS

3. AD

4. CF

5. CPT

Copyright © 2003, 1999 Mosby, Inc. All rights reserved.

6. CPAP

7. EPAP

8. FET

9. HFCWC

10. HZ

11. ICP

12. IPV

13. MI-E

14. PDPV

15. PEP

▶ AIRWAY CLEARANCE

Normal lungs generate a modest amount of mucus from the goblet cells, glands, and Clara cells. The mucociliary escalator whips that stuff up and out in no time. You

Copyright © 2003, 1999 Mosby, Inc. All rights reserved.

hardly even notice. Of course, things go wrong—that's where we come in.

16. Name the four phases of the normal cough. Give examples of impairments of each (Table 37-1).

      Phase   *Impairments*

A. _____ _____
                   _____

B. _____ _____
                   _____

C. _____ _____
                   _____

D. _____ _____
                   _____

17. Compare the effects of full and partial airway obstruction caused by retained secretions.

18. Name at least three conditions that can cause internal obstruction or external compression of the airway lumen.
    A. _____
    B. _____
    C. _____

19. Just for fun, state the airflow velocities and increase in lung pressure created by a good strong cough.
    A. Expiratory velocity
    B. Pleural/alveolar pressure

20. Name two obstructive lung diseases that result in excessive secretion of mucus and impairment of normal clearance.
    A. _____
    B. _____

21. List four neurologic or musculoskeletal conditions that impair cough.
    A. _____
    B. _____
    C. _____
    D. _____

▶ **BRONCHIAL HYGIENE: GOALS AND INDICATIONS**

Getting the gunk out of the lungs is the main idea, but there's more to it, of course. The big picture is made up of acute conditions, chronic disorders, prevention, and assessment.

22. Name four acute conditions in which bronchial hygiene is indicated (see Box 37-2).
    A. _____
    B. _____
    C. _____
    D. _____

23. Explain why you think bronchial hygiene is not useful in managing most cases of pneumonia or uncomplicated asthma.

24. Discuss bronchial hygiene therapy for chronic lung conditions. How much sputum needs to be produced daily for the therapy to be useful? What diseases are managed?

Copyright © 2003, 1999 Mosby, Inc. All rights reserved.

25. Describe the two well-documented preventive, or prophylactic, uses of this type of therapy.
    A.

    B.

26. To determine the need for bronchial hygiene therapy, you would assess the patient and the medical record. Give a brief explanation of the significance of each factors listed below (Box 37-3).

	Factor	Significance
A.	History	_____
		_____
B.	Airway	_____
		_____
C.	Chest radiograph	_____
		_____
D.	Breath sounds	_____
		_____
E.	Vital signs	_____
		_____

▶ BRONCHIAL HYGIENE METHODS

There are five general noninvasive approaches to managing secretion problems. Within each general approach are several choices. You will need to customize therapy for each patient on the basis of cost, effectiveness, clinical condition, and ability to participate in therapy.

Postural Drainage

27. Kinetic therapy has many pulmonary benefits. Name two nonpulmonary benefits.
    A. _____
    B. _____

28. Postural drainage therapy includes up to four components, not counting cough:
    A. _____
    B. _____
    C. _____
    D. _____

29. List two absolute and two relative contraindications to turning.
    A. Absolute
       1. _____
       2. _____
    B. Relative
       1. _____
       2. _____

30. What does your book mean by "plumbing problems"?

31. Describe prone positioning. What is it used for? What is the benefit?

32. How long should you wait to schedule postural drainage after a patient eats? Why?

Copyright © 2003, 1999 Mosby, Inc. All rights reserved.

33. What is the minimum range of time for effective application of postural drainage therapy?

34. Give two recommended interventions for each of the complications of postural drainage listed below (see Table 37-2).

Complication	Interventions
A. Hypoxemia	_____
	_____
B. Increased ICP	_____
	_____
C. Acute hypotension	_____
	_____
D. Pulmonary bleeding	_____
E. Vomiting	_____
	_____
F. Bronchospasm	_____
	_____
G. Cardiac dysrhythmias	_____
	_____

35. Discuss cough in relation to postural drainage.

36. How long does it take to determine the effectiveness of postural drainage? If therapy is effective, how often should you reevaluate in the hospital? In the home?
   A. How long?
   B. Reevaluate hospital patients
   C. Reevaluate home patients

37. Describe at least five factors that must be documented after each postural drainage treatment.
   A. _____
   B. _____
   C. _____
   D. _____
   E. _____

38. Describe percussion and vibration as techniques to loosen secretions. Are they effective?

39. Compare manual and machine methods of percussion and vibration.

Exercise: Learn Those Pesky Positions!

I wish I could tell you an easy way to learn the positions for chest drainage. Here are some suggestions. Photocopy Figure 37-3. Cut out each position and cut off the heading that names the position. Tape the picture to the front of a 3 × 5 index card and the title (lung segment) to the back. My

Copyright © 2003, 1999 Mosby, Inc. All rights reserved.

students find this an effective way to make flash cards. A good visual learning tool.

Maybe you are more of a kinetic learner. Get a partner (two partners works better) and a hospital bed (could be in the lab or the medical center). One person should name a lung segment. Position your victim in what you think is the correct position. Check the position to see if you got it right, or have a third person check. This way you will physically learn the positions and have to move someone around, add pillows, etc. Because there are approximately 12 positions for the 18 lung segments, you will need to spend 30 to 45 minutes on this exercise. You will need to repeat this at least two or three times before you have the positioning and related segments rock solid in your memory. I am sure this will pay off when you are tested.

P.S. If you don't have a partner, use a mannequin.

Coughing Techniques

Bronchial hygiene therapy is frustrating and sometimes useless if you can't get the patient to make an effective cough. Directed cough, cough staging, huff coughing, autogenic drainage, and active cycle of breathing are all good tools you'll want to have in your bag of tricks. Each patient may need a combination of hygiene and coughing techniques.

40. How would you position a patient (ideally) for an effective cough?

41. Standard directed cough must frequently be modified. Give three examples of patients who may need modified cough techniques.
    A. _____
    B. _____
    C. _____

42. What is splinting?

43. What special form of cough assistance is used in the care of patients who have neuromuscular conditions?

44. Describe the forced expiratory technique (FET).

45. Describe the three repeated cycles of the active cycle of breathing (ACB) technique.
    A.

Copyright © 2003, 1999 Mosby, Inc. All rights reserved.

B.

C.

46. What is the primary problem with autogenic drainage?

47. Describe the two cycles of mechanical in-exsufflation (MI-E) in terms of time and pressure.
A. Inspiratory

B. Expiratory

Positive Airway Pressure

48. Positive airway pressure is a popular way to help mobilize secretions. What are the four indications for PAP adjuncts according to the AARC CPG?
A. _____
B. _____
C. _____
D. _____

49. What type of monitoring is essential regardless of the equipment used to deliver PAP to help mobilize secretions?

High-Frequency Compression/Oscillation of the Chest Wall

50. Describe the two general approaches to oscillation.
A.

B.

51. What do you think are the primary problems with vests and shells? What group of patients most commonly use the ThAIRapy vest?

Copyright © 2003, 1999 Mosby, Inc. All rights reserved.

52. Describe at least four of the benefits or advantages of the flutter valve as a secretion management tool.

A.

B.

C.

D.

Mobilization and Exercise

Early mobilization and frequent position changes are standards of care in preventing pulmonary complications after surgery or trauma.

53. Describe the benefits of adding exercise as a mobilization technique.

54. What should you specifically monitor when exercising patients with lung problems?

▶ **CASE STUDIES**

Use the algorithm (Figure 37-13) to assist you in answering the following questions.

Case 1

Dr. Abraham Dock is a 60-year-old professor who has undergone colon resection for an intestinal tumor. He is receiving IS to help expand his lungs. You are asked to assess Dr. Dock for retained secretions. Auscultation reveals coarse rhonchi present bilaterally in the upper lobes. A few scattered crackles are heard in the bases. SpO_2 on room air is 94%. The patient states he is unable to cough up anything "because it hurts too much."

Copyright © 2003, 1999 Mosby, Inc. All rights reserved.

55. What technique could you use to decrease the pain associated with cough in a postoperative patient?

56. What cough techniques are options for this patient?

Case 2

Mabel Horowitz is a 75-year-old woman with bronchiectasis who states she coughs up "cups of awful mucus every day." She is admitted with a diagnosis of pneumonia.

57. What therapy is indicated while Mabel is in the hospital?

As you provide the therapy, you find out that Mrs. H is a widow who lives alone. She takes albuterol treatments via SVN when she has difficulty breathing.

58. What therapy alternatives can you recommend for home use?

▶ **WHAT DOES THE NBRC SAY?**

The Board says, "Study hard and listen to Uncle Steve so you can pass your boards!" Well, OK, what it really says is this (Entry Level examination matrix):

"B. Conduct therapeutic procedures to . . .
2. Remove bronchopulmonary secretions:

a. perform postural drainage, perform percussion and/or vibration . . .
d. instruct and encourage bronchopulmonary hygiene techniques [e.g., coughing techniques, autogenic drainage, positive expiratory pressure device (PEP), intrapulmonary percussive ventilation (IPV), Flutter, High Frequency Chest Wall Oscillation (HFCWO)]"

Here's a sample of what you can expect:

59. During the initial treatment, a PEP device is set to deliver a pressure of 15 cm H_2O. The patient reports dyspnea and can maintain exhalation for only a short time. Which of the following should the respiratory therapist recommend?
    A. Decrease the PEP level to 10 cm H_2O
    B. Increase the PEP level to 20 cm H_2O
    C. Discontinue the PEP therapy
    D. Add a bronchodilator to the PEP therapy

Copyright © 2003, 1999 Mosby, Inc. All rights reserved.

60. A patient is lying on her left side, one quarter turn toward her back, with the head of the bed down. What division of the lung is being drained?
    A. Lateral segments of the right lower lobe
    B. Right middle lobe
    C. Left upper lobe, lingular segments
    D. Posterior segment of the right upper lobe

61. A patient is receiving postural drainage in the Trendelenburg position. The patient begins to cough uncontrollably. What action should the respiratory therapist take at this time?
    A. Encourage the patient to use a huff cough
    B. Administer oxygen therapy
    C. Administer a bronchodilator
    D. Raise the head of the bed

62. In explaining the therapeutic goal of PEP therapy to a patient, it would be most appropriate to say
    A. "This will help prevent pneumonia"
    B. "This will increase your intrathoracic pressure"
    C. "This will help you cough more effectively"
    D. "This will prevent atelectasis"

63. A COPD patient with left lower lobe infiltrates is unable to tolerate a head-down position for postural drainage. What action would you recommend?
    A. Perform the drainage with the head of the bed raised
    B. Do not perform the therapy until 2 hours after the last meal
    C. Administer a bronchodilator before the postural drainage
    D. Notify the physician and suggest a different secretion management technique

64. Active patient participation is an important part of which of the following procedures?
    I. Postural drainage
    II. Directed cough techniques
    III. Airway suctioning
    IV. Positive expiratory pressure (PEP)
    A. I and II only
    B. II and IV only
    C. I, III, IV only
    D. I, II, and IV only

65. A respiratory therapist is preparing a patient with bronchiectasis for discharge. Which of the following techniques would be most appropriate for self-administered therapy in the home?
    A. IPPB
    B. Flutter
    C. Suctioning
    D. Percussion and postural drainage.

▶ **FOOD FOR THOUGHT**

66. How does hydration affect secretion clearance? What respiratory therapy modality can augment hydration of the airway?

Copyright © 2003, 1999 Mosby, Inc. All rights reserved.

67. Your text mentions never clapping directly over the spine or clavicles. Can you think of other places you should not clap? Use your imagination. (Could you get fired for clapping on certain parts of the anatomy?) So where *exactly* should you clap?

Oh, one more thing. When a patient has lung disease in only one lung, or "unilateral lung disease," positioning is very important. The rule of thumb is *down with the good lung*. When you put the good lung down, gravity takes the blood flow to the best ventilation. If you put the bad lung down, perfusion goes to the bad lung, and oxygenation can worsen dramatically. There are some exceptions: Lung abscess, pulmonary interstitial emphysema, and internal bleeding may necessitate that you put the bad lung down. Otherwise, watch your patients for signs of distress if you turn them so the diseased lung is down.

▶ INFORMATION AGE

High-frequency oscillation delivered via a vest is a hot new therapy being used for more than just patients with cystic fibrosis. There are hundreds of possible uses, such as amyotrophic lateral sclerosis, muscular dystrophy, and transplantation care. Check it out at **www.thevest.com**

Another innovation is vibratory PEP devices. Check out "Quake" at **www.methapharm.com/CANADA/Quake.htm**

and Acapella at **www.dhd.com**

They make TheraPEP as well.

If you're looking for a wide selection of information, I suggest you go to your search engine and type in "bronchial hygiene" or "secretion management." You'll get a lot of useful sites with these keywords.

Copyright © 2003, 1999 Mosby, Inc. All rights reserved.

Respiratory Failure and the Need for Ventilatory Support

"There's no success like failure, and
failure's no success at all."

Bob Dylan

Chapter 38 is short, sweet, and essential to your understanding of why patients need mechanical ventilation. Remember, 36% of all patients with a diagnosis of acute respiratory failure die in the hospital. When you understand the material in this chapter, you will be ready to tackle the complex subject of mechanical ventilation and critical care.

► **"LOOK OUT, KID, YOU'RE GONNA GET HIT WITH . . . ACRONYMS!"**

Here's a short, sweet crossword puzzle to help you get over your fear of small words.

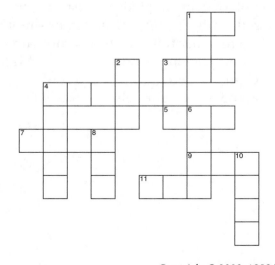

ACROSS

1. Preset minimum rate, patient can trigger breaths with set volumes
3. Maximum voluntary ventilation
4. Inability to maintain normal oxygen delivery to the tissues
5. Mode of ventilatory support designed to augment spontaneous breathing
7. Ventilatory support which patient breathes spontaneously at an elevated baseline
9. Measure of the output of respiratory muscles in cm H_2O pressure
11. Ventilator mode that uses high respiratory rates

DOWN

1. Another name for AC
2. Opposite of MIP
3. Also called NIF and MIF
4. Respirarory failure indicated by CO_2 greater than 50 in an otherwise healthy individual
6. Mode of support where spontaneous breaths are allowed between patient-triggered machine breaths
8. Mode of support in which breaths are delivered at a preset inspiratory pressure
10. Pressure above atmospheric during exhalation of a mechanical ventilator breath

Copyright © 2003, 1999 Mosby, Inc. All rights reserved.

▶ SO, WHAT COULD GO WRONG?

1. Complete this sentence: "Put simply, respiratory failure is the

2. What are the blood gas criteria for respiratory failure?
   A. $P5aO_2$

   B. $PaCO_2$

3. What are the two general types of respiratory failure based on the type of physiologic impairment?
   A. Type I is

   B. Type II is

▶ LET'S REVIEW

Egan's lists six causes of hypoxemia. Of these, decreased FIO_2, diffusion defect, and perfusion/diffusion impairment are not commonly seen in the acute care setting. Ventilation/perfusion ($\dot{V}/\dot{Q}$) mismatch, shunt, and hypoventilation are common.

- Ventilation/perfusion mismatch usually is a result of poor ventilation of areas that still get blood flow. A typical example would be bronchospasm.
- Shunt occurs when there is no ventilation at all. A typical example would be pneumonia or ARDS.
- Hypoventilation occurs in an essentially normal lung when CO_2 displaces O_2. A typical example would be a drug overdose.

It's not too difficult to tell these conditions apart.

- Ventilation/perfusion mismatch responds to oxygen therapy.
- Shunt does not respond to oxygen therapy.
- Hypoventilation manifests with a normal alveolar-arterial (A – a) gradient and responds to ventilation.

4. What is the classic blood gas presentation of acute hypoxemic respiratory failure due to $\dot{V}/\dot{Q}$ mismatch or shunt? (Remember this one. It will show up to haunt you on the boards. See the Mini Clini "Differentiating Causes of Hypoxemia" for help.)

Copyright © 2003, 1999 Mosby, Inc. All rights reserved.

▶ TELL ME MORE, TELL ME MORE

5. What is the relation between Pa_{CO_2} and alveolar ventilation?

6. *Egan's* states that three major disorders are responsible for acute hypercapnic respiratory failure (type II). Give two examples of disorders representative of each category. Table 38-1 provides a complete list.
   A. Decreased ventilatory drive
      1. _____
      2. _____
   B. Respiratory muscle fatigue/failure
      1. _____
      2. _____
   C. Increased work of breathing
      1. _____
      2. _____

7. Give an example of a condition that could cause greatly increased CO_2 production.

▶ ACUTE-ON-CHRONIC RESPIRATORY FAILURE

8. How does the body compensate for chronically elevated CO_2 levels associated with COPD or obesity hypoventilation syndrome?

9. What happens to the normal blood gas classification of respiratory failure in the care of patients with chronic respiratory failure?

10. Identify the five most common factors that lead to acute-on-chronic failure.
    A. _____
    B. _____
    C. _____
    D. _____
    E. _____

11. What are the four main treatment goals for this group of patients?
    A. _____
    B. _____
    C. _____
    D. _____

Copyright © 2003, 1999 Mosby, Inc. All rights reserved.

12. Complications of the management of acute respiratory failure are as life-threatening as the failure itself. Identify the likely causes of these pulmonary complications.
    A. Emboli

    B. Barotrauma

    C. Infection

13. Give one example of each of these non-pulmonary complications of life in the ICU.
    A. Cardiac

    B. Gastrointestinal

    C. Renal

14. Oh, go ahead, tell me three more complications associated with prolonged visits to the unit.
    A. _____
    B. _____
    C. _____

▶ TUBE 'EM

15. What is the primary goal of mechanical ventilation?

Copyright © 2003, 1999 Mosby, Inc. All rights reserved.

16. Your board exams will expect you to identify these classic criteria for mechanical ventilation. Remember that no one criterion mandates ventilation (except apnea). See Table 38-2.

Mechanism	Critical Value
A. Pa_{CO_2}	_____
B. pH	_____
C. Vital capacity (VC) (mL/kg)	_____
D. Maximal inspiratory pressure (MIP)	_____
E. MVV	_____
F. Minute ventilation ($\dot{V}_E$)	_____
G. V_{DS}/V_T	_____
H. Alveolar-arterial difference in partial pressure of oxygen $[P(A-a)O_2]$ on 100%	_____
I. Ratio between Pa_{O_2} and fractional concentration of inspired oxygen (P/F)	_____

I'm not kidding. You need to learn these values!

17. Oxygenation values such as P/F ratio and A – a gradient are useful in determining the severity of failure. What is the limitation of these methods?

18. Why is it useful to consider pH in evaluation of CO_2 levels to determine the need for intubation and ventilation?

19. Identify the two common causes of decreased ventilatory drive.
   A. _____
   B. _____

20. Name four less common potential causes of decreased drive.
   A. _____
   B. _____
   C. _____
   D. _____

21. Respiratory *muscle weakness* is most likely to occur in what patient group?

22. Name three conditions that frequently lead to respiratory *muscle fatigue*.
   A. _____
   B. _____
   C. _____

23. List three objective tests that can be performed to assess respiratory muscle strength at the bedside.
   A. _____
   B. _____
   C. _____

Copyright © 2003, 1999 Mosby, Inc. All rights reserved.

24. What will blood gas analysis show (one more time!) in full-blown ventilatory failure?

25. What is the cardinal sign of increased WOB?

▶ STRATEGIES

26. State the modes of support indicated for each of the following causes of respiratory failure. See Table 38-3.

    A. Rapidly reversible hypoxemic failure
    _____

    B. Slowly reversible hypoxemic failure
    _____
    _____

    C. Acute alveolar hypoventilation
    _____
    _____

    D. Chronic alveolar hypoventilation
    _____
    _____

    E. Altered mental status
    _____
    _____

    F. Acute muscle fatigue
    _____
    _____

    G. Chronic muscle fatigue
    _____
    _____

27. Give two strategies for preventing overdistention of alveoli in ARDS.
    A. _____
    B. _____

28. What mode of ventilation is most commonly used to guarantee $\dot{V}_E$ in patients with acute alveolar hypoventilation?

29. In terms of blood gases, what is the treatment goal for ventilation of patients with chronic hypoventilation?

30. Patients who need intubation for respiratory muscle fatigue (not weakness!) generally need what type of support (and for how long) to rest their muscles?
    A. Type of support _____
    B. How long? _____

▶ SPECIAL CASES

31. How does hyperventilation result in reduced ICP in head injury?

Copyright © 2003, 1999 Mosby, Inc. All rights reserved.

32. What is the target Pa_{CO_2} in these cases?

33. What is the chief concern regarding use of PEEP to increase oxygenation in patients with acute head injury?

34. Air trapping, or hyperinflation, as a result of obstructive lung disease (COPD, asthma) causes what two complications in mechanically ventilated patients?

    A. _____

    B. _____

35. How are V_T and flow rate manipulated to reduce complications in mechanically ventilated COPD patients?

    A. Tidal volume

    B. Flow rate

36. What surprising technique was found by MacIntyre to reduce auto-PEEP?

► **CHAPTER HIGHLIGHTS**

37. Acute respiratory failure is identified by a Pa_{CO_2} > _____ mm Hg and/or a Pa_{O_2} < _____ mm Hg in an otherwise healthy person (at sea level).

38. _____ respiratory failure usually is due to $\dot{V}/\dot{Q}$ mismatch, intrapulmonary _____, or _____.

39. _____ respiratory failure results from inadequate drive, respiratory muscle _____, or excessive work of _____.

40. Chronic respiratory failure may be represented by ABG values demonstrating _____ with evidence of metabolic compensation or _____ reflecting chronic hypoxemia.

41. The _____ status of the patient is the most important factor determining the need for ventilator support.

42. Excessive _____ is the most common cause of respiratory muscle fatigue.

Copyright © 2003, 1999 Mosby, Inc. All rights reserved.

43. Only patients with rapidly reversible conditions should undergo _____ ventilation in the acute setting.

44. The goal of therapy in acute hypercapnic respiratory failure is to guarantee a set _____ ventilation.

► CASE STUDIES

Case 1

Wendy Baldo is an alert, anxious 25-year-old woman who arrives in the emergency department with chills, fever, and shortness of breath. An ABG sample is drawn on room air with these results:

pH	7.45
Pa_{CO_2}	32 mm Hg
Pa_{O_2}	50 mm Hg
HCO_3	23 mEq/L

45. Interpret these blood gas results.

46. What is the A – a gradient?

47. What type of respiratory failure is present?

48. What do you recommend for initial respiratory treatment?

Case 2

Anne Town is a 27-year-old brought to the emergency department by paramedics after a drug overdose. She is obtunded. Blood gases are drawn on room air:

pH	7.24
Pa_{CO_2}	60 mm Hg
Pa_{O_2}	65 mm Hg
HCO_3	26 mEq/L

49. Interpret these blood gas results.

50. What is the A – a gradient?

51. What type of respiratory failure is present?

Copyright © 2003, 1999 Mosby, Inc. All rights reserved.

52. What is the appropriate initial respiratory treatment in this case?

56. What initial respiratory treatments are indicated? What are we trying to avoid?

Case 3

Danny Lang is an alert 56-year-old man with a history of COPD. He arrives in the emergency department reporting dyspnea that has worsened over the last few days. A blood gas sample is drawn on room air:

pH	7.26
Pa_{CO_2}	70 mm Hg
Pa_{O_2}	50 mm Hg
HCO_3	32 mEq/L

53. Interpret these blood gas results.

54. What is the A – a gradient?

55. What type of respiratory failure is present?

► WHAT DOES THE NBRC SAY?

Stop. Do not pass Go. Do not collect $200! The information presented in Chapter 38 is the basis of our understanding of respiratory failure. It is highly complex, combining blood gases, pathophizz, and more. The NBRC is passionate about your understanding of this material and will present you with many similar situations. Assess. Interpret. Recommend. Treat. Modify. Wow! When you are working on these problems, always start by interpreting the ABG results. Do this in the context of the patient's history. A history of COPD should raise a red flag that suggests you think hard before you interpret or act. Here are some examples.

57. A respiratory care practitioner is asked to evaluate a lethargic 50-year-old woman who is in respiratory distress after abdominal surgery. She is breathing spontaneously with a 50% air-entrainment mask at 32 breaths/min. ABG results show

pH	7.28
Pa_{CO_2}	55 mm Hg
Pa_{O_2}	60 mm Hg
HCO_3	26 mEq/L

On the basis of this information what would you recommend?

Copyright © 2003, 1999 Mosby, Inc. All rights reserved.

A. Intubation and mechanical ventilation
B. Increase the F_{IO_2} to 1.0
C. Administer IPPB
D. Administer bronchodilator therapy via SVN

58. An alert, anxious 60-year-old man with a history of CHF presents in the emergency department with respiratory distress. Auscultation reveals bilateral inspiratory crackles. He has peripheral edema. Arterial blood gas results drawn on partial rebreathing mask show

pH	7.45
Pa_{CO_2}	35 mm Hg
Pa_{O_2}	40 mm Hg
HCO_3	23 mEq/L

The most appropriate therapy for improving oxygenation would be
A. Intubation and mechanical ventilation
B. Administration of oxygen therapy via nonrebreathing mask
C. Administration of oxygen therapy via CPAP
D. Administration of bronchodilator therapy via SVN

59. An adult male patient is being mechanically ventilated immediately after surgery for a closed head injury. Settings are

Tidal volume	700 mL
Rate	10
Mode	AC
F_{IO_2}	0.40
PEEP	0

ABGs show

pH	7.37
Pa_{CO_2}	44 mm Hg
Pa_{O_2}	86 mm Hg
HCO_3	24 mEq/L

Which of the following ventilator changes would you recommend at this time?
A. Increase the F_{IO_2}
B. Decrease the volume
C. Increase the rate
D. Increase the PEEP

60. An adult patient is being mechanically ventilated after respiratory failure. Settings are

Tidal volume	800 mL
Rate	12
Mode	AC
F_{IO_2}	0.60
PEEP	2 cm H_2O

ABGs show

pH	7.37
Pa_{CO_2}	41 mm Hg
Pa_{O_2}	43 mm Hg
HCO_3	22 mEq/L

Which of the following ventilator changes would you recommend at this time?
A. Increase the F_{IO_2}
B. Decrease the volume
C. Increase the rate
D. Increase the PEEP

Copyright © 2003, 1999 Mosby, Inc. All rights reserved.

61. A patient with a history of hypercapnia and COPD is intubated and placed on the ventilator after respiratory failure. Twenty-four hours later the patient is alert and breathing spontaneously. Settings are

Tidal volume	800 mL
Rate	12
Mode	AC
FIO_2	0.30
PEEP	0 cm H_2O

ABGs show

pH	7.48
$PaCO_2$	41 mm Hg
PaO_2	60 mm Hg
HCO_3	30 mEq/L

Which of the following ventilator changes would you recommend at this time?
A. Decrease the FIO_2
B. Decrease the volume
C. Change to pressure-control ventilation (PCV)
D. Change to synchronized intermittent mandatory ventilation (SIMV)

62. A 77-year-old man with COPD is admitted with acute bronchitis. Room air blood gas results show

pH	7.52
$PaCO_2$	45 mm Hg
PaO_2	40 mm Hg
HCO_3	36 mEq/L

What intervention would be appropriate at this time?
A. CPAP with 24% oxygen
B. 28% air-entrainment mask
C. Nasal cannula at 5 L/min
D. Simple mask at 8 L/min

63. CPAP is indicated for treatment of patients with
A. Respiratory failure secondary to shunting
B. Apnea
C. Ventilatory failure with hypercapnia
D. Hypoxemia secondary to $\dot{V}/\dot{Q}$ mismatch

Between the cases, the chapter, and these questions you should be getting the general idea.

▶ **FOOD FOR THOUGHT**

Remember Table 38-2, the one about measurable indications for ventilatory support? I didn't forget about that one. Your boards expect you to know this information as part of the decision to intubate and ventilate or as part of the decision to wean.

64. What clinical situation or condition suggests use of ABGs to evaluate the need to intubate and ventilate? Compare this with situations better assessed with measures such as VC and MIP. We'll come back to this again in Chapter 44 when we talk about weaning.

▶ **INFORMATION AGE**

Let's go to virtual hospital for an overview of acute respiratory failure:
www.vh.org/adult/provider/ emergencymedicine/ARF/ AcuteRespiratoryFailure.html

A good overview of CPAP and BiPAP in the treatment of failure:
www.theberries.ns.ca/Archives/CPAP.html

Another good overview at emedicine:
www.emedicine.com/MED/topic2011.htm

Copyright © 2003, 1999 Mosby, Inc. All rights reserved.

CHAPTER 39

Mechanical Ventilators

"Just bag 'em till I get there."
Florida Society for RC T-Shirt

CMV PSV PCV AMV MMV VAPS ZEEP NEEP PEEP Bleep . . . Brain reeling. Neuronal meltdown. Must try to understand Chapter 39 . . . must remain conscious.

Once upon a time there were only three modes of ventilation. Control, assist control (AC), and the new kid, intermittent mandatory ventilation (IMV). Ventilators were driven by pistons or bellows, and an occasional light bulb glowed or buzzer sounded when there was a problem. Volume cycled, pressure limited was, well, exactly what it sounded like. Times have changed. Ventilators cost more than new cars, and microprocessors have allowed engineers to fulfill their wildest dreams. Whether the explosion of technology in ventilator design has improved healthcare has yet to be determined, but you, dear student, will have to try to make sense of it anyway.

▶ VENTILATOR VERBIAGE

Match these definitions to the key terms in the beginning of the chapter.
1. _____ Breath initiated by the ventilator
2. _____ Causes a breath to end

3. _____ Manipulated by machine to cause inspiration
4. _____ Controls the magnitude of inspiration
5. _____ Combination of machine and spontaneous breaths
6. _____ Machine breaths only, no spontaneous
7. _____ Pressure above the baseline in the expiratory phase of a machine breath
8. _____ Causes a breath to begin
9. _____ Breath initiated and ended by the patient

A. Spontaneous breath
B. Control variable
C. Limit variable
D. Cycle variable
E. Intermittent mandatory ventilation
F. Trigger variable
G. Continuous mandatory ventilation
H. Positive end-expiratory pressure
I. Mandatory breath

▶ HOW VENTILATORS WORK

10. What is a ventilator?

Copyright © 2003, 1999 Mosby, Inc. All rights reserved.

11. Describe the desired output of the ventilator in terms of the patient.

12. Identify at least three settings in which ventilators use direct current back-up power sources.
    A. _____
    B. _____
    C. _____

13. How are most modern intensive care ventilators powered?

14. Identify one setting in which electrical power is undesirable.

15. What other mechanisms are used to drive a ventilator besides compressed gas?

▶ **I'M IN CONTROL**

16. What does the output control valve do?

17. Setting an appropriate expiratory time (at least three time constants) is clinically important to avoid what dangerous condition?

18. What are the three variables that ventilators control?
    A. _____
    B. _____
    C. _____

19. Identify the five types of control circuits used in ventilators.
    A. _____
    B. _____
    C. _____
    D. _____
    E. _____

20. State two advantages of fluidic control circuits.
    A. _____
    B. _____

Copyright © 2003, 1999 Mosby, Inc. All rights reserved.

21. Control variables are how a ventilator manipulates inspiration. Fill in the blanks below to show what is constant and what changes for each control variable.

Control Variable	Constant	Varies with Changes in Lungs
A. Pressure	_____	_____
B. Volume	_____	_____
C. Flow	_____	_____

▶ PHASED OUT

22. Describe the basic purpose of the following phase variables in terms of the breathing cycle.

Phase Variable	Portion of Breathing Cycle Controlled
A. Trigger variable	_____
B. Limit variable	_____
C. Cycle variable	_____
D. Baseline variable	_____

23. Name the three ways to trigger the ventilator.
    A. _____
    B. _____
    C. _____

24. Time triggering divides each minute into segments allotted for each breath. This is the total cycle time. If the rate is 12 breaths/min, what is the total cycle time? (Hint: Divide the minute into 12 equal parts.)

25. What is the normal setting range for pressure triggering? Flow triggering?
    A. Pressure _____ to _____ cm H_2O
    B. Flow _____ to _____ below baseline flow

26. Pressure-support ventilation (PSV) is an example of a mode that has a limit (pressure) but is cycled off by another variable (flow). Define the term limit variable.

27. Define the term cycle variable.

28. What is the most common application of pressure cycling?

29. What lung inflation therapy entails use of a pressure-cycled machine?

Copyright © 2003, 1999 Mosby, Inc. All rights reserved.

30. Try to explain the difference between pressure limiting and pressure cycling.

31. What is the usual cycling value for PSV?

32. Define the term baseline variable.

33. What baseline variable is used on all modern ventilators?

34. Explain what is meant by these acronyms. Which is the default value for ventilators?
    A. ZEEP

B. NEEP

C. PEEP

► **A LA MODE**

35. Define the phrase mode of ventilation.

36. You need to decide on a control variable to end inspiration. What are the two primary ways to end inspiration?
    A. _____
    B. _____

37. What does dual control mean?

Copyright © 2003, 1999 Mosby, Inc. All rights reserved.

38. Define spontaneous and mandatory breaths. Give another term for each.
   A. Spontaneous

   B. Mandatory

B. CSV

C. IMV

39. Explain the basic sequence of ventilation represented by each of these terms.
   A. CMV

Are you sitting down? Take a slow, deep breath and let it out. Now look at Table 39-2. Oh boy. These are the most common modes in use today. Egan's points out, in Table 39-2, that ventilator companies do not standardize names of modes. So two identical modes have different names on different machines. The five ventilators shown have 36 different names for just a few modes. What's a student to do?

Copyright © 2003, 1999 Mosby, Inc. All rights reserved.

	Acronym	Full Name	Pattern	Ventilator
A.	CMV	_____	VC-CMV	Drager
B.	A/C	_____		Hamilton
C.	PC-CMV	Pressure control–continuous mandatory ventilation	PC-CMV	840
D.	TC	_____	PC-CSV	840
E.	SIMV+	_____	VC-IMV	All vents
F.	CPAP	_____	PC-CSV	Drager
G.	PCAC	Pressure control–assist control	_____	_____
H.	PC-SIMV	_____		Hamilton 840
I.	CPAP+PS	Continuous positive airway + pressure support	PC-CSV	_____
J.	APRV	Airway pressure release vent	_____	_____
K.	MMV	_____	_____	_____
L.	VS	_____	DC-PSV	Servo
M.	Bi-Level	_____	_____	840

40. To start learning this material, you need to know the basic acronyms used for various modes. Later, when you are working, you may need to know only those used on the vents at your hospital. I'll help you fill this in (use Table 39-2 as well).

Let's recap:

- All ventilators offer a mode that intermixes spontaneous breaths with ventilator breaths. This is called synchronized intermittent mandatory ventilation (SIMV).
- All ventilators offer a mode that is machine breaths only. Common names are continuous mandatory ventilation (CMV) and assist control (AC).
- All ventilators offer the choice of volume-controlled ventilator breaths (VC) and pressure-controlled ventilator breaths (PC) for any mode that offers a machine breath.
- All ventilators have a mode that is spontaneous breathing without machine breaths. This is called spontaneous or continuous positive airway pressure (CPAP).
- All ventilators offer a way to augment spontaneous breaths with a pressure boost. This is called pressure support (PS or PSV).
- A few ventilators offer a spontaneous mode that switches between two baseline pressures above 0 cm H_2O. This is called airway pressure release ventilation (APRV) or bilevel ventilation.

▶ RIDE THE WAVES

Ventilator waveforms have been around for a long time, but when I was a student we couldn't really see them in action. Most modern ventilators are capable of displaying waveforms graphically so you can apply them clinically. For example, if you see that expiratory flow does not return to baseline before the next breath starts, you know that the patient is not able to exhale completely.

Copyright © 2003, 1999 Mosby, Inc. All rights reserved.

You can then adjust the ventilator to allow complete exhalation or try to manage the problem (by giving a bronchodilator, for example). I know only two ways to help you learn waveforms. One method of learning this difficult subject is to practice drawing the waveforms. The other way is to go to a ventilator in the classroom or lab. Attach the ventilator to a test lung, turn on the graphics, and adjust the ventilator to deliver different settings and look at the waveforms produced. It will help you if an instructor is handy to guide you through this procedure. Once you learn to identify the various waveforms, you can move on to the next step, which is to learn the problem pictures, what they mean clinically, and how to fix the problem. Egan's covers this area in Chapter 39.

41. Draw these flow patterns.
    A. Rectangular _____
    B. Ascending ramp _____
    C. Descending ramp _____
    D. Sinusoidal _____

Most ventilators allow the therapist to select the flow waveform from at least three of these four patterns. The pressure waveform will be determined by the mode you select.

▶ PICK A MODE, ANY MODE: CLINICAL APPLICATION OF VENTILATOR MODES

Continuous Mandatory Ventilation

Continuous mandatory ventilation allows the operator to greatly reduce patient WOB and control minute volume. Pretty good if the patient is apneic or exhausted or you want a specific $PaCO_2$ level.

42. Pressure or volume may be used as the control variable for machine breaths. What happens to volume and airway pressure when compliance decreases?

Control Variable	Volume	Airway Pressure
A. Pressure	_____	_____
B. Volume	_____	_____

43. Why is manipulation of mean airway pressure clinically important?

44. What is the primary goal of CMV?

45. What are three potential harmful effects of excess triggering in CMV?
    A. _____
    B. _____
    C. _____

46. Use of VC-CMV allows the clinician fairly precise control over what values?

Copyright © 2003, 1999 Mosby, Inc. All rights reserved.

47. When is PC-CMV indicated?

48. Why does PC improve patient comfort and ventilator synchrony?

49. What value has to be closely monitored in PC to avoid volutrauma or ventilator-induced hypoventilation?

50. Dual-control CMV may be useful when a patient has unstable or changing pulmonary mechanics. The ventilator makes small adjustments in pressure to maintain a good tidal volume. Pressure-regulated volume control (PRVC) is one example of dual-control CMV (DC-CMV). Give an example of a clinical situation in which DC-CMV could be useful.

Synchronized Intermittent Mandatory Ventilation

The most popular mode in the country, SIMV often is used for weaning (although it can be a bit slow). Synchronized intermittent mandatory ventilation also provides work for the respiratory muscles and other benefits of spontaneous breathing. You set the level of support by determining how many machine breaths you want to give each minute.

51. What is the potential cardiac benefit of the spontaneous breaths in SIMV?

52. Patients with Guillain-Barré syndrome usually have normal lungs and a drive to breathe. What mode would you select?

53. Pressure-control IMV (PC-IMV) or DC-IMV (if you have it) could be useful in what clinical situation involving COPD or asthma? Why?

Copyright © 2003, 1999 Mosby, Inc. All rights reserved.

Spontaneous Ventilation

In this mode the patient begins and ends each breath. You can set the level of support the ventilator gives during the spontaneous breath. There are many spontaneous breathing modes, but CPAP and PSV are the common terms used throughout our profession.

54. Give an example of initial pressure levels for CPAP mode.

55. What does this accomplish physiologically?

56. Pressure support is popular because of its many attributes. List at least four.
    A. _____
    B. _____
    C. _____
    D. _____

► CASE STUDIES

Case 1

Dane Lopez, a 21-year-old patient, is placed on a ventilator after a closed head injury. The physician desires to control this patient's ventilation to achieve a specific CO_2 level in the arterial blood.

57. What level of CO_2 is desirable in this situation?

58. What would you recommend if the patient's breathing pattern were out of synch with the ventilator?

Case 2

Martha Gomes is a 35-year-old woman with a neuromuscular disease. She is placed on a Puritan-Bennett 840 ventilator in CMV mode. The ventilator is set for AC volume-cycled ventilation at a rate of 10 breaths/min, but the machine is triggering at a rate of 28 breaths/min. Martha looks pretty scared.

59. What is the most likely cause of the excess ventilator triggering?

60. What mode of ventilation does Egan's suggest you use to solve this problem?

Copyright © 2003, 1999 Mosby, Inc. All rights reserved.

▶ WHAT DOES THE NBRC SAY?

The following modes of ventilation are listed in the examination matrices.

- PCV
- SIMV
- PS or PSV
- CPAP
- PCV
- AC
- Adjust ventilator mode (nonspecific)

For the more common traditional modes you are expected to be able to recommend, initiate, adjust, etc, in other words, everything! We'll get into this more in Chapter 41, so don't worry. The less common modes, such as APRV, are not specifically mentioned, but you still need to know a little general information, such as when to recommend these modes.

61. A patient with ARDS is being ventilated with the following settings:

Mode	AC
V_T	800 mL
Rate	14 breaths/min
FIO_2	80%
PEEP	15 cm H_2O

Peak pressure is unacceptably high while oxygenation remains poor. Which of the following changes may be beneficial in this situation?
A. Change the PEEP to 20 cm H_2O
B. Increase the FIO_2 to 100%
C. Initiate pressure control ventilation
D. Place the patient on BiPAP by mask

62. A patient being ventilated in SIMV mode is making spontaneous efforts with a tidal volume of 150 mL. What modification would you recommend?
A. Initiate PEEP
B. Initiate PSV
C. Change to CPAP mode
D. Change to CMV mode

63. A patient with COPD and CO_2 retention is intubated after respiratory failure. The physician states she wants to avoid overventilation and air trapping. Which of the following modes would you recommend?
A. SIMV
B. AC
C. CPAP
D. APRV

64. A patient in the early stages of ARDS is intubated. The physician states he wishes to minimize the possibility of volutrauma or barotrauma. Which of the following modes would you recommend?
A. Volume-control ventilation
B. Manual ventilation
C. CPAP
D. Pressure-control ventilation

65. An 80-kg (176 lb) patient is being ventilated in pressure control mode. During a ventilator check, the therapist notes that the compliance has decreased from 40 mL/cm H_2O to 35 mlL/cm H_2O. What effect will this change in compliance have on the patient-ventilator system?
A. No effect
B. Increased peak airway pressure
C. Decreased mean airway pressure
D. Decreased tidal volume

Copyright © 2003, 1999 Mosby, Inc. All rights reserved.

▶ FOOD FOR THOUGHT

Not all modes are used in all parts of the country. What are your hospitals using? Does practice vary between community hospitals and the trauma center? A good starting point for the new practitioner is to learn about the modes most commonly used in current practice where you live and where you do your clinical training. For example, if you are being assigned to do clinical in a small hospital where CMV and AC are the main modes, don't go in with the idea that you will implement PC-IRV. Instead, learn as much as you can about the art of using CMV. The best respiratory therapists can make the best of whatever mode is used in their institutions while acting as resources to the nurses and physicians. Therapists pull the other modes out of their bags of tricks when the opportunity arises. But only after making themselves experts. Introducing a new ventilator or new mode of ventilation is fraught with hazards if in-service training doesn't come along with the changes.

▶ INFORMATION AGE

A nice tutorial on the differences between APRV, bilevel, and other advanced modes with pressure control is found at **www.ccmtutorials.com/rs/mv/page13.htm**

A short and fairly clear explanation of some of the newer modes of ventilation is found on ISPUB, the Internet journal of anesthesia at **www.ispub.com/ostia/index.php?xmlFile Path=journals/ija/vol4n4/ventilation.xml**

Here's another thought for you. Go on-line to **www.medscape.com** and register. It's free. This will give you access to more than 100 on-line journals and other resources. I found lots of articles on mechanical ventilation.

Copyright © 2003, 1999 Mosby, Inc. All rights reserved.

Physiology of Ventilatory Support

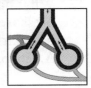

"Life is like riding a bicycle. You don't fall
off unless you stop pedaling."
Author unknown

Mechanical ventilation can be a life-sustaining procedure. But it is not natural.
There are physiological consequences to
applying positive pressure to the lungs and
chest. For better or for worse, we're currently married to this technology, and you
will need to understand what happens
when you connect the patient to the
machine.

► WORD POWER

There aren't too many new words to learn
in Chapter 40. Look up the definitions in
the glossary and write them out next to the
six words I've listed below.

1. Barotrauma _____
   _____

2. Time constant _____
   _____

3. Intrinsic PEEP _____
   _____

4. Transrespiratory pressure _____
   _____

5. Ventilator asynchrony _____
   _____

6. Work of breathing _____
   _____

7. Mean airway pressure _____
   _____

8. Transpulmonary pressure _____
   _____

► LIFE UNDER PRESSURE

9. Which pressure is responsible for
   maintaining normal alveolar inflation?

10. Which pressure gradient is required
    to expand the lungs and chest wall
    together?

11. Which pressure causes airflow in the
    airways?

Copyright © 2003, 1999 Mosby, Inc. All rights reserved.

12. What happens to transpulmonary pressure during normal inspiration? Exhalation?
    A. Inspiration

    B. Exhalation

13. What happens to transpulmonary pressure during inspiration with a negative pressure ventilator? Exhalation?
    A. Inspiration

    B. Exhalation

14. What is "tank shock"?

15. What happens to the airway and pleural pressures during inspiration with a positive pressure ventilator?

▶ WHAT ABOUT OXYGENATION?

Remember type I failure? The mechanical ventilator can be used to improve oxygenation through a variety of methods.

16. Explain how mechanical ventilation improves oxygenation for each of the following causes of hypoxemia:
    A. Hypoventilation

    B. Ventilation/perfusion mismatch

    C. Shunt

Copyright © 2003, 1999 Mosby, Inc. All rights reserved.

17. State the formula for D_{O_2}. Explain how PEEP may decrease D_{O_2}.

18. I know we had this before, but tell me again what is meant by "optimal PEEP."

► EFFECTS OF MECHANICAL VENTILATION

There are so many effects of mechanical ventilation that we need to break them down into little pieces to understand what happens when you attach that circuit to the ET tube! Let's start with

► VENTILATION

19. State the formula for minute ventilation ($\dot{V}_E$).

20. What is the normal range of tidal volume during spontaneous breathing?

21. It's important to set a tidal volume on the ventilator that is based on pathophysiology. What volume would you set for a patient with
    A. ARDS
    B. COPD
    C. Normal lungs
    D. Neuromuscular disease

22. Besides increasing the volume, how can you increase $\dot{V}_E$ with the ventilator?

23. What effect does $\dot{V}_E$ have on Pa_{CO_2}?

24. Where is gas distributed by a normal spontaneous breath? What about a positive pressure breath?
    A. Spontaneous _____
    B. PPV _____

Copyright © 2003, 1999 Mosby, Inc. All rights reserved.

25. How does perfusion, or blood flow, in the lung change during positive-pressure ventilation (PPV)?

26. What's the net effect of all this redistribution on the $\dot{V}/\dot{Q}$ ratio?

27. How would poor ventilator management result in respiratory acidosis?

28. There are several ways you could assess this problem. Explain results for each of the following.
    A. Draw arterial blood

    B. Check electrolytes

C. Check ECG

29. How would poor ventilator management result in respiratory alkalosis?

30. There are several ways you can assess this problem. Explain results for each of the following.
    A. Draw arterial blood

    B. Check electrolytes

    C. Check ECG

Copyright © 2003, 1999 Mosby, Inc. All rights reserved.

► LUNG MECHANICS

31. How long does it take for 95% of the alveoli in a normal lung to fill with air?

32. What are the two major factors that affect alveolar time constants?
    A. _____
    B. _____

33. Compare a restrictive disorder such as ARDS and an obstructive problem such as COPD in terms of the time it takes for alveolar filling and emptying.
    A. ARDS needs _____ inspiratory time and _____ expiratory time.
    B. COPD needs _____ inspiratory time and _____ expiratory time.

34. You could help prolong the inspiratory phase by making adjustments:
    A. Inspiratory time should be _____
    B. Inspiratory flow should be _____

35. You could help prolong the expiratory phase by making adjustments:
    A. Inspiratory flow should be _____
    B. Mandatory ventilator rate should be _____
    C. Tidal volume should be _____

36. What is meant by the term peak inspiratory pressure? What's the abbreviation?

37. What is meant by the term *plateau pressure?* What's the symbol?

38. We can protect patients' lungs from damage caused by pressure by maintaining plateau pressures at less than _____ to _____ cm H_2O.

39. See if you know how to adjust mean airway pressure. It's a little complicated. Circle "T" if the choice increases mean airway pressure.

    A. Increase peak pressure   T   F
    B. Decrease inspiratory time   T   F
    C. Synchronized IMV   T   F
    D. Increase PEEP levels   T   F
    E. Constant pressure pattern   T   F
       (PC mode)

40. OK, now tell me how increasing mean airway pressure affects FRC and oxygenation.
    A. FRC

Copyright © 2003, 1999 Mosby, Inc. All rights reserved.

B. Oxygenation

41. Does PPV by itself increase FRC? What do you need to add to improve this lung capacity?

42. What effect does PPV have on dead space?

► WHAT ABOUT WOB?

Ventilators are intended to decrease WOB. Many patients in respiratory failure are exhausted, and their breathing muscles need a break to recover.

43. What happens to the diaphragm if the ventilator does the work for too long?

44. What type of triggering reduces WOB?

45. What inspiratory maneuver can be added to SIMV to reduce WOB through the ET tube and ventilator circuit?

46. Rapid, shallow breathing index (RSBI) is a simple way to look at WOB at the bedside. What's the formula for RSBI and what value is predictive of a workload consistent with weaning from the vent?

► MINIMIZING ADVERSE EFFECTS OF THE VENTILATOR ON THE LUNG

Mechanical ventilation is life-saving. Unfortunately, it can also damage the lung. The respiratory therapist is the advocate for the patient's lung tissue.

Copyright © 2003, 1999 Mosby, Inc. All rights reserved.

47. Although there is no absolute maximum, *Egan's* suggests keeping PIP less than what value?

48. What about plateau pressure (P_{plat}) (I know, I already asked this but it's important)?

49. Look at Table 40-2 and give two negative pulmonary effects of too much PEEP.
    A. _____
    B. _____

50. Why is PEEP a problem with severe unilateral lung disease?

51. Identify two potential harmful effects of controlled CMV.
    A. _____
    B. _____

52. Name two advantages of IMV.
    A. _____
    B. _____

53. What is the primary reason for using PC-CMV?

54. What are some of the possible benefits of APRV?

55. What is PSV designed to accomplish?

56. *Egan's* says PSV will result in four beneficial effects. Name them
    A. _____
    B. _____
    C. _____
    D. _____

57. What is the effect of CPAP on ventilation?

Copyright © 2003, 1999 Mosby, Inc. All rights reserved.

58. Identify the important physiological effect of CPAP.

59. Bilevel CPAP was originally developed for management of OSA. It also has been shown to be useful in acute care settings. Explain.
    A. COPD

    B. ARDS

60. Automatic tube compensation is not a mode of ventilation. What is it?

61. Patients with unilateral lung disease benefit greatly from what type of positioning?

62. What unique position improves oxygenation in ARDS?

▶ NOT JUST THE LUNGS!

Amazingly enough, PPV affects almost every important organ system in the body. Heart, kidney, liver, brain, and gastrointestinal (GI) tract. And you thought you would just put the patient on the ventilator!

63. Briefly explain the negative effects of PPV on the heart.

64. Compare the cardiovascular effects of positive pressure in patients with compliant lungs, noncompliant lungs, and noncompliant chest walls. Give examples of these conditions.
    A. Emphysema (compliant lung)

    B. ARDS (stiff lung)

Copyright © 2003, 1999 Mosby, Inc. All rights reserved.

C. Kyphoscoliosis (stiff chest)

65. Healthy persons can easily compensate for moderate increases in airway pressure. What patients are especially sensitive to the cardiovascular effects of PPV?

66. How can you use the ventilator to temporarily manage increased ICP?

67. Explain the mechanism behind the drop in urine output in ventilated patients.

68. There is a high incidence in GI bleeding among ventilator patients, usually owing to stress ulceration of the gastric mucosa. Name the two pharmacologic agents used to protect the GI tract.
A. _____
B. _____

69. Increased ICP is not the only central nervous system (CNS) problem associated with mechanical ventilation. The ICU experience can cause fear, anxiety, and pain. Name one sedative and one analgesic that may help.
A. Sedative
B. Analgesic

We'd like to get the patient to level 2 or 3 on the Ramsay scale.

► WHAT ELSE COULD GO WRONG?

Everything to do with the ventilator, circuit, and the airway, of course. I won't bore you with the details, just highlight some things that might be important on your board exams.

70. Chest cuirass and poncho-type negative pressure ventilators are still used in some settings. Hypoventilation can result from what two problems?
A. _____
B. _____

71. Positive pressure ventilation has long been associated with barotrauma. List three of the clinical signs of pneumothorax.
A. Chest motion
B. Percussion note
C. Breath sounds

72. Tension pneumothorax is life-threatening in a ventilated patient. How and where is this managed?
A. How

Copyright © 2003, 1999 Mosby, Inc. All rights reserved.

B. Where

73. What is volutrauma, and how is it prevented?

74. Air trapping in ventilator patients can result in what condition?

75. Oxygen toxicity can damage lung tissue. Every effort should be made to reduce the FIO_2 to what value?

76. List three ways to reduce the risk of ventilator-associated pneumonia.
    A. Positioning
    B. Circuit changes
    C. Reduce condensates

and, of course, the essential antiinfection procedure . . .

▶ **CHAPTER HIGHLIGHTS**

Fill in the blanks, thanks.

77. Positive physiological effects of PPV include improved _____ and ventilation and decreased _____ of breathing.

78. No single _____ pattern has been demonstrated to be more physiologically effective than another.

79. Research indicates better ventilator synchrony and gas exchange with the _____ flow pattern than with the _____ flow pattern.

80. _____ triggering appears to be a better choice than _____ triggering when it is available on the ventilator.

81. Positive end-expiratory pressure is applied to restore _____ in restrictive disease and _____ the airways in obstructive disease.

82. Positive end-expiratory pressure allows the respiratory therapist to decrease _____, thereby avoiding the complications of _____ toxicity.

83. Positive pressure ventilation is detrimental to the $\dot{V}/\dot{Q}$ ratio primarily by shifting _____ to areas that are less _____.

84. Positive pressure ventilation PPV can decrease venous _____ and cardiac _____.

Copyright © 2003, 1999 Mosby, Inc. All rights reserved.

85. Positive pressure ventilation PPV can cause hepatic and GI malfunction primarily owing to decreased _____ of those _____ beds.

► CASE STUDIES

Case 1

The condition of Willie Wilson, a trauma patient, is stabilized after a motor vehicle accident. Willie is intubated and transported to the ICU, where you place him on ventilator. As soon as you put him on the machine, Mr. Wilson's blood pressure falls dramatically.

86. What should you do (right away!)?

87. What is the most likely cause of hypotension in a trauma patient who has been placed on PPV?

Case 2

Two days later, poor lung compliance and hypoxemia associated with noncardiogenic pulmonary edema (ARDS) have developed. The patient is being ventilated with AC, 12 breaths/min, 900 mL, +15 cm H_2O PEEP, and FIO_2 70%. Blood gases show pH, 7.37; $PaCO_2$, 38 mm Hg; PaO_2, 55 mm Hg. Peak inspiratory pressure is 60 cm H_2O; P_{plat} is 50 cm H_2O.

88. There are two serious problems here. Identify them.
   A. Serious problem 1

   B. Serious problem 2

89. What change(s) in ventilator strategy would you suggest?

► WHAT DOES THE NBRC SAY?

Not much, actually. Nothing new, that is. Of course, you need to be able to recognize the harmful effects of PPV. If pneumothorax develops, you assess, recognize, and recommend treatment. Chapter 40 reviews each of the common modes of ventilation, and the board exams are quite clear that you should be familiar with them, as I mentioned in Chapter 39. Let's move on.

Copyright © 2003, 1999 Mosby, Inc. All rights reserved.

▶ FOOD FOR THOUGHT

90. If the newest modes of ventilation are not proved to alter patient outcome, why should we use them?

91. Patients on ventilators have a high incidence of GI bleeding. Why is GI bleeding such a big deal to respiratory therapists?

▶ INFORMATION AGE

One place you might look is
www.ards.org

This sight has information in plain English and has some application if you'd like to learn more about managing this condition. For a more scientific approach, there is a good on-line bibliography at
www.novametrix.com/library/bib_vm.htm

or check out this good article at emedicine
www.emedicine.com/emerg/topic788.htm

ARDSnet is another good site:
hedwig.mgh.harvard.edu/ardsnet

Finally, don't forget Dr. Sharma's great website:
www.ssharma.com

I find good information on ventilator stuff under each disease category. Oh, I could go on and on, but you are getting sleepy, very sleepy. Now you will go to sleep, and when you wake up you will remember the physiology of ventilator support.

Copyright © 2003, 1999 Mosby, Inc. All rights reserved.

Initiating and Adjusting Ventilatory Support

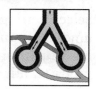

> "Paralyze resistance with persistence."
>
> **Woody Hayes**

A long time ago, in an ICU far, far away, we used a one size fits all approach to mechanical ventilation. It was easier that way, but we did not realize how this could harm the patient. Chapter 41 is one of the best and most important chapters in *Egan's* because it details a clear-cut plan for initiating and managing the ventilator in terms of what's wrong with the patient. Custom-made ventilation. The concept of pathophysiology-based mechanical ventilation is so important the NBRC included an article on the concept in its newsletter. So whether you are talking about board exams or clinical practice, it's the way to go.

▶ FIRST THINGS FIRST

I'll share my approach, and you can see whether it works for you. First, I read the chapter and highlighted key points with one of those fluorescent yellow markers. Took 2 hours and four cups of coffee. Next, I mapped out a plan. Looks like this:

Step 1

Decide whether to use positive or negative pressure. Easy because negative pressure is pretty much used for long-term neuromuscular problems and chest wall disorders. Used in the hospital only if the patient brings it in.

Step 2

Full ventilator support or partial support? I'll pick full support for patients who are apneic or paralyzed by drugs, or if they are exhausted from struggling to breathe. I'll remember to use this modality for a short time to avoid muscle atrophy. Partial support is good for patients with a drive to breathe, for patients being weaned, or for minimization of adverse effects of positive pressure.

Step 3

Select volume or pressure control. Volume control works pretty well and is especially good when you want to control minute ventilation and Pa_{CO_2}. Pressure control is great when you need to keep pressure low to prevent lung injury with ARDS or ALI. Pressure control also is good when you want to let the patient control flow and volume. It's more comfortable and flexible.

Step 4

Pick a mode. Assist control (CMV) and SIMV are the most common and best understood of all the modes. Pressure support is almost always added to SIMV to help reduce WOB.

Copyright © 2003, 1999 Mosby, Inc. All rights reserved.

Step 5

Select settings for ventilation. Rate, volume, FIO_2, and PEEP should be set according to pathophysiology. Alarm settings are pretty standardized.

Step 6

Assess the patient after you initiate your choices. Make changes to meet your goals for the patient. Comfort and synchrony, gas exchange and hemodynamics. That's what you want to look at.

▶ IS THERE AN ACRONYM IN THE HOUSE?

I feel really bad about all these acronyms. Lucky for you we already covered every one of these babies. Besides, I'm saving my strength for vocabulary in Chapter 42.

▶ CASE STUDIES

We're nearing the end of this book. At this point, I think you would benefit from less traditional workbook questions and fill-in problems. Let's go right to the cases and find out whether you understand how to initiate and adjust ventilatory support. I found four basic types of lungs and 10 specific disorders that make up almost every case of mechanical ventilation.

▶ LUNG FUN

Box 41-15 is dynamite! It covers most of the bases. Your four basic types of lungs are

- Normal lungs, such of those of a young patient with obstructive disease, 10 to 12 mL/kg for V_T
- Normal lungs, such as those of a patient with neuromuscular disease, 12 to 15 mL/kg

- Obstructed lungs, such as those affected by acute exacerbation of COPD or asthma, 8 to 10 mL/kg
- Stiff lungs, such as those affected by ARDS/ALI, 8 mL/kg; can go lower to keep pressure down

Let's get to work! You will need Tables 41-6 and 41-8, and Box 41-15 to help with the cases.

Case 1

Yvonne Robertson is a 5′5″ tall, 132-lb (60 kg), young woman who attempted suicide by drug overdose. She is unconscious and breathing slowly and shallowly. The emergency department physician elects to intubate Ms. Robertson.

1. What size ET tube would be appropriate for an adult woman?
   A. 6.0 mm inside diameter (ID)
   B. 7.0 mm outside diameter (OD)
   C. 7.5 mm ID
   D. 8.0 mm ID

2. In the emergency setting, how will you assess proper tube placement?
   I. Auscultate the chest
   II. Auscultate the epigastrium
   III. Attach an exhaled CO_2 monitor
   IV. Observe chest wall motion
   A. I, II only
   B. I, III only
   C. II, III, IV only
   D. I, II, III, IV

After intubation is completed, a small amount of white secretions is suctioned from the airway. The physician requests room air ABG analysis at this point. Results show

pH	7.25
$PaCO_2$	60 mm Hg
PaO_2	55 mm Hg
HCO_3	26 mEq/L

Copyright © 2003, 1999 Mosby, Inc. All rights reserved.

Vital signs are

Heart rate	115 beats/min
Blood pressure	125/75 mm Hg
Respiratory rate	26 breaths/min
Temperature	37° C

A chest radiograph is obtained that reveals the tip of the ET to be 4 cm above the carina with no sign of pneumothorax.

3. What action would you recommend in regard to ET tube placement?
  A. Advance the tube 2 to 3 cm
  B. Withdraw the tube 2 to 3 cm
  C. Maintain current placement
  D. Remove the tube and insert a laryngeal mask airway

4. The ABG results are interpreted as
  A. Metabolic acidosis with severe hypoxemia
  B. Respiratory acidosis with moderate hypoxemia
  C. Partially compensated respiratory alkalosis with mild hypoxemia
  D. Partially compensated metabolic alkalosis with moderate hypoxemia

Ms. Robertson is transported to the ICU. The physician requests that you initiate mechanical ventilation.

5. Calculate ideal body weight. The formula for women is 105 + 5 (Height in centimeters − 60).
  A. 45 kg
  B. 59 kg
  C. 65 kg
  D. 130 kg

6. Which of the following volumes would you recommend?
  A. 475 mL
  B. 600 mL
  C. 900 mL
  D. 1000 mL

7. What mode and rate would you select?
  A. SIMV 10
  B. AC (CMV) 16
  C. SIMV 6
  D. AC (CMV) 8

8. What type of humidification system would you recommend for this patient?
  A. Heated wick humidifier set at 35° C.
  B. HME
  C. Heated passover humidifier
  D. Bubble humidifier

One week later, Ms. Robertson is alert, and weaning is initiated. When the rate is decreased to 5 breaths/min, however, the patient's spontaneous respiratory rate increases to 30 breaths/min, and V_T decreases to 200 mL.

9. To help solve this problem, you might recommend initiation of
  A. CMV
  B. AC
  C. PSV
  D. APRV

Case 2

Diana Olivera is a 5′2″ tall, 110-lb (50-kg), 65-year-old woman with a history of COPD. Paramedics bring her to the emergency department for management of dyspnea. She is wearing a nasal cannula set at 2 L/min. ABGs are drawn. Results show

pH	7.30
Pa_{CO_2}	70 mm Hg
Pa_{O_2}	45 mm Hg
HCO_3	34 mEq/L

Vital signs are

Copyright © 2003, 1999 Mosby, Inc. All rights reserved.

Heart rate	100 beats/min
Blood pressure	100/70 mm Hg
Respiratory rate	34 breaths/min
Temperature	39° C

Noninvasive positive pressure ventilation (NPPV) is attempted with bilevel ventilation, but the patient is unable to tolerate the mask and fights the system. A decision is made to intubate and initiate mechanical ventilation. Mrs. Olivera is given a small amount of sedation and intubated nasally with a 6.5-mm ID tube. Settings are

Mode	SIMV
Rate	8 breaths/min
V_T	450 mL
FIO_2	28%
PEEP	0
Peak flow	20 L/min
Sensitivity	1.5 cm H_2O below baseline

10. How long should you wait before drawing an ABG to assess the results of these settings?
    A. 5 minutes
    B. 10 minutes
    C. 20 minutes
    D. 30 minutes

11. What is the maximum desirable P_{plat} during mechanical ventilation?
    A. 15 cm H_2O
    B. 25 cm H_2O
    C. 35 cm H_2O
    D. 45 cm H_2O

During your first ventilator check, the following observations are made:

PIP	45 cm H_2O
Plateau	35 cm H_2O
Set rate	8 breaths/min
Total rate	34 breaths/min
Exhaled V_T	440 mL
Spontaneous $V_T (V_{Tsp})$	120 mL
Ratio of inspiratory time to expiratory time (I:E ratio)	1:1.5

12. What high-pressure alarm limit should you set?
    A. 35 cm H_2O
    B. 45 cm H_2O
    C. 55 cm H_2O
    D. 65 cm H_2O

13. What value should you set for the low-$\dot{V}_E$ alarm?
    A. 3.5 L
    B. 6.0 L
    C. 7.2 L
    D. 8.0 L

14. Which of the following would result in a lower WOB for this patient?
    I. Addition of 100 mL mechanical dead space
    II. Initiation of PSV at 5 cm H_2O
    III. Changing to flow-triggering 3 L/min
    IV. Addition of 10 cm H_2O PEEP
    A. I, II only
    B. II, III only
    C. I, III only
    D. II, III, IV

15. What action should you take to increase the I:E ratio ?
    A. Increase the peak flow
    B. Increase the V_T
    C. Increase the set rate
    D. Increase the FIO_2

Copyright © 2003, 1999 Mosby, Inc. All rights reserved.

16. According to *Egan's,* what is the minimum I:E ratio for COPD patients to provide sufficient time for exhalation and prevent auto-PEEP?
    A. 1:1
    B. 1:2
    C. 1:4
    D. 1:8

Case 3

Lynette Cooler is a 5'6" tall woman who weighs 220 lb (100 kg). She is in the ICU after surgery for multiple injuries sustained in a motor vehicle accident. An arterial line and a pulmonary arterial catheter are in place. The chest radiograph shows bilateral infiltrates consistent with ARDS. The ET tube is in good position. Current ventilator settings are

Mode	VC-CMV
V_T	1000 mL
Rate	12 breaths/min
FIO_2	70%
PEEP	5 cm H_2O
Peak flow	60 L/min
Sensitivity	1.0 cm H_2O below baseline

17. What is this patient's approximate ideal body weight?
    A. 50 kg
    B. 60 kg
    C. 80 kg
    D. 100 kg

18. What set V_T would you recommend to prevent further lung injury?
    A. 480 mL
    B. 600 mL
    C. 720 mL
    D. Maintain current setting

The following data are obtained:

Heart rate	110 beats/min, normal sinus rhythm with occasional PVCs
Blood pressure	110/75 mm Hg
SpO_2	88%
Pulmonary arterial pressure	38/8 mm Hg
PCWP	12 mm Hg
Cardiac output	5.8 L/min
Mixed venous oxygen saturation ($S\bar{v}O_2$)	59%

19. With regard to the patient's oxygenation, what action would you recommend?
    A. Increase the FIO_2
    B. Increase the PEEP
    C. Add mechanical dead space
    D. Maintain current settings

A PEEP trial is conducted with the following results:

PEEP (cm H_2O)	Static Compliance	PaO_2	Cardiac Output (L/min)
5	22	57	5.8
10	25	66	5.7
15	30	72	5.9
20	35	77	5.2
25	32	85	4.8

20. What PEEP level would you recommend?
    A. 5 cm H_2O
    B. 10 cm H_2O
    C. 15 cm H_2O
    D. 20 cm H_2O
    E. 25 cm H_2O

Ms. Cooler's condition continues to deteriorate over the next 2 days. Her compliance and PaO_2 have decreased, and PIP has increased to 60 cm H_2O for maintenance of a normal $PaCO_2$.

Copyright © 2003, 1999 Mosby, Inc. All rights reserved.

21. Which of the following ventilator modes could be considered as alternatives?
    I. PC-CMV
    II. VC-SIMV
    III. APRV
    IV. CSV-CPAP
    A. I, III only
    B. II, III only
    C. II, IV only
    D. I, IV only

22. Which of these techniques is used in ARDS to reduce lung injury or improve oxygenation?
    I. Expiratory retard
    II. Prone positioning
    III. Permissive hypercapnia
    IV. Unilateral lung ventilation
    A. I, II only
    B. II, III only
    C. I, II, III
    D. II, III, IV

Case 4

Kim Young is a respiratory student who fell down the stairs while reading *Egan's* and suffered a closed-head injury. Kim is 5'5" tall and weighs 132 lb (60 kg). Intracranial pressure and blood pressure are elevated. She is being ventilated with these settings:

Mode	Controlled CMV
Rate	12 breaths/min
V_T	700 mL
Fio2	30%
PEEP	0

Blood gases on these settings are

pH	7.40
Pa_{CO_2}	40 mm Hg
Pa_{O_2}	55 mm Hg
HCO_3	24 mEq/L

23. These blood gas results should be interpreted as
    A. Normal with moderate hypoxemia
    B. Respiratory alkalosis with mild hypoxemia
    C. Compensated respiratory acidosis with severe hypoxemia
    D. Compensated metabolic alkalosis with moderate hypoxemia

24. With regard to the oxygenation, what change would you suggest?
    A. Increase the PEEP
    B. Increase the rate
    C. Change to APRV
    D. Increase the F_{IO_2}

25. With regard to ventilation, what change would you suggest?
    A. Increase the rate
    B. Increase the V_T
    C. Change to SIMV
    D. Add mechanical dead space

26. What is the formula for calculating the rate needed to produce a desired change in Pa_{CO_2}?
    A. Pa_{CO_2} measured × Set rate ÷ Pa_{CO_2} desired
    B. Pa_{CO_2} desired × Set rate ÷ Pa_{CO_2} measured
    C. Pa_{CO_2} measured × Pa_{CO_2} desired ÷ Set rate
    D. Pa_{CO_2} measured × Pa_{O_2} measured ÷ Set rate

27. What rate would you suggest for this patient if the desired Pa_{CO_2} is 30 mm Hg?
    A. 8 breaths/min
    B. 10 breaths/min
    C. 14 breaths/min
    D. 16 breaths/min

Copyright © 2003, 1999 Mosby, Inc. All rights reserved.

28. How long should you maintain a head injury patient in a hyperventilated state?
    A. 2 to 4 hours
    B. 6 to 8 hours
    C. 12 to 24 hours
    D. 24 to 48 hours

Case 5

Nancy Hoe is a 27-year-old, 5'7" tall woman who weighs 140 lb (63 kg). She has a long history of asthma, including previous intubation and mechanical ventilation. She arrives in the emergency department with high-pitched, diffuse wheezing. She is barely able to talk because of dyspnea. She has not responded to two consecutive SVN treatments with 5 mg of albuterol and 0.5 mg of ipratropium bromide (Atrovent). Peak flow is not measurable, and SpO_2 is 92% on 2 L via nasal cannula. Ms. Hoe is using her accessory muscles to breathe and has some intercostal retractions on inspiration. Treatment with IV cyclosporine (Solu-Medrol), continuous bronchodilator therapy, and ECG monitoring is begun. One hour later the patient is lethargic, and breath sounds are almost absent. You draw an ABG with the following results:

pH	7.32
$PaCO_2$	45 mm Hg
PaO_2	64 mm Hg
HCO_3	23 mmol/L (23 mEq/L)
SaO_2	90%

29. What action would you recommend at this time?
    A. Continue the present therapy
    B. Oral intubation with No. 7.5 ET tube and mechanical ventilation
    C. Trial of NPPV via bilevel mask ventilation
    D. Tracheostomy and mechanical ventilation

30. The emergency department physician elects to intubate Ms. Hoe and move her to the medical ICU as soon as her condition is stabilized. You assist in the transport. In the ICU, you are asked to set up the ventilator. You would select
    A. SIMV 10, 500, 1.0 FIO_2, +3 PEEP, +5 PSV
    B. AC (CMV) 12, 750, +5 PEEP, 0.40 FIO_2
    C. APRV high PEEP 30, low PEEP 20, 0.60 FIO_2, 1-second release time
    D. CPAP (CSV) +10 PEEP, 0.30 FIO_2

31. What pharmacologic agent is recommended at this time?
    A. Inhaled corticosteroids
    B. Sedation with midazolam
    C. Paralysis with tubocurarine
    D. Respiratory stimulus with doxapram

32. Bronchodilator therapy also is indicated. How do you need to adjust the dosage for administration to a ventilated patient?
    A. Give the standard dose
    B. Increase the dose to 2 to 4 times normal amount
    C. Decrease the dose by half the normal amount
    D. Give the standard dose IV

33. Which of the following are major concerns in ventilation of patients with severe asthma?
    I. Pulmonary barotrauma
    II. Development of auto-PEEP
    III. Ventilator asynchrony
    IV. High airway pressure
    A. I, II
    B. I, III, IV
    C. II, III, IV
    D. I, II, III, IV

Copyright © 2003, 1999 Mosby, Inc. All rights reserved.

34. An appropriate peak flow and flow pattern for this patient would include
    A. 60 L/min with a decelerating flow waveform
    B. 30 L/min with a square flow waveform
    C. 100 L/min with a sine wave flow pattern
    D. 50 L/min with an accelerating flow waveform

35. What alteration in the mode of ventilation might be useful to prevent barotrauma and improve comfort?
    A. Addition of mechanical dead space
    B. Use of a heated humidifier
    C. Switching to pressure control
    D. Use of IRV

Case 6

Mr. Mal Corasone is a 66-year-old, 6-foot-tall, 180-lb (82 kg) man who has been brought to the SICU after CABG surgery. He has no history of lung disease. Mr. C. is intubated with a No. 8 oral ET tube. The anesthesiologist asks you to select ventilator settings.

36. What V_T is appropriate for a postoperative patient?
    A. 500 mL
    B. 650 mL
    C. 700 mL
    D. 950 mL

37. Why should you add a small amount of PEEP to the system?
    A. To prevent auto-PEEP
    B. To prevent atelectasis
    C. To prevent cardiogenic pulmonary edema
    D. To prevent barotrauma

38. What is your primary goal for this patient?
    A. Prevent ventilator-associated barotrauma
    B. Prevent ventilator-associated pneumonia
    C. Control air trapping
    D. Wean and extubate as quickly as possible

OK. We did six of the common situations you need to be able to manage. The other four are

- Unilateral lung disease
- Neuromuscular disorders
- CHF
- Bronchopleural fistula

See if you can identify the main concerns for each of these situations.

▶ WHAT DOES THE NBRC SAY?

The examination matrix is quite clear on this subject. You should be able to

- Initiate and adjust ventilators when settings are specified (and when they're not)
- Initiate and adjust AC, SIMV, PSV, and PCV
- Select appropriate V_T, $\dot{V}_E$, and respiratory rate

You should also know when to modify

- Mode
- V_T
- FIO_2
- Inspiratory plateau
- PEEP and CPAP levels
- Pressure support and pressure control
- Alarm settings
- Mechanical dead space
- Mean airway pressure
- IRV

Copyright © 2003, 1999 Mosby, Inc. All rights reserved.

The list goes on. The Written Registry exam adds more difficult questions and

- Independent lung ventilation
- High-frequency ventilation
- Application of computer technology (waveforms)

There also may be questions similar to those on the Entry Level exam but at a higher difficulty level. So even if you don't do APRV anywhere in your state, you still need to know the basic idea. Remember that these exam matrices change approximately every 5 years, and the last one was 1999!

If you can understand and apply the material in this chapter, you are well on your way to passing your boards and becoming a great therapist!

▶ FOOD FOR THOUGHT

39. What is the single most common ventilator strategy currently in use in the United States?

40. What are the common ventilator modes (and adjuncts such as PEEP and PSV) where you are training or working?

41. How can you determine correct pressure and inspiratory time when you switch from volume-controlled to pressure-controlled ventilation?

▶ INFORMATION AGE

One way to approach this topic on the Internet is to search for the specific diseases you are interested in, such as "mechanical ventilation of COPD patients." I found this overview at
www.rcjournal.com/contents/03.02/03.02.0247.asp

Of course this is only a summary. To get the real info you will need to leave the Internet and get the journal *Respiratory Care* for March and April 2002. The journal summarizes a 2-day conference on mechanical ventilation with the world's greatest experts. I can't think of a better way for you to supplement the material in Chapter 41 than to read these two issues of the journal. You can't go wrong with this one.

Or you can do a general search on "ventilator management." One site I found was ventworld.com. They have some case studies:
www.ventworld.com/education/casestudies.asp

Finally, you might consider another way to use the computer to learn. Most schools have good collections of clinical simulations on CD-ROM. These are great ways to study, learn, and test your knowledge. Good for getting ready for the Clinical Simulation exams, too!

Copyright © 2003, 1999 Mosby, Inc. All rights reserved.

Noninvasive Positive Pressure Ventilation

> **"Thou knows't the mask of**
> **night is on my face"**
> **William Shakespeare**

Noninvasive positive pressure ventilation by mask has been used in home care for many years, especially in the management of sleep-disordered breathing. Other forms of noninvasive ventilation, such as rocking beds and pneumobelts, have been around since the 1930s. In the 1970s and 1980s, we ventilated many a patient with IPPB and mask to try to avoid intubation. But it was not until 1989 that serious efforts were made to use NPPV as a means of managing acute respiratory failure. Increased technology in NPPV ventilators and advances in mask design have enabled the modern RCP to put noninvasive ventilation on the front lines of acute respiratory care in the management of COPD, asthma, and cardiogenic pulmonary edema. Noninvasive positive pressure ventilation is even used in the chronic care setting to relieve symptoms of hypoventilation and improve quality of life.

▶ GOALS AND INDICATIONS

1. The three main goals of NPPV in the acute care setting are
   A. Avoid
   B. Relieve
   C. Enhance

2. In the acute care setting, NPPV is indicated for nine conditions. Name at least five.
   A. _____
   B. _____
   C. _____
   D. _____
   E. _____

3. Noninvasive positive pressure ventilation also is indicated in the chronic care setting. List three conditions.
   A. _____
   B. _____
   C. _____

4. Noninvasive positive pressure ventilation should be reserved for use in COPD patients who are at risk of needing what invasive procedure?

Copyright © 2003, 1999 Mosby, Inc. All rights reserved.

5. Patients with status asthmaticus experience a high degree of complications when intubated and mechanically ventilated. What were the results of the study by Meduri et al on NPPV in the management of status asthmaticus?

6. Compare mask CPAP with mask ventilation in the management of acute cardiogenic pulmonary edema.

7. Noninvasive positive pressure ventilation should be used for what group of patients with community-acquired pneumonia?

8. Should NPPV be used to manage hypoxemic respiratory failure?

9. List four other indications for noninvasive ventilation in the acute care setting.
   A. _____
   B. _____
   C. _____
   D. _____

10. What three criteria does the rule of thumb say should be met before implementation of NPPV in acute respiratory failure?
    A. _____
    B. _____
    C. _____

▶ **SELECTION AND EXCLUSION CRITERIA**

11. How is the need for ventilatory assistance established?
    A. Respiratory rate
    B. Dyspnea
    C. Pa_{CO_2}
    D. pH
    E. P/F ratio

12. Many patients are expected to benefit from NPPV but are excluded because we know it won't work for them. Name at least four of these criteria.
    A. _____
    B. _____
    C. _____
    D. _____

Bottom line: The acute respiratory failure must be reversible within a few days!

13. Once you put the patient on the noninvasive ventilator, some predictors of success can be measured. Give the values for
    A. Respiratory acidosis _____
    B. pH _____
    C. Improvement in gas exchange_____

Copyright © 2003, 1999 Mosby, Inc. All rights reserved.

▶ TOOLS OF THE TRADE

Masks

You get to play with a lot of masks in non-invasive ventilation: nasal, full-face, and total face. The straps are fun too.

14. Which type of mask is better tolerated? Which one makes a better seal?

15. How can you pick the correct mask size—besides plain old trial and error?

16. The oral mask has a lot of potential problems. List at least four.
    A. _____
    B. _____
    C. _____
    D. _____

17. In spite of all the problems with face masks, what huge advantage do they have in the critical care setting?

Ventilators

Positive pressure ventilators to ventilate critically ill patients via ET usually need a sealed system to operate. Noninvasive ventilators are made to work with leaks. It will help if you understand the following terms:

- CPAP: Breathing at an elevated baseline pressure during inspiration and exhalation
- EPAP: Elevated pressure at exhalation
- IPAP: Elevated pressure during inspiration

Figure 42-9 illustrates these three concepts.

18. What happens to tidal volume when you increase the EPAP without increasing the IPAP?

19. What are some of the problems with using standard critical care ventilators to deliver mask ventilation?

▶ START ME UP

Once you've chosen a ventilator and a mask that fits, you have to select mode and settings just as you do for invasive mechanical ventilation.

Copyright © 2003, 1999 Mosby, Inc. All rights reserved.

20. How should you position the patient?

21. What mode is recommended?

22. Give initial settings for use with a non-invasive ventilator:
    A. IPAP
    B. EPAP
    C. Back-up rate

23. Give initial settings for critical care ventilator with mask:
    A. Mode
    B. PS
    C. PEEP
    D. Trigger

24. You won't be setting a tidal volume, but you still want a good one. What volume would you like to achieve? Which control do you increase if the volume is too low?
    A. Goal
    B. Adjust

25. What two adjustments can be made to improve oxygenation?

Table 42-1 gives a clear overview of the controls to manipulate to get the results you need. You have to do a little fine-tuning to make this work. Don't forget to encourage and reassure the patient.

26. Although you can initiate NPPV any-where, in which unit should the patient be while NPPV is in use?

▶ **WHAT COULD GO WRONG?**

27. Use Table 42-2 to help you find out what could go wrong and how to fix it!

Side Effect	*Occurrence*	*Remedy*
Mask		
A. Discomfort	_____	_____
		_____
B. Claustrophobia	_____	_____
		_____
C. Skin breakdown	_____	_____
		_____
Flow		
D. Congestion	_____	_____
		_____
E. Sinus pain	_____	_____
		_____
F. Dryness	_____	_____
		_____
G. Air leak	_____	_____
		_____

Copyright © 2003, 1999 Mosby, Inc. All rights reserved.

Bad Stuff

H. Aspiration _____ _____
   _____

I. Low blood _____ _____
   pressure _____

J. Pneumo- _____ _____
   thorax _____

_____

▶ WHAT DOES THE NBRC SAY?

This subject is not a big part of the exams because it is relatively new. I expect to see a growing number of questions in the future. Here's what the matrix says you should know.

Registered Respiratory Therapist: Written Registry

- Select, assemble, etc, noninvasive positive pressure ventilators
- Initiate and adjust CPAP, PEEP, and noninvasive ventilation

▶ CERTIFIED RESPIRATORY THERAPIST

- Select, assemble, etc, noninvasive positive pressure ventilators
- Initiate nasal and mask ventilation
- Initiate and adjust CPAP, PEEP, and noninvasive ventilation

So for the exams, it's really three things:

- Do you know when to recommend a trial of NPPV?
- Can you state the initial vent settings?
- What should you change if O_2 is low? CO_2 is high?

▶ INFORMATION AGE

Of course the Internet is good for this subject because it is hot, hot, hot.

Another great sources is our own *Respiratory Care:*
www.rcjournal.com/ contents/11.00/ contents.asp

This article is found in the November 2000 issue and is devoted to the subject of NPPV at the end of life.

University Hospital in Newark, NJ, has a center for noninvasive ventilation:
www. theuniversityhospital.com/ventilation/ index.html

• • •

I like the total face mask. It's too cool. Put me on that one please!

Copyright © 2003, 1999 Mosby, Inc. All rights reserved.

Monitoring and Management of the Patient in the ICU

"The best monitor is a knowledgeable, observant and dedicated healthcare professional."
Donald F. Egan, MD

You didn't think I'd finish this book without a quote from Dr. Egan did you? Truer words were never spoken. Monitoring in the ICU has reached a level of complexity that is as dazzling as it is expensive. The amount of data available to the critical care clinician is staggering. The key to success in this endeavor is to combine appropriate information gathering with sound clinical assessment. You can't learn that from a book! What you can do is learn the basics: normal values, waveforms, terms, and most common problems and situations you will encounter. When you go out into the clinical setting you can learn to apply this new information. I'm going to make you work hard in this chapter, but then you are near the end of the book, and you need to put this all together.

▶ MONITORING MATCH

Match these key terms to the definitions that follow.

1. _____ Afterload
2. _____ Swan-Ganz catheter
3. _____ Point-of-care testing
4. _____ APACHE score
5. _____ V_{DS}/V_T
6. _____ Pressure-volume curve
7. _____ Preload
8. _____ Capnometry
9. _____ Glasgow score
10. _____ Artifacts

A. Pressure the ventricle has to contract against
B. Pressure stretching the ventricle at the onset of contraction
C. Unreal events seen on monitors often caused by movement
D. Popular system for measuring neurologic impairment
E. Hemodynamic monitoring device placed in the pulmonary artery
F. Amount of wasted ventilation per breath
G. Ventilator graphic used to assess compliance and inflection points
H. Popular acute illness index
I. Measuring CO_2 at the airway
J. Analyzers brought to the bedside

▶ RESPIRATORY MONITORING

Quick, memorize Table 43-1 on p. 1096! Just kidding, you probably already know this stuff. Right?

Copyright © 2003, 1999 Mosby, Inc. All rights reserved.

11. Gas exchange at the lung is best monitored with what test?

12. Why is pulse oximetry the standard for continuous monitoring of oxygenation?

13. What is the most serious clinical limitation of using pulse oximetry to assess respiratory status?

14. Pulse oximetry is affected by lots of factors. Name four. (See Box 43-2)
    A. _____
    B. _____
    C. _____
    D. _____

15. What is the value for normal oxygen consumption?

16. State the Fick equation for cardiac output (Qt).

17. Pa_{O_2}/F_{IO_2} ratio is the most reliable index of gas exchange. What is the normal ratio? What ratio suggests ALI? ARDS?
    A. Normal
    B. ALI
    C. ARDS

18. The most accurate and reliable measure of pulmonary oxygenation efficiency is direct calculation of shunt. State the classic shunt equation.

19. What two blood gas samples are needed for calculation of shunt?
    A. _____
    B. _____

▶ MONITORING VENTILATION

20. What is the standard of reference for assessing the adequacy of ventilation?

Copyright © 2003, 1999 Mosby, Inc. All rights reserved.

21. Efficiency of ventilation is assessed by measurement of physiologic dead space. State the modified Bohr equation.

22. List the normal and critical values for dead space to tidal volume (V_{DS}/V_T) ratio.

Normal   Critical

_____   _____

23. What is the formula for measuring minute ventilation?

24. What is the difference between arterial and end-tidal CO_2 in healthy persons?

25. Capnometry is extremely useful in two emergency situations. Name them.
   A. _____
   B. _____

26. What test has to be done to validate the CO_2 value of a capnometer?

► MONITORING CHEST WALL MECHANICS

27. The pressure-volume curve is a ventilator graphic that can show compliance and lower inflection points. The lower inflection point may help you set what ventilator value?

28. The upper inflection point may point out what problem?

Compliance

29. Compliance shows stiffness of the lungs. What is the formula for calculating compliance? (Be sure to subtract PEEP).

30. What is normal compliance?

Copyright © 2003, 1999 Mosby, Inc. All rights reserved.

31. Low compliance in a patient with ARDS may decrease to what values?

Resistance

32. What is the formula for calculating airway resistance?

33. What is normal airway resistance? What's normal for a vent patient?
    A. Normal _____
    B. Ventilated patients _____

34. Resistance calculations for ventilated patients should be performed with the inspiratory flow set to what pattern?

35. Effects of what therapy can be measured by resistance changes?

Peak and Plateau Pressures

36. What is the maximum safe PIP?

37. What is the maximum safe P_{plat}?

Increases in peak pressure are due to either increased resistance or decreased compliance. Look at the peak and plateau pressures. When they increase together, the problem is compliance. When the peak pressure increases and the plateau stays the same, the problem is airway resistance. Box 43-7 gives common clinical conditions that alter compliance and resistance.

Auto-PEEP

Auto-PEEP occurs when lungs don't empty well (obstructive disease) or when there is a high minute ventilation (ARDS). Auto-PEEP causes all kinds of problems from difficulty in triggering the ventilator to hemodynamic compromise.

38. What ventilator maneuver unmasks auto-PEEP?

Copyright © 2003, 1999 Mosby, Inc. All rights reserved.

Work of Breathing

Research hospitals have several methods of measuring WOB, including use of esophageal balloons.

39. What is the simplest way to monitor WOB?

40. What score for RSBI is a good predictor of weaning success?

▶ **MONITORING MUSCLE STRENGTH**

41. What two values are measured at the bedside?
    A. _____
    B. _____

42. What is a normal VC? What VC indicates poor muscle strength?
    A. Normal _____
    B. Poor _____

43. What are the benefits of measuring MIP compared with measuring VC?
    A. _____
    B. _____

44. How long should you measure MIP?

45. Why should you use one-way valves when you measure MIP?

▶ **MONITORING THE PATIENT-VENTILATOR SYSTEM**

Most hospitals require ventilator checks every 2 hours. You need to record a number of values, assess the patient, and evaluate the information gathered so you can make any necessary changes.

46. Briefly discuss the five areas you need to check.
    A. Airway

    B. Vent settings

    C. Gas exchange

    D. Respiratory mechanics

Copyright © 2003, 1999 Mosby, Inc. All rights reserved.

E. Alarms

47. Ventilator graphics allow rapid deter-
mination of a number of variables.
Look at Box 43-8, and list five of the
parameters you can check.
A. _____
B. _____
C. _____
D. _____
E. _____

▶ MATHEMAGIC

Stop right there. A lot of important math
problems are presented in the last section of
Chapter 43. Before we go on to the dreaded
hemodynamics section, I want to make sure
you can do the voodoo.

Shunt

You will at best have to recognize the classic
shunt equation. At worst, be able to calculate it (even though we use computers in the
clinical setting). Let's see if you can estimate
shunt using the formula from *Egan's*. Let's
do it together first.

A patient is breathing 100% oxygen. The
Pa_{O_2} is 200 mm Hg. What is the estimated
shunt?

Pa_{O_2} = (760 – 47) × 1.0 – Pa_{CO_2} (assume
40 mm Hg). Say 673 mm Hg for Pa_{O_2}.
Now plug the numbers into the formula.
673 – 200 gives a 473 mm Hg difference
between A and a. If there is a 5% shunt for
each 100 mm Hg difference, the estimated
shunt is 473/100 × 5, or 24%.

Your turn.

48. A patient is breathing 100% oxygen.
Barometric pressure is 747 mm Hg
(conveniently), Pa_{CO_2} is 47 mm Hg
(goody), and Pa_{O_2} is 300 mm Hg.
Estimate the shunt.

A. Pa_{O_2} =

B. A – a =

C. Shunt =

Fick

Fick was *the* physiologist. You can use his
equation to calculate cardiac output or oxygen consumption. This isn't used much in
the clinical setting, but it can be on your
boards. Let's do one together.

What is cardiac output for a patient who
has oxygen consumption ($\dot{V}_{O_2}$) of 250
mL/min, arterial oxygen content (Ca_{O_2}) of
19 vol% (mL O_2/100 mL), and mixed
venous oxygen consumption ($C\bar{v}_{O_2}$) of 14
vol%?

Plug the numbers into the formula:

$$Qt \text{ (total perfusion or cardiac output)} = \dot{V}_{O_2}/Ca_{O_2} - C\bar{v}_{O_2} \times 10$$

or

$$Qt = 250/19 - 14 \times 10 = 250/5 \times 10 = 250/50 = 5 \text{ L/min}$$

49. What is cardiac output for a patient
who has a $\dot{V}_{O_2}$ of 200 mL/min, a
Ca_{O_2} of 20 vol%, and a $C\bar{v}_{O_2}$ of
16 vol%?

A. Formula _____
B. Calculation _____
C. Answer _____

Copyright © 2003, 1999 Mosby, Inc. All rights reserved.

You could rearrange this to calculate $\dot{V}O_2$ if you knew the cardiac output. For example, what is the $\dot{V}O_2$ for a patient who has a cardiac output of 4 L/min, CaO_2 of 17 vol%, and $C\bar{v}O_2$ of 13 vol%?

$\dot{V}O_2 = 4 \times 17\text{-}13$, or 160 mL/min.

You can keep on rearranging all you like.

Minute Ventilation

That was fun, now try an easy one. Exhaled $\dot{V}_E$ is respiratory rate multiplied by tidal volume: $\dot{V}_E = f \times V_T$. For example, a patient has a respiratory rate of 12 breaths/min and a V_T of 500 mL, so the exhaled $\dot{V}_E$ is 6000 mL, or 6 L.

50. What is the $\dot{V}_E$ for a patient who has a respiratory rate of 8 breaths/min and a V_T of 400 mL?
    A. Formula _____
    B. Calculation_____
    C. Answer _____

What about a patient who has ventilator breaths and spontaneous breaths (SIMV)?

51. A patient has a set rate of 6 breaths/min and a machine volume of 700 mL. The patient has 10 spontaneous breaths at 300 mL. What is the total $\dot{V}_E$?

Bohr

Egan's is correct in giving you the precise version of the modified Bohr equation. You need to be careful to be accurate and include all factors when performing this procedure on ventilated patients. The board exams are kinder, ask you only to recognize the main equation:

$$V_D/V_T = PaCO_2 - PETCO_2/PaCO_2$$

First we'll calculate the physiologic dead space to tidal volume ratio (V_{DS}/V_T), then use it in combination with $\dot{V}_E$. For example, what is the V_{DS}/V_T for a patient who has an arterial CO_2 of 40 mm Hg and an exhaled (end tidal) CO_2 (PETCO_2) of 30 mm Hg?

$40 - 30/40 = 10/40$, or 25%. Normal.

52. Your turn. Calculate V_{DS}/V_T for a patient who has an arterial CO_2 of 40 mm Hg and an exhaled CO_2 of 20 mm Hg.
    A. Formula _____
    B. Calculation_____
    C. Answer _____

Now let's combine this with the minute volume equation to calculate *alveolar* $\dot{V}_E$. Let's use respiratory rate of 12 breaths/min, V_T of 500 mL, $PaCO_2$ of 40 mm Hg, and PETCO_2 of 30. The new formula is

$$V_A = f(V_T - V_D)$$

Dead space is 25%. So multiply the V_T by 0.25 to get V_{DS}:

$$500 \times 0.25 = 125 \text{ mL}$$

Now plug in the numbers:

$$V_A = 12 (500 - 125), \text{ or } 12 \times 375 = 4500 \text{ mL}$$

53. Calculate alveolar $\dot{V}_E$ for a patient who has a rate of 10 breaths/min, V_T of 500 mL, arterial CO_2 of 40 mm Hg, and PETCO_2 of 28 mm Hg.
    A. Formula _____
    B. Calculation_____
    C. Answer _____

Copyright © 2003, 1999 Mosby, Inc. All rights reserved.

Expect some combination of this material on your board exams!

Compliance

Like dead space, compliance calculations are simplified on the board exams. We'll do it both ways here. First, static effective compliance the simple way. A patient has an exhaled volume of 600 mL. The P_{plat} is 35 cm H_2O, and the PEEP is 5 cm H_2O. Compliance is 600/35 − 5, or 600/30 = 20 mL/cm H_2O. You try.

54. Calculate static effective compliance for a patient who has an exhaled volume of 1000 mL, P_{plat} of 35 cm H_2O, and PEEP of 10 cm H_2O.
    A. Formula _____
    B. Calculation_____
    C. Answer _____

In clinical practice it is important to subtract the compressed volume with some ventilators. A comparison will make this clear. The patient in Question 54 has a volume of 600 mL and compliance of 20 mL/cm H_2O. But if the PIP is 40 cm H_2O and the circuit expansion factor is 5 mL/cm H_2O, then the volume lost to expansion is 200 mL (factor × PIP). The new compliance calculation is

$$(600 - 200)/(35 - 5), \text{ or } 400/30 = 13 \text{ mL/cm } H_2O.$$

You try:

55. Calculate compliance for a patient who has a V_T of 800 mL; PIP, 50; P_{plat}, 35 cm H_2O; and PEEP, 5 cm H_2O. The circuit factor is 4 mL/cm H_2O.
    A. Formula _____
    B. Calculation_____
    C. Compliance _____

Some ventilators compensate for tubing compliance, and you don't need to do this step.

Resistance

A look at the difference between PIP and P_{plat} is useful for clinical estimates of airway resistance. First, you need to use a square or constant flow pattern on most modern ventilators. Next, you need to determine the flow rate in liters per second, not liters per minute. Here is an example:

Calculate resistance for a patient who has a PIP of 50 cm H_2O, plateau of 40 cm H_2O, and flow rate of 60 L/min. Sixty liters per minute converts to liters per second this way: 60 L/min divided by 60 seconds per minute = 1 L/s. Now calculate

$$PIP - Plateau \div Flow = 50 - 40 \div 1 = 10 \text{ cm } H_2O \text{ per liter per second.}$$

Now your turn.

56. Calculate airway resistance for a patient who has a peak pressure of 50 cm H_2O, P_{plat} of 40 cm H_2O, and flow rate of 30 L/min.
    A. Convert flow to liters per second
    B. Resistance formula
    C. Calculation
    D. Airway resistance is

If you are doing patient care, you may not have to calculate to see that resistance or compliance has changed. Look at the difference between peak pressure and plateau pressure. If the difference has increased and all else is stable, then the resistance also has increased. Some ventilators perform compliance and resistance calculations for you. The manual calculations give answers slightly different from the ventilator values.

Copyright © 2003, 1999 Mosby, Inc. All rights reserved.

Policy will determine the way you do the numbers at a any particular hospital.

Remember, if the patient is actively breathing spontaneously, it will be very difficult to make accurate calculations. These calculations are intended for full ventilatory support.

► ASSESSMENT OF HEMODYNAMICS

We're here at last. The dreaded hemodynamics. Strikes terror into the hearts of respiratory care students everywhere, but it will be okay. We'll break it down into small pieces: indications, complications, normal values, equipment, and waveforms. You can do it! Let's start with invasive arterial monitoring.

"Oooh, I Heard It through the Art Line . . ."

57. Identify the two main sites for arterial cannulation in adults.
    A. _____
    B. _____

58. What are the two indications for an indwelling arterial line?
    A. _____
    B. _____

59. List the normal values for these systemic arterial values. Check Table 43-3.
    A. Systolic
    B. Diastolic
    C. Mean

When the art line values don't agree with manual measurements, the manual method is safer. One problem may be that the pressure transducer is not at the level of the heart. A transducer that is above the

heart results in *lower* pressure on the monitor.

Another problem may be a "dampened" tracing. This means the waveform is flattened out. Clots and air bubbles in the system are common causes of a dampened tracing.

Equipment

One more area you need to become familiar with is the basic parts of the system. Take a look at this picture.

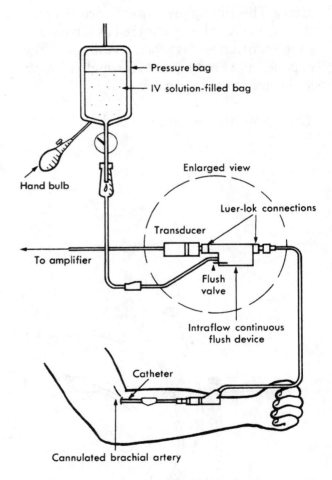

Use of pressurized IV fluid bag and Intraflow flush device for optimal maintenance of arterial catheter patency. Stopcocks may be placed on each side of the flush device for room air reference and blood sampling. *(From Schroeder JE, Daily EK: Techniques in bedside hemodynamic monitoring, St Louis, 1976, Mosby.)*

Copyright © 2003, 1999 Mosby, Inc. All rights reserved.

Starting at the top, you see a *pressurized IV bag* that may also contain heparin to help reduce the chance of clotting. The main thing is the pressure. Without it, blood from the patient could back up into the system, and we wouldn't be able to *flush,* or wash out blood back into the artery. The *transducer* converts the arterial pressure waveform to an electronic signal that can be sent to the amplifier and displayed on the monitor.

Special *stiff, or noncompliant, IV tubing* connects the transducer and continuous flush device to the catheter that is in the artery. This tubing prevents the arterial pressure wave from being damped as it passes up to the transducer (as when ventilator tubing expands as a breath passes through it and we lose some in the expansion).

There now, that wasn't too bad.

▶ PULMONARY ARTERIAL PRESSURE MONITORING

Flow-Directed, Balloon-Tipped, Pulmonary Arterial Catheter . . Oh, Let's Just Call It a Swan

Dr. Swan and Dr. Ganz are credited with developing this nifty tube for looking at pressure inside the heart and lungs, so many people still call it a "Swan" or "Swan-Ganz" catheter. *Pulmonary arterial catheter* (PAC) is more generic. Pulmonary arterial monitoring *is* a complex subject, but you can make it much simpler if you start by learning certain basic pieces of information. (You can also pass your boards.)

60. Name six conditions that suggest insertion of a PAC.
    A. _____
    B. _____
    C. _____
    D. _____
    E. _____
    F. _____

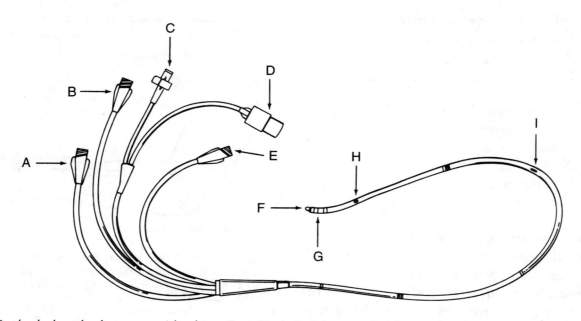

Quadruple-channel pulmonary arterial catheter. *(From Martin L: Pulmonary physiology in clinical practice, St Louis, 1987, Mosby.)*

Copyright © 2003, 1999 Mosby, Inc. All rights reserved.

61. Let's look at the catheter itself. Identify the labeled parts.

A. _____
B. _____
C. _____
D. _____
E. _____
F. _____
G. _____

H. _____
I. _____

Pneumopnugget

A picture is not the best way to learn this, but it is okay. Either get a catheter from one of your instructors or look at one in the ICU that is in a box, then in a patient. You really should learn the parts.

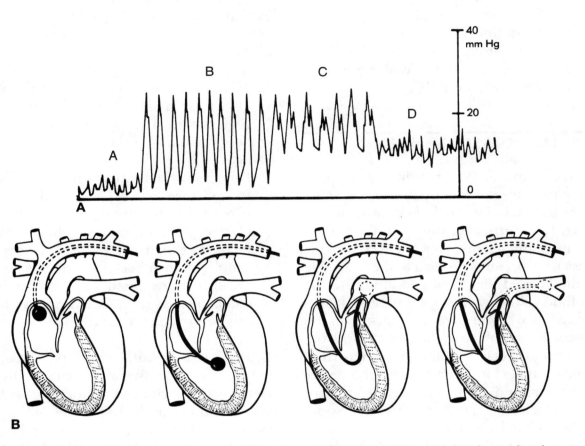

A, pressure tracings. **B,** Pulmonary arterial catheter position in heart. *(From Martin L: Pulmonary physiology in clinical practice, St Louis, 1987, Mosby.)*

62. Now label the following four wave-forms.

A. _____
B. _____
C. _____
D. _____

Pneumopnugget

These are the four patterns seen on insertion and during normal monitoring. Very useful. As in ECGs, there are abnormal patterns, too, but don't worry about them yet. Each of the normal waveforms corresponds to an anatomical location. If, for example, the catheter is supposed to be in

Copyright © 2003, 1999 Mosby, Inc. All rights reserved.

the pulmonary artery, but you see a right ventricular waveform, you know something is wrong (maybe it is pulled back too far). Or if the waveform appears wedged when it isn't supposed to be, perhaps the catheter has migrated too far forward.

63. List the normal values for these pressures (see Table 43-3).
   A. Central venous (CVP)
   B. Right atrial
   C. Pulmonary arterial
      1. Systolic
      2. Diastolic
   D. Pulmonary arterial wedge pressure (PWP, PCWP, PAWP)

▶ WHAT DOES IT ALL MEAN?

Interpretation of PAC readings is a pretty complex subject. I want you to learn some of the basics, so I will deliberately be simplifying. Right atrial pressure and CVP often are used interchangeably. Central venous pressure represents preload to the right side of the heart. It can be a good indicator of the fluid volume status of the patient. It also can tell us whether there is a backup in the system between the right atrium and the left atrium, such as pulmonary hypertension, a blood clot, heart failure, or a defect in the tricuspid valve. The wedge pressure does much the same for the left side. Under normal circumstances it shows us the left ventricular preload. Considered along with CVP, wedge pressure helps us decide about fluid balance. If both CVP and PWP are low, you should consider hypovolemia.

Here is where the RCP must really think. Because both CVP and PWP are measured inside the chest, and PPV increases intrathoracic pressure, it is possible for the ventilator to affect the readings. The pressure tracings will move up and down with positive pressure breaths, and you may be able to detect this by watching the tracing increase and decrease as the ventilator cycles. But PEEP causes a constant increase in pressure, and PEEP levels above 10 cm H_2O, especially in hypovolemic patients, can artificially elevate the values, especially wedge pressure. A high value means the patient has too much fluid, so someone might conclude a patient needs to lose fluid when really the patient is dry. A complete explanation of what to do about this would keep us here a long time, but here are some ideas:

1. Measure pressure values from the PAC at end exhalation. You will need to run off a printed strip to do this, because the digital values on the monitor are averaged.
2. Do not take the patient off the ventilator to measure values, especially if the patient is receiving a high level of PEEP.
3. Correct the PAC values if the patient is receiving a high level of PEEP. This is not simple—remember that the degree of pressure transmitted depends on lung compliance as well, so learn more about this before you try it.

You can use the catheter to look at other things besides overall fluid balance. Diagnosis of certain conditions is aided by information from the PAC. Table 43-4 provides a look at some of these conditions. For example, compare ARDS with left-ventricular failure. The pulmonary arterial pressure may increase in both conditions, the radiograph shows infiltrates, and breath sounds may reveal crackles. Both patients have hypoxemia and decreased lung compliance. But the failing left ventricle causes the wedge pressure to increase whereas ARDS does not. Combine this information with patient history and results of other assessments and you get the big picture. Certain other values can be meas-

Copyright © 2003, 1999 Mosby, Inc. All rights reserved.

ured besides pressure, so let's look at those next.

64. List the normal values for these measurements. (see Table 43-3)
    A. Cardiac output (CO)
    B. Cardiac index (CI)
    C. Systemic vascular resistance (SVR)
    D. Pulmonary vascular resistance (PVR)

With the Swan, cardiac output is measured by thermodilution. Very helpful information, especially in administration of drugs that support cardiac function. Or if you want to know whether changes in the ventilator are affecting the heart. The problem is, cardiac output is not personal enough. For example, you would expect a sumo wrestler to have a greater cardiac output than an elderly woman, but both would have values technically within the normal range at 5 L/min of output. If you divide the output by body surface area, you derive CI, and this is more useful, because everyone should have the same range for CI. Anyone who drops below 2.5 is in trouble.

Another useful calculation is vascular resistance. It's just like airway resistance (PIP – $P_{plat/}$Flow), only now we want to know how much pressure drop occurs when we push the blood through the vessels. Let's look at the PVR formula, because you might have to calculate this on your boards.

$$PVR = MPAP - PAWP/CO$$

If we have a patient with a mean pulmonary arterial pressure (MPAP) of 12 mm Hg, CVP of 4 mm Hg, and CO of 4 L/min, we get 12 – 4/4 = 2 mm Hg/L per minute for resistance. Sometimes this number is multiplied by 80 to convert it to dynes. Either way, PVR is normally quite low.

65. What common respiratory problem results in vasoconstriction, or elevated vascular resistance in the pulmonary vessels? (*Hint:* It's the first one on the list in Table 43-3.)

66. Calculate PVR for a patient who has an MPAP of 15 mm Hg, CVP of 3 mm Hg, and cardiac output of 5L/min.

Sometimes you need to be able to calculate mean arterial pressure so you can work the resistance problem. Remember that MAP = Systolic pressure + (2 × Diastolic)/3.

67. Calculate MPAP if systolic pulmonary arterial pressure is 25 mm Hg and diastolic pulmonary arterial pressure is 10 mm Hg.

By now, your brain must be getting tired. Remember to learn the basics and normal values. When you are looking at the data, think about where in the heart or lungs the pressure is being measured. That will help give you a clue about what part of the system has become abnormal. To increase your expertise you will have to go to the clinical setting and look at the patient data

Copyright © 2003, 1999 Mosby, Inc. All rights reserved.

from the PAC and learn interpretation at the bedside.

▶ MANAGEMENT OF THE PATIENT-VENTILATOR SYSTEM

I think that checking the system every 2 hours is a sort of national average (not a standard of care), but I have worked at hospitals where formal checks were made every hour and some where it was done only every 4 hours. What you do during the check also varies widely according to where you work. For example, sometimes you don't routinely analyze F_{IO_2}, you use the pulse oximeter to see what is going on with the patient. Analysis is done only when the ventilator is tested. There are lots of possibilities of just how to do this procedure. The main point is to ensure patient safety through early identification of potential problems.

Troubleshooting

68. Troubleshooting revolves around what two general problem areas (Box 43-12)?
    A. _____
    B. _____

69. Use Table 43-7 to help you identify common problems.

Clue	Possible Problem	Corrective Action
A. Sudden increase in PIP	1. _____	_____
	2. _____	_____
B. Gradual increase in PIP	1. _____	_____
C. Sudden decrease in PIP	1. _____	_____
	2. _____	_____
D. Decreased minute or tidal volume	1. _____	_____
	2. _____	_____
E. Increased minute or tidal volume	1. _____	_____
	2. _____	_____

70. Use Box 43-12 to help you identify four patient-related causes of sudden respiratory distress.
    A. _____
    B. _____
    C. _____
    D. _____

71. List four ventilator-related causes of sudden respiratory distress.
    A. _____
    B. _____
    C. _____
    D. _____

Copyright © 2003, 1999 Mosby, Inc. All rights reserved.

72. Regardless of the source of the problem, what is always the first priority?

73. If there is any doubt as to the cause or solution of a problem, what action should you take (see Box 43-13)?

74. How can you check the airway?

75. As a last resort, when all other options have been ruled out, it may be necessary to sedate or paralyze the patient. Give examples of drugs in the following classes:
    A. Tranquilizing agents
        1. _____
        2. _____
        3. _____
    B. Narcotic analgesics
        1. _____
        2. _____
    C. Neuromuscular blocking agents
        1. Long-term (nondepolarizing)
        2. Short-acting (depolarizing)
    D. Sedative hypnotics/miscellaneous
        1. _____
        2. _____

The flavor of the month for this one is propofol (Diprivan). We like to call this stuff "milk of amnesia." Looks like milk. Rapid acting and has a short half-life, so it's easy to get out of the system when the nurses turn off the IV.

▶ WHAT ABOUT THOSE BOARD EXAMS?

After reviewing several practice exams, I have concluded that any given Written Registry exam can have as many as 10 questions on hemodynamic monitoring alone. The material in this chapter could include even more. The CRT exam has some basic hemodynamics as well.

Let me be specific:

Review the chart:

- Cardiac output, PCWP, pulmonary arterial pressure, CVP
- Shunt studies
- Fluid balance (intake and output)
- V_D/V_T ratio

Recommend

- Shunt studies
- Insertion of arterial or central venous lines
- Cardiac output

Perform and interpret results of bedside procedures:

- V_D/V_T
- Shunt
- PCWP
- Mixed venous sampling
- $P(A - a)O_2$
- Lung compliance
- Cardiac output
- $C(a - v)O_2$
- Airway resistance

Copyright © 2003, 1999 Mosby, Inc. All rights reserved.

Assemble and check equipment for proper function:

- Hemodynamic monitoring devices: Swan-Ganz, arterial catheters
- Ventilators

Modify mechanical ventilation in every way imaginable.

You can clearly see that the information in Chapter 43 is vital. Because entire textbooks are devoted to hemodynamic monitoring or ventilator management, *Egan's* cannot possibly give you everything you need. It is a great place to start and clearly summarizes the main points. Chapter 43 will make an excellent reference when you go to prepare for the tests. Here are some sample questions.

76. A 42-year-old patient with a cervical spinal injury is being mechanically ventilated in control mode. As you enter the room, the low-pressure alarm is sounding. The patient is connected to the ventilator, but you do not see his chest moving. Your first action would be to
    A. Manually ventilate the patient with the resuscitation bag
    B. Check the alarm settings
    C. Observe the exhaled volumes
    D. Manually ventilate the patient with the mechanical ventilator

77. After insertion of a Swan-Ganz catheter via the left subclavian vein, a patient's compliance quickly drops. The high-pressure alarm on the ventilator is activated. Breath sounds are absent over the left chest, and the trachea is deviated to the right side. The patient appears extremely anxious. What action should the respiratory care practitioner take?
    A. Use a capnometer to assess ventilation noninvasively
    B. Recommend administration of midazolam (Versed)
    C. Call for a portable chest radiograph
    D. Recommend a chest tube

78. A 38-year-old woman with a diagnosis of myasthenia gravis is being mechanically ventilated. As you enter the room the high-pressure alarm is sounding. The patient appears anxious. Auscultation reveals coarse bilateral rhonchi. What action should you take at this time?
    A. Manually ventilate the patient.
    B. Check the alarm setting
    C. Recommend sedation
    D. Suction the patient

79. An 89-year-old woman with emphysema is being mechanically ventilated. The high-pressure and high-rate alarms are being activated. Breath sounds are clear. Pulse oximetry and vital sign values are within normal limits. Hemodynamics are normal. The patient is very agitated, and her respiratory rate is 32 breaths/min. What are your recommendations?
    A. Administer diazepam (Valium)
    B. Increase the alarm limit
    C. Suction the patient
    D. Call for a portable chest radiograph

Copyright © 2003, 1999 Mosby, Inc. All rights reserved.

80. The data below are reported for a patient:

PCWP	19 mm Hg
Pulmonary arterial pressure	40/24 mm Hg
CI	1.9 L/min per square meter

These data suggest which of the following?

A. Noncardiogenic pulmonary edema
B. Cardiogenic pulmonary edema
C. Pulsus paradoxus
D. Hypovolemia

81. When properly placed, the distal tip of the Swan-Ganz catheter will be located in the
A. Left atrium
B. Right atrium
C. Right ventricle
D. Pulmonary artery

Questions 82 to 84 refer to the following situation. A patient is intubated and placed on the ventilator after she respiratory failure develops after hip replacement surgery. The following values are recorded:

Pa_{CO_2}	50 mm Hg
Pa_{O_2}	60 mm Hg
FI_{O_2}	0.40
PET_{CO_2}	10 mm Hg
Tidal volume	800 mL
Respiratory rate	20 breaths/min

82. These data indicate a dead space to tidal volume ratio of
A. 20%
B. 40%
C. 60%
D. 80%

83. What is the exhaled minute volume?
A. 8.0 L
B. 12.0 L
C. 16.0 L
D. 20.0 L

84. What is the alveolar minute volume?
A. 3.2 L
B. 11.2 L
C. 12. 8 L
D. 16.0 L

85. The following information is recorded for a patient:

$\dot{V}_{O_2}$	200 mL/min
Ca_{O_2}	16 vol%
$C\bar{v}_{O_2}$	12 vol%

What is the cardiac output?

A. 2.0 L/min
B. 3.0 L/min
C. 4.0 L/min
D. 5.0 L/min

86. The hemodynamic data below are recorded for a patient who is being mechanically ventilated:

Cardiac output	3.5 L/min
Pulmonary arterial pressure	16/8 mm Hg
PWP	4 mm Hg
CVP	2 mm Hg
Heart rate	125 beats/min

These data probably indicate

A. Hypovolemia
B. Pulmonary hypertension
C. Fluid overload
D. Pulmonary embolism

Copyright © 2003, 1999 Mosby, Inc. All rights reserved.

87. A pressure waveform obtained from a radial artery catheter is dampened. Possible causes of this problem include all of the following *except*
    A. An air bubble in the tubing
    B. A blood clot on the tip of the catheter
    C. The transducer is lower than the heart
    D. Use of standard IV tubing

Well, I could go on like this forever, but I think you get the picture.

▶ FOOD FOR THOUGHT

An editorial in the journal *Respiratory Care* a few years ago was titled something like this: "The Pulmonary Artery Catheter: It Goes in through Your Arm and You Pay through the Nose." I want you to think about three questions in relation to this idea.

First, do you think it is important to use top-of-the-line technology in every setting? Second, if your loved ones were ill, what would you want for them? Third, do you think the average person understands the complexity of "the high cost of medicine"?

▶ INFORMATION AGE

Nurse Bob's Critical Care site has some basic overviews that might help you: **rnbob.tripod.com/index.htm**

Don't forget Dr. Sharma. His website has a slide show on hemodynamics: **www.ssharma. com/presentations/ hemodynamic/index.htm**

If you're looking for more respiratory care information on ventilator monitoring and you have PowerPoint, you might try downloading **www.sw.vccs.edu/rth/RTH_132/ mvmonit.ppt**

This is a good overview done by a respiratory care program. Ventworld also has some interesting items **http://www.ventworld.com/education/edu cation.asp**

Copyright © 2003, 1999 Mosby, Inc. All rights reserved.

Discontinuing Ventilatory Support

"I'm losing."
**Reported as the last
words of Frank Sinatra**

It's relatively easy to initiate mechanical ventilation, and some patients are equally easy to get back off again. Unfortunately, there is no magic number that tells you a patient will be successfully weaned or removed from support. You will have to customize the job for each patient. Sometimes this task takes all our skills and resources to accomplish. Sometimes, it can't be done.

▶ I'M SPEECHLESS

It looks as if you already know all the key terms in this chapter. Take a break.

▶ FIRST THINGS FIRST

1. What's the difference between weaning and discontinuing ventilator support?

2. So you're thinking about taking your patient off the vent. Patients will pretty much fall into what three general categories?
   A. _____
   B. _____
   C. _____

3. What has to happen before you can get the patient off the ventilator?

▶ CAUSES OF VENTILATOR DEPENDENCE

4. Patients may need mechanical ventilation for what three general reasons?
   A. _____
   B. _____
   C. _____

5. State the four factors that determine total ventilatory workload.
   A. _____
   B. _____
   C. _____
   D. _____

Copyright © 2003, 1999 Mosby, Inc. All rights reserved.

6. What do fever, shivering, agitation, trauma, and sepsis have in common?

7. List two causes of increased dead space ventilation.
   A. _____
   B. _____

8. Name four common causes of decreased lung compliance.
   A. _____
   B. _____
   C. _____
   D. _____

9. Name three causes of decreased thoracic compliance.
   A. _____
   B. _____
   C. _____

10. State three causes of increased airway resistance.
    A. _____
    B. _____
    C. _____

11. Why are artificial airways implicated in increased airway resistance?

12. Give examples of conditions that adversely affect ventilatory capacity.
    A. CNS drive
       1. _____
       2. _____
       3. _____
       4. _____
    B. Muscle strength
       1. _____
       2. _____
       3. _____
       4. _____

13. Once ventilatory muscles are fatigued, how long should they be rested before any attempt at weaning?

Now you have this giant list of things that could make removal from the ventilator difficult. Sometimes one thing, such as reduced drive to breathe from drugs, is the problem. That's easy to solve. You can give an antidote (e.g., naloxone [Narcan] for heroin or morphine), cleanse the blood (dialysis, for example), or wait for the effects to wear off (anesthesia, for instance). Or you might run into something a little more complicated, such as a depressed patient with COPD and CHF who has a small ET tube, bronchospasm, malnutrition, CO_2 retention, and electrolyte disorders along with the lung infection that put him on the vent in the first place. That's a plate full of issues to be resolved before weaning. See Box 44-3 if you need this to get more complicated.

Copyright © 2003, 1999 Mosby, Inc. All rights reserved.

▶ PATIENT EVALUATION

Careful, systematic assessment is an especially important part of your approach to ventilator discontinuance.

14. What is the first thing you should evaluate whether you are considering weaning or taking the patient off the ventilator?

15. What are the four questions you should ask?
    A. _____
    B. _____
    C. _____
    D. _____

Once the patient's condition is stable and things are looking up, you can take a look at the weaning indexes. I told you (Chapter 38, Table 38-2) these things would return to haunt you. Do they work? Like everything else—sometimes. Even though indexes have limitations, we still need to gather the information because it helps quantify the patient's overall status.

16. Your board exams will expect you to identify these classic criteria for weaning from mechanical ventilation. Remember that no one criterion mandates that you wean or don't wean. Use Table 44-1 to help out with this question.

	Measurement	Critical Value
A.	Pa_{CO_2}	_____
B.	pH	_____
C.	VC (mL/kg)	_____
D.	V_{Tsp}	_____
E.	Spontaneous rate (f_{sp})	_____
F.	$\dot{V}_E$	_____
G.	MVV	_____
H.	MIF (NIF, MIP)	_____
I.	V_{DS}/V_T	_____
J.	$P(A-a)O_2$ on 100%	_____
K.	P/F ratio	_____
L.	Pa_{O_2}	_____
M.	Qs/Qt	_____
N.	FI_{O_2}	_____
O.	f/V_T	_____
P.	Compliance	_____

Another giant menu to memorize then apply to clinical. (If it seems overwhelming, break it down into small pieces, and learn a few at a time. Then chant this mantra, "I want to be a really good RCP, I want to be a really good RCP.")

17. Describe the breathing patterns that can cause problems with weaning or discontinuance.

Copyright © 2003, 1999 Mosby, Inc. All rights reserved.

18. Physical assessment of respiratory muscles can be useful. Describe what you are looking for in this area.

19. Rapid shallow breathing index may be the best overall predictor of weaning outcome. Calculate the index for a patient who has a spontaneous rate of 25 breaths/min with a spontaneous volume of 350 mL. What is the criterion for success?
    A. Calculation

    B. Criterion

20. How could you modify the criterion to be a better predictor with elderly patients?

21. What do you have to do with the ventilator patient to get the RSBI?

22. Give the Pa_{O_2} and FI_{O_2} values that should be met before weaning.
    A. Pa_{O_2}

    B. FI_{O_2}

23. What is the effect of excessive carbohydrate administration?

24. Identify the critical values for confirming cardiovascular stability (Table 44-2).

Measurement	Values Inconsistent with Weaning
A. Heart rate	_____
B. Systolic pressure	_____
C. Diastolic pressure	_____
D. Hemoglobin	_____
E. CI	_____

Copyright © 2003, 1999 Mosby, Inc. All rights reserved.

25. Describe the three ways renal function can affect weaning.

A.

B.

C.

26. Describe the ideal CNS status you'd like to see.

27. How is ability to be weaned different from ability to be extubated?

28. Because many factors are associated with success, weaning indexes are becoming more popular. What is a weaning index? Which one is the most useful?

▶ PREPARING THE PATIENT

A quick glance at Box 44-6 should amuse you—or scare you. Respiratory care practitioners should start by optimizing the parts of the patient's medical condition they have direct control over and focus on psychological and environmental factors they can influence.

29. Name two drug therapies the RCP can use to reduce airway resistance.

A. _____

B. _____

30. How else can the RCP improve conditions in the airway?

31. What time of day should weaning activities be conducted?

Copyright © 2003, 1999 Mosby, Inc. All rights reserved.

32. What percentage of patients may develop "ICU psychosis" or other psychological disturbances after a few days in the unit?

33. How can the RCP help the patient get adequate sleep?

34. Describe the environmental considerations that may improve patient well-being.

35. What three methods does *Egan's* identify for helping patients communicate?
    A. _____
    B. _____
    C. _____

▶ WEANING METHODS

When the original problem is resolving, the indices look good, and you've optimized as many factors as possible, you must get down to the business of discontinuing ventilation. Rapidly or slowly, you have several methods to choose from.

36. List the four basic methods of discontinuing support.
    A.

    B.

    C.

    D.

37. Instead of putting the patient on a T piece with an aerosol, you could use one of the spontaneous (CSV) ventilator modes. Name these two modes and suggest appropriate levels of support.

Copyright © 2003, 1999 Mosby, Inc. All rights reserved.

A.

B.

38. Describe the specific advantage of using the ventilator instead of the T tube.

39. What is the typical minimum length of time for a T-tube trial when you are going for rapid discontinuance?

40. How should you position the patient before the trial breathing period?

Rapid discontinuance works really well on patients who have been on the ventilator for a short time. A postop patient, a patient with obstructive disease who is now awake, that sort of thing. Wouldn't it be nice if more patients fell into this category? For the more difficult customer, you basically have three choices: T piece, SIMV, or spontaneous breathing trial (SBT).

41. Describe the T piece (T tube) trial for gradual weaning (see Box 44-8)

42. What F_{IO_2} is ideal for T-piece weaning?

43. What happens at night?

44. Describe the variation of this method in which the patient is kept on the ventilator.

Copyright © 2003, 1999 Mosby, Inc. All rights reserved.

45. What are the biggest drawbacks of T-piece weaning?

46. Compare T-piece with IMV weaning.

47. Why do you think IMV (SIMV) is the predominant weaning method in the United States?

48. What are the typical initial settings when SIMV is used for full ventilatory support?
    A. Tidal volume
    B. Respiratory rate

49. What is the typical amount the rate is adjusted at any one time in SIMV weaning?

50. When is partial support an unwise ventilator strategy?

51. Describe pressure support ventilation (PSV).

52. What is PSVmax?

53. From what level of PSV may a patient be extubated?

54. *Egan's* gives a formula for estimating the level of pressure support needed to overcome WOB. Calculate the level needed for a patient who has a PIP of 50 cm H_2O, plateau pressure of 30 cm H_2O, ventilator flow rate of 60 L/min, and a spontaneous inspiratory flow rate of 30 L/min. (You can look at the Mini Clini "Setting Pressure Support Levels" for help.)
    A. Formula _____
    B. Calculation _____
    C. Answer _____

Copyright © 2003, 1999 Mosby, Inc. All rights reserved.

If you're just trying to overcome WOB through the ET tube, it's a lot easier to use the "tube compensation" modes found on newer ventilators. The machine does the calculating for you. Other times you want to set PSV to achieve a desired tidal volume, either in milliliters or in milliliters per kilogram. Another way to set PSV is to increase the pressure until spontaneous rate drops to a desirable level.

► SPONTANEOUS BREATHING TRIALS

Spontaneous breathing trials are the hottest of the hot for ventilator discontinuance. Remember, an SBT should be done formally and systematically by the therapist. The first SBT is a brief screening trial.

55. How long is the first SBT?

56. The patient must meet two of the following three criteria to continue:

Assessment	Criterion for Success
A. Spontaneous V_T	_____
B. MIP	_____
C. Respiratory rate	_____

57. A formal SBT is at least _____ minutes and no longer than _____ minutes.

58. An SBT must be performed with a T piece or, if the patient stays on the vent, with PSV of _____ cm H_2O or CPAP of ≤ _____ cm H_2O.

59. Monitor the patient during the trial. You should stop the SBT if distress occurs.

Assessment	Signs of Serious Distress
A. Mental status	_____
B. Respiratory rate	_____
C. Heart rate	_____
D. Blood pressure	_____
E. SpO_2	_____

If the SBT fails, put the patient back on the ventilator with *full support* for 24 hours. Try to figure out why the trial failed and fix the problem. For example, perform more aggressive bronchial hygiene. If the SBT is successful, keep the patient off the ventilator for a little while longer and consider extubation.

60. When should you repeat the SBT if the first trial fails?

61. Describe mandatory minute ventilation (MMV).

62. What specific patient population would be at risk when using MMV?

Copyright © 2003, 1999 Mosby, Inc. All rights reserved.

63. Mandatory minute ventilation systems compare $\dot{V}_{Esp}$ with desired $\dot{V}_E$. How do they adjust the ventilation delivered by the machine?

64. What is the main advantage of flow-triggering over pressure triggering?

65. Volume support, volume-assured pressure-supported ventilation (VAPS), adaptive support ventilation (ASV), proportional assist ventilation (PAV), and proportional pressure support (PPS) are new methods of approaching ventilation. What is the basic idea behind these modes?

66. Discuss the role of NPPV in weaning.

Table 44-4 summarizes the pros and cons of the various weaning methods.

▶ MONITORING THE PATIENT

Whew, that last section was long. But we're not done yet!

67. What are the two easily monitored and reliable indicators of patient progress during weaning?
   A. _____
   B. _____

68. What is the single best index of ventilation?

69. What is the simplest way to monitor oxygenation during weaning?

70. Give the expected and excessive changes for each of the following parameters.

Parameter	Expected	Deleterious
A. Respiratory rate	_____	_____
B. Pa_{O_2}	_____	_____
C. Pa_{CO_2}	_____	_____
D. Heart rate	_____	_____
E. Blood pressure	_____	_____

The NBRC expects you to know these changes well. So do your instructors. So does the patient.

Copyright © 2003, 1999 Mosby, Inc. All rights reserved.

▶ EXTUBATION

Weaning and extubation are separate issues. We know this, but other clinicians may not be as clear, so the RCP has to be a strong advocate in the decision to remove or maintain the artificial airway. Failed extubation may be hazardous to your patient's health. Results of a study published in the July 1999 issue of *Respiratory Care* indicated that a failure rate (patient's needing reintubation) of 10% to 20% was acceptable in the medical ICU population. In the surgical ICU (uncomplicated postop status) a failure rate of less than 5% is reasonable. Failure rates above 20% probably mean you are not assessing the patients carefully enough. Failure rates below 10% probably mean you are keeping the patient on the ventilator too long.

71. What is the important thing to remember about the presence of the artificial airway in terms of weaning? What can be done about it? (See Table 44-7.)

72. What is the minimum ability required for personnel performing routine extubation?

73. What is the minimum ability required for personnel performing high-risk extubation?

74. What are common patient complaints after extubation?

75. Describe the cuff leak test. See Box 44-16.

76. Identify the appropriate management of postextubation stridor.
    A. Mild

    B. Moderate

Copyright © 2003, 1999 Mosby, Inc. All rights reserved.

C. Severe

77. What patients are at risk of aspiration after extubation? How can you minimize the risk?

▶ FAILURE TO WEAN

As much as we all want to get the patient off the vent, it doesn't always work.

78. Identify two common causes of weaning failure for each of the following areas.
    A. Oxygenation
        1. _____
        2. _____
    B. Ventilation
        1. _____
        2. _____
    C. Cardiovascular factors
        1. _____
        2. _____

79. The ICU is no place for the long-term ventilator patient. It's too expensive, and the staff usually is not trained to deal with the issues. What are the alternative care sites?

80. Table 44-8 is a monster! Identify strategies for each of the following problems.

Problem	Management Strategy
A. Anemia	_____
	_____
B. Tube-related WOB	_____
	_____
C. Bronchospasm	_____
D. Secretions	_____
	_____
E. Dyspnea	_____
	_____
F. Muscle fatigue	_____
	_____
G. Hemodynamics	_____
	_____
H. Infection	_____
	_____
I. Metabolic factors	_____
J. Nutrition	_____
	_____
K. Exercise	_____
	_____
L. Psychological factors	_____
	_____
M. Sleep	_____
	_____
	_____
N. Pain	_____
	_____

Copyright © 2003, 1999 Mosby, Inc. All rights reserved.

Many of these techniques are useful once the patient is removed from the ICU and placed in an alternative site. A skilled, multidisciplinary approach is needed for patients who need long-term ventilation. Some patients remain on the machine for life.

81. Who should be involved in the decision to terminate life support?

82. Who does *Egan's* suggest perform the actual termination?

► CASE STUDIES

Case 1

Melba T. is an alert 61-year-old placed on the ventilator because of respiratory failure due to CHF and COPD. Twenty-four hours later, the physician asks for your recommendation regarding weaning. Breath sounds reveal coarse crackles in both bases. Pedal edema is present as well. The following information is obtained.

f_{sp}	28 breaths/min
V_{Tsp}	0.2 L
MIF	−18 cm H_2O
VC	0.6 L
Heart rate	116 beats/min
Blood pressure	90/60 mm Hg
pH	7.33
Pa_{CO_2}	35 mm Hg
Pa_{O_2}	65 (on FIO_2 0.5)
CI	2.3

83. What is your assessment of the respiratory status?

84. Has the primary problem been solved?

85. What is the RSBI?

86. Explain your recommendation regarding initiating weaning? If you recommend weaning, also recommend the method.

Copyright © 2003, 1999 Mosby, Inc. All rights reserved.

Case 2

Ed McM. is a 61-year-old placed on the ventilator after open heart surgery. Twelve hours later the patient is awake, and the physician asks for your recommendation regarding weaning. The following information is obtained.

f_{sp}	14
V_{Tsp}	0.2 L
MIF	−35 cm H_2O
VC	1.2 L
Heart rate	116 beats/min
Blood pressure	90/60 mm Hg
pH	7.37
$PaCO_2$	35 mm Hg
PaO_2	85 mm Hg (on FIO_2 0.35)

87. What is your assessment of the patient's respiratory status?

88. Has the primary problem been solved?

89. What is the RSBI?

90. Explain your recommendation regarding initiating weaning. If you recommend weaning, also recommend a technique.

Case 3

E. Benedict is a 61-year-old placed on the ventilator after an acute episode of Guillain-Barré syndrome. Twenty-one days later the patient is regaining strength and movement in his limbs. The physician asks for your recommendation regarding weaning. The following information is obtained.

f_{sp}	22
V_{Tsp}	0.22 L
MIF	−20 cm H_2O
VC	1.0 L
Heart rate	116 beats/min
Blood pressure	90/60 mm Hg
pH	7.38
$PaCO_2$	37 mm Hg
PaO_2	70 mm Hg (on FIO_2 0.40)

91. What is your assessment of the patient's respiratory status?

Copyright © 2003, 1999 Mosby, Inc. All rights reserved.

92. Has the primary problem been solved?

93. What is the RSBI?

94. Explain your recommendation regarding initiating weaning. If you recommend weaning, also recommend a technique.

95. What would you recommend at this time?

96. What is the RSBI?

97. How long does the patient need to succeed on the trial before you would consider extubation?

Case 4

C. Suzette is a 5'2" tall, 110-lb (50 kg), 80-year-old woman who has been on the ventilator for 2 days because of hemodynamic instability after open-heart surgery. The vital signs are now stable. Dr. Schultz wants you to conduct an SBT. You suction Ms. Suzette and sit her up for trial. Pretrial respiratory rate is 22 breaths/min, MIP is −45 mm Hg, and V_{Tsp} is 400 mL. She is placed on a T piece for 3 minutes with 40% oxygen. After 3 minutes, f is 25; MIP, −40; and V_{Tsp}, 420 mL.

▶ WHAT DOES THE NBRC SAY?

I guess it's clear from the number of questions I've put in this chapter that weaning and discontinuance are important topics. But is weaning really specified in the exam matrices? The Entry Level examination matrix states that you should, "Initiate and modify weaning procedures" and "wean or change weaning procedures and extubation." The Written Registry matrix specifically mentions extubation, but not weaning. The key to understanding this subject is in the ways mechanical ventilation is applied. Modes such as PSV, SIMV, IMV, CPAP, and PEEP are frequently cited in different areas of these test preparation tools. It is difficult to know exactly how many questions on weaning will be on an

Copyright © 2003, 1999 Mosby, Inc. All rights reserved.

individual test. It could vary from a few (2 or 3) to many (5-7)! Spontaneous breathing trials and RSBI are not in the matrices, yet. I bet these two concepts are coming to an examination soon. Here are some examples for your thinking pleasure.

98. Which of the following would you evaluate before initiating T-piece weaning?
    I. PaO_2
    II. Gag reflex
    III. Spontaneous respiratory rate
    IV. Minute ventilation
    A. I, II only
    B. I, III only
    C. II, III, IV only
    D. I, III, IV only

99. A patient being assessed for readiness to wean has the following values:

pH	7.36
$PaCO_2$	42 mm Hg
PaO_2	67 mm Hg (FIO_2 40%)
MIP	−25 cm H_2O
Heart rate	105 beats/min
Respirations	20 breaths/min
Vital capacity	12 mL/kg

    What action should the respiratory care practitioner recommend at this time?
    A. Initiate a T-piece trial
    B. Continue with mechanical ventilation
    C. Initiate breathing exercises to strengthen ventilatory muscles
    D. Repeat the vital capacity maneuver

100. Which of the following indicates a readiness to wean?
    A. Spontaneous rate of 28
    B. Spontaneous tidal volume of 200 mL
    C. Negative inspiratory force of 18 cm H_2O
    D. Minute volume of 8 L/min

101. An alert patient is being mechanically ventilated. Settings are

Mode	SIMV
Rate	2
Tidal volume (set)	800
FIO_2	0.30
PEEP	5 cm H_2O

    ABG results 30 minutes after initiating these settings are

pH	7.37
$PaCO_2$	38 mm Hg
PaO_2	75 mm Hg

    What should the RCP recommend at this time?
    A. Increase the set rate to 4
    B. Discontinue mechanical ventilation
    C. Decrease the PEEP to 0 cm H_2O
    D. Decrease the FIO_2 to 0.21

Copyright © 2003, 1999 Mosby, Inc. All rights reserved.

102. A 70-year-old, 70-kg (154 lb) patient with a history of COPD is being mechanically ventilated. The patient is alert but making no spontaneous efforts.

Mode	AC
Rate	12
Tidal volume (set)	800
FIO_2	0.40
PEEP	3 cm H_2O
pH	7.51
$PaCO_2$	38 mm Hg
PaO_2	95 mm Hg
HCO_3	36 mEq/L

Which of the following should the RCP recommend?

   I. Change to SIMV mode
  II. Decrease the FIO_2
 III. Decrease the set rate
 IV. Decrease the PEEP
A. I, II only
B. I, III only
C. I, II, III only
D. I, III, IV only

103. A patient is being ventilated in the SIMV mode with a rate of 8 breaths/min, volume of 800 mL, and FIO_2 of 0.40. ABG results show

pH	7.47
$PaCO_2$	33 mm Hg
PaO_2	88 mm Hg
HCO_3	23 mEq/L

What action should the RCP recommend in response to these findings?
A. Increase the tidal volume
B. Increase the FIO_2
C. Change to AC mode
D. Reduce the rate

104. A patient on SIMV experiences difficulty each time you try to reduce the rate below 6. The patient becomes tachypneic with a rate of 28 and a spontaneous volume of 200. Which of the following modifications would be *least* useful in this situation?
A. Adding pressure support ventilation
B. T-piece weaning
C. A trial of extubation
D. Changing to flow-by or flow triggering

It's not too difficult to wean patients on paper. If you know your values. Watch out for COPD patients who are being overventilated or overoxygenated by the machine.

▶ FOOD FOR THOUGHT

Your book mentions weaning indices but doesn't really mention the details. Here's the scoop. Simplified weaning index (SWI) and CROP (compliance, rate, oxygenation, and PI_{max}[aka MIP]) are two of the better methods.

$$SWI = \frac{fmv(PIP - PEE)}{MIP} \times \frac{PaCO_2mv}{40}$$

$$CROP = \frac{Cdyn \times MIP \times \dfrac{PaO_2}{PAO_2}}{f}$$

Copyright © 2003, 1999 Mosby, Inc. All rights reserved.

105. What is the single best approach to weaning?

► **INFORMATION AGE**

David Walker, RRT, presents an overview of this subject at **home.earthlink.net/~firstbreath/ventxt. htm**

You could also go to **www.umdnj.edu/rspthweb/bibs/ weaning.htm**

if you are interested in a comprehensive bibliography of just about every article ever written on the subject!

For expert information on long-term ventilation, you might like to try Barlow Hospital. The site is **www.barlow2000.org/research/default. htm**

Copyright © 2003, 1999 Mosby, Inc. All rights reserved.

Neonatal and Pediatric Respiratory Care

"Any sufficiently advanced technology is indistinguishable from magic."
Arthur C. Clarke

If you actually knew me, you'd understand that I really don't like taking care of sick babies or kids. I have always been an adult care practitioner. Not that I haven't bagged my fair share of babies, or managed croup, or cystic fibrosis, or even epiglottitis. When I had to.

In general, I leave kids to those who like to care for them. On my boards, however, neonatal and pediatrics were my best area. I knew that I was clinically weak, so I made an extra effort to know the subject well. Whether you dream of working with this special population or in a community hospital, where you will need the skills and knowledge periodically, or just want to do well on your boards, you will find Chapter 45 is just what the doctor ordered. It's a comprehensive and comprehensible overview of the care and feeding of little ones who can't breathe. I'll warn you right now that this is a very long chapter, packed with a huge amount of information, so make an extra large pot of coffee for this one. (If you need a refresher on fetal lung development and anatomic differences between kids and adults, you'll find it in Chapter 7.)

► LITTLE WORDS

I guess you've noticed that I think medical terminology is important and that I like crosswords. There's a final puzzle on p. 456 to help you build up your baby talk.

► FETAL FUN AND GAMES

1. Assessment of the newborn begins with maternal history. Identify three conditions likely to result in a baby that is small for gestational age (see Table 45-1).
   A. _____
   B. _____
   C. _____

2. Identify five maternal factors likely to lead to premature delivery (see Table 45-1)
   A. _____
   B. _____
   C. _____
   D. _____
   E. _____

3. What maternal condition is likely to result in an infant that is large for gestational age?

Copyright © 2003, 1999 Mosby, Inc. All rights reserved.

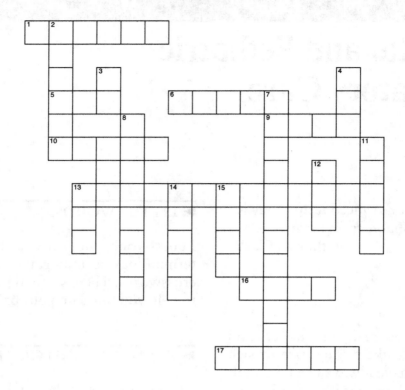

ACROSS

1. Four part cardiac disorder
5. Baby hemoglobin
6. This hole connects the right and left atria
9. Persistent hypertension
10. Premature babies are prone to this breathing pattern
13. Inflammation of the small airways
16. Mysterious fatal disorder of newborns
17. _____ fibrosis, a lethal genetic disorder

DOWN

2. Common obstructive disease of chidren
3. Short for 65 roses
4. Rapid breathing that comes and goes
7. Life-threatening infection of airway cartilage
8. Fetal doo-doo
11. Flaring means distress
12. Neutral thermal environment
13. Lung disease in IRDS and ventilator survivors
14. Viral upper airway infection that results in a barking cough
15. Infant respiratory distress syndrome

4. The fetus can be assessed by a variety of methods. Discuss each of the following tests.
   A. Ultrasonography

B. Amniocentesis

Copyright © 2003, 1999 Mosby, Inc. All rights reserved.

C. Fetal heart rate monitoring

D. Fetal blood gas analysis

5. What L/S ratio indicates lung maturity? When does this usually occur?

6. What is the relation between fetal scalp gases and ABGs?

▶ ASSESSING THE LITTLE DARLINGS

7. When are Apgar scores taken?

8. You really need to learn the Apgar scoring system, so . . . (see Table 45-2)

Sign	0	1	2
A. Heart rate	_____	_____	_____
B. Respiration	_____	_____	_____
C. Muscle tone	_____	_____	_____
D. Reflex	_____	_____	_____
E. Color	_____	_____	_____

(You could make up some kind of mnemonic to help you remember the five signs, such as "Heart Rate Must Really Count," if it helps you.)

9. What term is used to describe the following weeks of gestation?
   A. Before 38 weeks
   B. 38 to 42 weeks
   C. After 42 weeks

10. Name the two common systems used for assessing gestational age on the basis of physical characteristics and neurological signs.
    A. _____
    B. _____

11. Explain the abbreviations and identify the weights that correspond to the following terms.

Abbreviation	Full Name	Weight Range
A. VLBW	_____	_____
B. LBW	_____	_____
C. AGA	_____	_____
D. LGA	_____	_____

12. Why does anyone care about birth weight and gestational age?

Copyright © 2003, 1999 Mosby, Inc. All rights reserved.

► HI-HO, SILVERMAN, AWAY. . . !

13. State the normal range for a term infant's vital signs.
    A. Heart rate
    B. Respiratory rate
    C. Blood pressure

14. Describe the usual way to measure an infant's heart rate.

15. Infants in respiratory distress typically exhibit one or more of these five signs. Explain the significance of each sign.
    A. Nasal flaring

    B. Cyanosis

    C. Expiratory grunting

D. Retractions

E. Paradoxical breathing

16. What scoring system is used to grade the severity of underlying lung disease?

17. What are the two usual sources for arterial blood in infants?
    A. _____
    B. _____

18. Name two alternative sources.
    A. _____
    B. _____

19. List the ABG values for preterm and term infants at birth and at 5 days (see Table 45-4)

Value	Preterm	Term	5 Days
A. pH	_____	_____	_____
B. Pa_{CO_2}	_____	_____	_____
C. Pa_{O_2}	_____	_____	_____

Copyright © 2003, 1999 Mosby, Inc. All rights reserved.

► WHAT'S THE BIG IDEA?

20. At what temperature does cold stress occur in newborns?

21. Identify five harmful consequences of cold stress or hypothermia in babies.
    A. _____
    B. _____
    C. _____
    D. _____
    E. _____

22. What is meant by *neutral thermal environment* (NTE)?

23. What is the usual range of ambient temperature needed to maintain NTE?

24. How are sick infants usually fed?

25. What is a major source of colonization by *Staphylococcus* and *Streptococcus* organisms in newborns?

► RESPIRATORY CARE TECHNIQUES

Back to Basics

26. Considering the hazards, we need to agree on the safe limits for oxygen therapy. Give the accepted ranges for these values.
    A. Pao_2 _____ to _____
    B. Fio_2 _____ to _____
    C. Spo_2 _____ to _____

27. Hyperoxia is associated with ROP and BPD in some infants. What do these acronyms stand for?
    A. ROP
    B. BPD

28. Name two other factors associated with ROP (see Box 45-1)
    A. _____
    B. _____

29. What is meant by the "flip-flop phenomenon"?

Copyright © 2003, 1999 Mosby, Inc. All rights reserved.

30. Name three factors that should be continuously monitored when administering oxygen to infants.
    A. _____
    B. _____
    C. _____

31. Compare the use of the following oxygen delivery devices (see Table 45-5)

Device	Age	Advantage	Disadvantage
A. AEM	_____	_____	_____
B. Cannula	_____	_____	_____
C. Incubator	_____	_____	_____
D. Hood	_____	_____	_____
E. Tent	_____	_____	_____

32. Name four conditions in which secretion retention is common in children.
    A. _____
    B. _____
    C. _____
    D. _____

33. Identify one other situation in which bronchial hygiene therapy may be useful.

34. Because infants can't cough on command, how will you get the mucus out once it is mobilized?

35. How long should you wait after feedings to perform postural drainage on infants and small children?

36. How can you help prevent hypoxemia during head-down positioning?

37. What are the hazards of overheating or underheating gases administered to newborns?
    A. Overheating
        1. _____
        2. _____
    B. Underheating
        1. _____
        2. _____
        3. _____

Copyright © 2003, 1999 Mosby, Inc. All rights reserved.

38. How is application of the nasal cannula different for adults and kids in terms of humidification?

39. Identify three reasons why continuous nebulization usually is avoided in infants.
    A. _____
    B. _____
    C. _____

40. How would you deliver a bronchodilator to a newborn? (See Table 45-6)

41. How would you deliver an MDI to an infant?

42. What is the dosage range for albuterol delivered by SVN? (See Table 45-7)

43. What are the dose range and frequency for racemic epinephrine?
    A. Dose
    B. Frequency

44. What are the dose and treatment schedule for nebulized budesonide?
    A. Dose
    B. Treatment schedule

45. Identify the correct ET tube size and suction catheter size for these kids (see Table 45-8).

Age/Weight	ET	Length (oral)	Suction
A. <1000 g	_____	_____	_____
B. 1000-2000 g	_____	_____	_____
C. 2000-3000 g	_____	_____	_____
D. >3000 g	_____	_____	_____
E. 2 y	_____	_____	_____
F. 6 y	_____	_____	_____

If this seems silly, don't laugh. Parts of Question 45 will appear on your board exams.

46. State the two formulas for calculating tube size (see Table 45-8)
    A. _____
    B. _____

47. Use the first formula to estimate the correct tube size for a 4-year-old.

48. Estimate the correct tube size for a child who is 122 cm (48 in) tall.

Copyright © 2003, 1999 Mosby, Inc. All rights reserved.

49. Which laryngoscope blade is usually used for infant intubation?

50. What is the main difference between infant or pediatric ET tubes and adult tubes?

51. What are the recommended vacuum pressures for suctioning infants and children?
    A. Infants
    B. Children

52. How should you preoxygenate newborns to avoid hyperoxia?

53. What is the duration of suctioning for newborns? How does this compare with suctioning for adults?

▶ NEONATAL RESUSCITATION

54. What is the first step of resuscitation immediately after delivery?

55. What action should be taken if meconium is visible in the larynx?

56. Identify the criteria for initiating chest compressions after delivery.

▶ ADVANCED FUN AND GAMES

57. Play with baby's FRC by applying CPAP. What is the specific indication for CPAP? Give the blood gas values.

Copyright © 2003, 1999 Mosby, Inc. All rights reserved.

58. Name four signs of respiratory distress that suggest the need for CPAP (see Box 45-5)
    A. _____
    B. _____
    C. _____
    D. _____

59. Discuss adjustment of CPAP in infants.

60. CPAP usually is administered to an infant via what type of delivery system?

61. Give the range of tidal volumes for infants.

62. Identify the inspiratory time ranges that should be set for these age groups.
    A. Low-birth-weight infants
    B. Term infants
    C. Toddlers
    D. Children

63. Ventilator rates should be adjusted to maintain what range of Pa_{CO_2}?

64. What PEEP levels are usually used in neonates?

65. Why would it be common to observe lower exhaled than inhaled volumes in pediatric patients?

66. Describe how to reduce the following values during weaning.
    A. F_{IO_2}

    B. PEEP

Copyright © 2003, 1999 Mosby, Inc. All rights reserved.

C. Rate

72. Oxygenation in HFV is adjusted through increases in mean airway pressure and F_{IO_2}, just as in adults. Elimination of CO_2 depends mainly on what factor? How is this different from standard adult ventilator therapy?

67. What ventilator settings suggest evaluation for extubation?
    A. Set rate
    B. PIP
    C. F_{IO_2}
    D. PEEP

68. Describe the leak test for upper airway edema.

▶ JUST SAY NO

Nitric oxide is an FDA-approved drug. When inhaled, this gas is called iNO. Nitric oxide selectively vasodilates pulmonary vessels surrounding the functional alveoli.

73. What effect does NO have on oxygenation?

▶ HIGH-FREQUENCY VENTILATION

69. List four clinical indications for initiating HFV.
    A. _____
    B. _____
    C. _____
    D. _____

74. Two big problems exist with NO inhalation. Explain.
    A. Rebound

70. Identify the three common characteristics of HFV.
    A. _____
    B. _____
    C. _____

71. What are the three most common types of HFV?
    A. _____
    B. _____
    C. _____

    B. Altered hemoglobin

Copyright © 2003, 1999 Mosby, Inc. All rights reserved.

You can read more about this gas in Chapter 35.

▶ HOURS OF BOREDOM, MOMENTS OF TERROR

A friend of mine who administers ECMO describes her job as pretty routine until something goes wrong. One of my students who is a flight attendant says the same thing about her job. Extracorporeal membrane oxygenation is a fascinating and vital form of therapy in which respiratory therapists play a leading role. More than 16,000 neonates have been treated with ECMO with a 78% survival rate.

75. What does ECMO do?

76. Describe the two basic forms of ECMO.
   A. VA

   B. VV

77. Give three examples of neonatal conditions in which ECMO is being used after conventional medical therapies fail.
   A. _____
   B. _____
   C. _____

▶ WHAT DOES THE NBRC SAY?

The exam matrices make detailed references to the material in Chapter 45. Here's a partial list:

Perinatal data:

- Maternal history
- Perinatal history
- Apgar scores
- Gestational age
- L/S ratio

Recommend procedures:

- Umbilical line
- Transcutaneous monitoring

Inspect the patient:

- Apgar score
- Gestational age
- Retractions
- Nasal flaring
- Transillumination of the chest

Equipment:

- Oxygen hoods and tents
- Specialized ventilators-oscillators, high frequency

The Clinical Simulation examination matrix makes it clear that you will have one pediatric and one neonatal problem. They list these cases as examples:

Copyright © 2003, 1999 Mosby, Inc. All rights reserved.

Neonatal:

- Delivery room management, resuscitation, infant apnea, meconium aspiration, respiratory distress syndrome, congenital heart defect

Although Chapter 45 covers some of this information, you would be wise to consider taking a Neonatal Advanced Life Support (NALS) and PALS course before you take the boards. Here are some sample multiple choice questions.

78. Which of the following tests would be useful in determining lung maturity?
    A. Sweat chloride
    B. L/S ratio
    C. Fetal hemoglobin
    D. Pneumogram

79. Calculate the Apgar score for a crying infant who has a heart rate of 120 beats/min, actively moves, and sneezes when a catheter is put in the nose but has blue extremities.
    A. 5
    B. 6
    C. 7
    D. 9

80. The simplest way to apply CPAP to manage hypoxemia in an infant is to use
    A. Nasal prongs
    B. Nasal mask
    C. Full face mask
    D. An oxygen hood

► FOOD FOR THOUGHT

If you choose to work in this field, it would be a good idea to take the Neonatal/Pediatric Specialty Examination to test your knowledge and demonstrate your competence in this specialty area.

► INFORMATION AGE

When you do a Google search for "neonatal respiratory care" the first three hits are books. Whole books are written on this subject, and you're going to need one to cover neonatal and pediatric respiratory care in depth. If you like the Internet, I'll make these suggestions:
www.vh.org/pediatric

Virtual children's hospital is a good site. Very useful to me as a teacher.

Another good source is
www.lungusa.org/diseases

Copyright © 2003, 1999 Mosby, Inc. All rights reserved.

Patient Education and Health Promotion

**"Quit worrying about your
health. It will go away."**
Robert Orben

1. Affective domain

2. Cognitive domain

3. Disease prevention

Teaching can be very satisfying—when learning is taking place. (I should know.) It's equally frustrating to try to learn when teaching is disorganized or the objectives are unclear. (You should know.) Client and community education go to the far ends of the spectrum. It is tremendously rewarding to help someone stop smoking or learn to be more independent or to teach children how to manage their asthma. *Real* victories in the battle for better health. On the other hand, you can go nuts trying to get your message across to some people. Chapter 46 provides you with valuable ideas on how to develop, conduct, and measure the outcome of a health education program. You can use this information in school, with patients, in the community, and in teaching coworkers. Let's go do some educatin'!

4. Health education

► TEACHER TALK

I want to make sure you have a good grasp of the key terms in this chapter before you apply them. Write out the definition for each of these terms. You can use the chapter or the glossary.

Copyright © 2003, 1999 Mosby, Inc. All rights reserved.

5. Health promotion

6. Psychomotor domain

▶ PATIENT EDUCATION

Respiratory care practitioners have always been on-the-spot instructors at the bedside, but the role of respiratory therapists as formal educators has increased dramatically in the past few years as healthcare delivery methods and settings have changed.

OVERVIEW

7. What are the five main causes of death in the United States?
   A. _____
   B. _____
   C. _____
   D. _____
   E. _____

8. Why is educating the public about these illnesses so important?

▶ WHAT'S IN A DOMAIN?

9. Why should you consider developing written objectives for patient teaching? (Isn't that just something teachers do to look good?)

10. How can you state an objective in measurable terms?
    A. Begin with a . . .

    B. Include a single patient . . .

11. Give an example of an objective for each of the following learning domains. (Oh, go ahead, take one out of *Egan's*.)

Domain	*Objective*
A. Cognitive	_____
B. Affective	_____
C. Psychomotor	_____

12. Which of the learning domains (*domaine* is a French word that means realm, estate, or property) should be evaluated before you proceed with patient education?

Copyright © 2003, 1999 Mosby, Inc. All rights reserved.

13. Maslow's hierarchy of needs (pretty useful if you apply it) explains why a dyspneic patient will not be very receptive to learning a new skill. How can you assess readiness to learn?

14. What is the key to motivating patients to learn?

15. What is the key to teaching psychomotor skills? How can you confirm that a patient or family member has learned a new skill?

16. Give an example from the text of how to relate psychomotor skills a patient uses every day to help the patient make the transition from everyday life to therapy.

► F.A.T. T.I.P.S*

*Forget Academic Theory. This Is Practical Stuff.

Now that you've reviewed some important ideas about teaching, let's take a look at . . .

Crystal Clear Classroom Commandments

I. Meet immediate patient needs first.
II. Create an educational setting.
III. Include hearing, seeing, touching, writing, and speaking.
IV. Keep sessions short.
V. Repeat, repeat, repeat.
VI. Allow plenty of time to practice skills.
VII. Spend time preparing for the session.
VIII. Organize your materials and presentation.
IX. Personalize and customize the learning experience.
X. Be enthusiastic.

If you think about your own learning experiences, you will have no difficulty believing in these powerful ideas for improving your teaching abilities. (Make a copy and mail them to someone!)

Teaching Children

17. How is teaching children different from teaching adults? How is it the same? (See Box 46-1.)

Copyright © 2003, 1999 Mosby, Inc. All rights reserved.

18. Where could you find resource materials to help in teaching children with asthma? (See the Mini Clini.)

19. What suggestions are given for rewarding performance?

Evaluation

20. What process answers the question, "Has the patient learned?" When should you begin to develop this process?

21. Describe some of the ways you can tell if a patient has met affective domain objectives.

22. When is it important to go outside the formal teaching mechanisms described above? What does *Egan's* call this situation?

▶ **HEALTH EDUCATION**

Naturally, respiratory therapists are expected to be role models who demonstrate healthy behaviors in public. Imagine giving a patient information about nicotine intervention when you smell like cigarettes yourself! Role models aren't enough, however, to achieve large-scale improvements in public health.

23. What is the primary goal of health education?

24. Learning activities must incorporate values and beliefs of the learner. What four factors need to be considered in this area?
    A. _____
    B. _____
    C. _____
    D. _____

Copyright © 2003, 1999 Mosby, Inc. All rights reserved.

CHAPTER 46 · Patient Education and Health Promotion 471

25. How do the personal characteristics of the educator affect learning?

▶ AN OUNCE OF PREVENTION IS WORTH...

26. State the four central, preventable causes among the major causes of death in the United States.
    A. _____
    B. _____
    C. _____
    D. _____

27. Compare the standard medical approach to health in the United States with the public health model.

28. Give goals and examples of each of the following levels of prevention.

Level	Goal	Example
A. Primary	_____	_____
	_____	_____
B. Secondary	_____	_____
	_____	_____
C. Tertiary	_____	_____
	_____	_____

29. Give examples of projects in which respiratory therapists can participate in organized health promotion activities targeted at primary, secondary, and tertiary goals.
    A. Primary _____
    B. Secondary_____
    C. Tertiary_____

30. Besides the hospital, name four other settings in which respiratory therapists would be likely to function as individual counselors or public health advocates.
    A. _____
    B. _____
    C. _____
    D. _____

▶ CASE STUDIES

Your text has several perfectly good cases in the form of Mini Clinis, so let's do something else. Suppose you had to teach your classmates how to use a peak flowmeter. Using behavioral terms, write three objectives for this topic for each domain.

31. Cognitive domain
    A. _____
    B. _____
    C. _____

32. Affective domain
    A. _____
    B. _____
    C. _____

33. Psychomotor domain
    A. _____
    B. _____
    C. _____

Copyright © 2003, 1999 Mosby, Inc. All rights reserved.

34. How long would your teaching session last?

35. Give examples of how you would involve the following senses in your session.
    A. Hearing
    B. Seeing
    C. Touching
    D. Writing
    E. Speaking

36. Give an example of how you would measure learning for each domain.
    A. Cognitive
    B. Affective
    C. Psychomotor

▶ WHAT DOES THE NBRC SAY?

Not much. You should be able to educate a patient. Here's an example.

37. The best way to ensure that a patient learned to properly administer a bronchodilator via MDI is to
    A. Ask the patient to answer questions regarding inhaler use
    B. Give the patient appropriate literature regarding MDI use
    C. Ask the patient to demonstrate how to use the inhaler
    D. Have the patient explain when he is to use the MDI

▶ FOOD FOR THOUGHT

38. Why do you think the public should be educated about the risk factors for the top five causes of death? After all, many respiratory therapists are employed taking care of patients who have ignored these risk factors.

39. How is teaching other caregivers different from teaching patients or family members?

▶ INFORMATION AGE

I often look for teaching materials that have already been designed by others. No point in reinventing the wheel, right? Here are some places where you can find material that is ready to use.

COPD resources:
www.aarc.org/klein

the AARC of course!
Asthma:
www.breatherville.org/breatherville.htm

A great asthma site!

Lung disease in general:
www.lungusa.org

Copyright © 2003, 1999 Mosby, Inc. All rights reserved.

The ALA. You can also go to your local chapter. Or go to National Jewish at **nationaljewish.org/understanding/ understanding_online.html**

The Hawaii Medical Library offers a consumer health information service at **www.hml.org/CHIS/topics/lung.html**

The Internet is at its finest in this area. I can get material on any subject from teaching tracheostomy care to ARDS. Literally anything.

Copyright © 2003, 1999 Mosby, Inc. All rights reserved.

Nutritional Aspects of Health and Disease

"To eat is human. To digest divine."
Mark Twain

I'm continually surprised at how little attention most of us give to what we eat. Hospitals put a tremendous effort into providing nourishing, specialized diets—with about as much public relations success as the airlines. When was the last time you heard anyone raving about the three-star meal she had after surgery? Dietary habits have far-reaching consequences in terms of overall health, so it should come as no surprise to you that nutrition plays a role in cardiopulmonary function (or that respiratory therapists would get involved).

▶ EAT YOUR WORDS

The language in Chapter 47 reads like a French menu—incomprehensibly. I guess you'll need to look up some of these terms before you can match them up with their definitions (I guess I will too!).

1. _____ Anergy
2. _____ Anthropometry
3. _____ Azotemia
4. _____ Basal metabolic rate
5. _____ Gluconeogenesis
6. _____ Indirect calorimetry
7. _____ Ketogenesis
8. _____ Kwashiorkor
9. _____ Marasmus
10. _____ Normometabolic
11. _____ Protein-energy malnutrition
12. _____ Resting energy expenditure (REE)

A. Excess nitrogenous waste in the blood
B. Formation of glycogen from proteins or fatty acids
C. Toxic byproduct of the breakdown of fat
D. Daily resting energy consumption
E. Impaired immune response
F. Science of measuring the human body
G. Hypercatabolic form of malnutrition
H. Hourly resting energy consumption after fasting
I. Energy measurement based on O_2 consumption and CO_2 production
J. Malnutrition associated with starvation
K. Calorimetry REE within 10% of predicted value
L. Wasting condition resulting from a deficient diet

▶ MEET THE OBJECTIVES

13. Describe the food pyramid (see Figure 47-1).

Copyright © 2003, 1999 Mosby, Inc. All rights reserved.

14. What do decks of cards have to do with daily protein requirements?

15. Name the three macronutrients (subgroups for each) that supply your body's energy requirements. State the calorie intake per gram for each *main* category.

	Macro	*Calories per gram*
A.	_____	_____
1.	_____	_____
2.	_____	_____
B.	_____	_____
1.	_____	_____
2.	_____	_____
C.	_____	_____
1.	_____	_____
2.	_____	_____
3.	_____	_____

16. What is meant by the terms MUFA, PUFA, and SFA?
    A. _____
    B. _____
    C. _____

17. Write the Harris-Benedict prediction equation for estimating REE. Calculate yours.
    A. Formula _____
    B. Calculation _____

18. How many calories will an average man who weighs 80 kg need per day to maintain his body weight?

19. State two benefits of soluble and insoluble fiber?
    A. Soluble
       1. _____
       2. _____
    B. Insoluble
       1. _____
       2. _____

20. What antioxidants have been shown to improve lung function?

21. Compare starvation and hypercatabolism malnutrition. Be sure to give at least two clinical examples of each that a respiratory therapist would encounter.
    A. Starvation

    B. Hypercatabolism

22. State the effect of decreases in the following micronutrients through disease or malnutrition. (Just a few examples—this is a really huge subject!)
    A. Zinc _____
    B. Magnesium _____
    C. Phosphate _____

23. What percentage of patients with acute respiratory failure have malnutrition?

Copyright © 2003, 1999 Mosby, Inc. All rights reserved.

24. Give two reasons why malnourished patients are difficult to wean from the ventilator.
    A. _____
    B. _____

25. Why are COPD patients often malnourished?

26. What are the consequences of malnutrition on respiratory muscles and response to hypoxia and hypercapnia?

27. Who normally conducts nutritional assessments in the hospital?

28. State the formula for calculating ideal body weight.
    A. Men _____
    B. Women _____
    C. Calculate your own ideal body weight: _____

29. Identify one condition that represents each of the following high-risk groups (see Box 47-5)
    A. Poor intake _____
    B. Nutrient loss _____
    C. Hypermetabolism _____
    D. Drugs _____

30. List three conditions in which indirect calorimetry may be indicated (see Box 47-7).
    A. _____
    B. _____
    C. _____

31. What are the contraindications to indirect calorimetry in the care of mechanically ventilated patients? (See the CPG.)

32. According to the AARC CPG, closed-circuit calorimeters can reduce alveolar volume or increase WOB. Explain how these two hazards occur.
    A. _____
    B. _____

33. What actions should be taken to prepare a patient for indirect calorimetry? (See Box 47-8.)
    A. 4 hours before the test
    B. 2 hours before the test
    C. 1 hour before the test

Copyright © 2003, 1999 Mosby, Inc. All rights reserved.

34. Describe the most serious problem in performing indirect calorimetry on mechanically ventilated patients.

35. Interpret the following respiratory quotients (RQs) and identify the general nutritional strategy (see Table 47-4).

Value	Inter-pretation	Strategy
A. >1.0	_____	_____
B. 0.9-1.0	_____	_____
C. 0.7-0.8	_____	_____

36. State the formula for calculating REE using a pulmonary arterial catheter.

37. What factors are used to adjust predicted REEs in patients? Give one example. (See Box 47-11).

38. Explain what happens when patients receive too much of the following substrates. Give a pulmonary example, please.
A. Protein

B. Carbohydrates

C. Fat

39. What do the terms *enteral* and *parenteral* mean?
A. Enteral

B. Parenteral

Copyright © 2003, 1999 Mosby, Inc. All rights reserved.

40. Explain what is meant by the following tube feeding regimens:
    A. Bolus

    B. Intermittent

    C. Drip

41. How would the RCP confirm suspected aspiration of tube feedings? How is this complication avoided?

42. Patients with COPD have special dietary problems. Identify four factors that lead to poor intake in these patients.
    A. _____
    B. _____
    C. _____
    D. _____

43. What diet is provided to the hypercapnic patient?

44. How and what should COPD patients eat to optimize nutrition?

▶ CHAPTER HIGHLIGHTS

45. The majority of daily calories should come from _____, fruits, and _____.

46. _____ nutrients supply the body's energy requirements.

47. _____ nutrients play essential roles in normal metabolism and physiology.

48. The _____ - _____ equations are used to estimate daily REE.

49. _____ is a state of impaired metabolism in which the intake of nutrients falls short of the body's needs.

50. For the patient with pulmonary disease, high _____ loads can increase CO_2 production.

Copyright © 2003, 1999 Mosby, Inc. All rights reserved.

51. Whenever possible, the _____ route should be used for supplying nutrients.

52. The likelihood of _____ during tube feedings can be minimized by _____ the head of the bed by _____.

► CASE STUDY

Case 1

John Barleycorn, a thin, undernourished COPD patient, tells you that he has difficulty eating because he gets tired and short of breath during meals.

53. What eating pattern should be emphasized to Mr. Barleycorn?

54. Make some suggestions for poor John B. that would increase his nutrient intake.

55. What nutritional supplement was specifically designed for COPD patients?

► WHAT DOES THE NBRC SAY?

Sorry folks, although muscle wasting and general appearance do show up in the matrix, and although respiratory therapists are very involved in indirect calorimetry in many institutions, this information has not made it to the boards yet. No, this is just practical stuff you can use in patient assessment and patient teaching.

► FOOD FOR THOUGHT

56. What type of nutritional strategy can help in weaning of COPD patients from the ventilator?

57. Why is it important to verify tube placement before beginning feeding?

► INFORMATION AGE

I found some good material on COPD and nutrition at **www.cheshire-med.com/services/dietary/ nutrinew/copdnut.html**

and **www.nlm.nih.gov/medlineplus/ copdchronicobstructivepulmonary disease.html**

All this talk of food is making me hungry. It must be time for a root beer float!

Copyright © 2003, 1999 Mosby, Inc. All rights reserved.

CHAPTER 48

Cardiopulmonary Rehabilitation

"No one is useless in this world who lightens the burden of another."
Charles Dickens

Alvan Barach first recommended reconditioning programs for COPD patients more than 40 years ago. Unfortunately, it was not until recently that these programs began in earnest around the nation. When I worked in home care in the 1980s, it was often up to the individual therapist to try to provide these concepts and encourage individual patients. Now there are many well-established inpatient and outpatient programs to meet the physical and psychosocial needs of our patients with chronic lung disease.

Although there are many good textbooks and patient teaching aids available, you will find that Chapter 48 provides an excellent overview of the subject. Even if you don't work in rehabilitation, you will be in a position to identify patients who can benefit from these services, and you can play a key role in improving the quality of your patient's lives. You may also wish to participate in one of the support groups founded by the ALA, local healthcare organizations, or chapter of the AARC.

▶ **CEREBRAL MUSCLE TRAINING**

You can build impressive mental muscles by adding these words to your vocabulary.

Match the following terms and acronyms to their definitions.

1. _____ ADL
2. _____ Borg scale
3. _____ CORF
4. _____ Hypoglycemia
5. _____ METS
6. _____ OBLA
7. _____ Reconditioning
8. _____ Respiratory quotient
9. _____ Target heart rate

A. Physical activities designed to strengthen muscles and improve O_2 utilization
B. Measure of an individual's ability to perform common tasks
C. Point at which there is insufficient O_2 to meet the demands of energy metabolism
D. Measure of an individual's perception of breathing difficulty
E. Cardiac goal for aerobic conditioning based on 65% of maximum O_2 consumption
F. Ratio of CO_2 production to O_2 consumption
G. Medicare-approved facility that provides ambulatory rehab services
H. Low blood sugar level
I. Indirect measure of physiologic work performed during exercise stress testing

Copyright © 2003, 1999 Mosby, Inc. All rights reserved.

► DEFINITIONS AND GOALS

Pulmonary rehabilitation is not the same animal as other types of rehab, although it can contain some of the same elements.

10. What is meant by the general term *rehabilitation*?

11. The definition of pulmonary rehabilitation is really long. Please put it into your own words.

12. What are the two specific objectives of pulmonary rehab according to the American Thoracic Society?
A.

B.

► SCIENTIFIC BASIS FOR PULMONARY REHAB

Exercise physiology plays an important role in our understanding of the benefits of reconditioning, but physiology alone is not sufficient to achieve desired outcome in the care of patients with COPD.

13. How do social sciences play a role in establishing ways to improve the patient's quality of life?

14. Why is MVV a useful PFT in regard to assessing physical activity?

15. How can you estimate MVV using simple spirometry?

16. Identify the three general ways that reconditioning will increase exercise tolerance.
A. _____
B. _____
C. _____

Copyright © 2003, 1999 Mosby, Inc. All rights reserved.

17. Compare the roles of psychosocial and physical methods in terms of outcomes of rehabilitation.

18. Describe the two-way relation between physical reconditioning and psychosocial support.

▶ PULMONARY REHABILITATION PROGRAMS

Program designs may vary, but the desired outcome and basic components are similar.

19. Why is it so important to have specific objectives for the program goals?

20. State five accepted benefits of exercise reconditioning (see Table 48-1).
    A. _____
    B. _____
    C. _____
    D. _____
    E. _____

21. Research literature clearly shows that rehabilitation has limits. Name two.
    A. _____
    B. _____

22. List one evaluation tool from each of the three categories shown in Box 48-2.
    A. Exercise tolerance
    B. Symptoms
    C. Other changes

23. State three potential hazards of physical reconditioning.
    A. _____
    B. _____
    C. _____

24. What is the first step in patient evaluation for a pulmonary rehab program?

25. Name four tests that should be included with the physical examination.
    A. _____
    B. _____
    C. _____
    D. _____

26. Two tests usually are conducted to assess cardiopulmonary status. State two purposes of these tests.
    A. Exercise evaluation
       1. _____
       2. _____
    B. Pulmonary function testing
       1. _____
       2. _____

Copyright © 2003, 1999 Mosby, Inc. All rights reserved.

27. List two contraindications to and two complications of exercise testing.
    A. Contraindications
       1. _____
       2. _____
    B. Complications
       1. _____
       2. _____

28. Identify four physiologic values that should be monitored during exercise testing.
    A. _____
    B. _____
    C. _____
    D. _____

29. Name two types of patients usually excluded from selection for rehab.
    A. _____
    B. _____

30. State the four general groups of patients included in pulmonary rehab programs.
    A. _____
    B. _____
    C. _____
    D. _____

31. What are the benefits of grouping patients on the basis of severity and overall ability?

32. Give one benefit and one drawback of the open-ended program model.
    A. Benefit _____
    B. Drawback _____

33. Give one benefit and one drawback to the traditional closed design.
    A. Benefit _____
    B. Drawback _____

34. Describe two ways to set target heart rate for patient exercise.
    A.

    B.

35. Describe a typical walking exercise program.

36. What is the basic concept behind ventilatory muscle training?

Copyright © 2003, 1999 Mosby, Inc. All rights reserved.

37. Briefly discuss the following high-priority educational components of a program.
    A. Breathing control

    B. Stress management

    C. Medications

    D. Diet

38. What is the ideal class size for a rehab program? What external factor affects this ideal?

39. Give specific examples of each of the following sources of program reimbursement.
    A. Nongovernmental health insurance

    B. Federal and state health insurance

    C. Ancillary insurance

    D. Other option

40. What is the most likely cause of lack of measurable improvement within a pulmonary rehab program?

Copyright © 2003, 1999 Mosby, Inc. All rights reserved.

► CASE STUDIES

Case 1

Bill Friendly is an alert 55-year-old man with long-standing asthma and COPD. He is admitted because of acute exacerbation of his illness following a "chest cold." This admission is Bill's fourth in the last 3 months. Mr. Friendly tells you that he has had to quit his job and take early retirement because of his lung problems.

41. What concerns does this situation raise?

42. Explain to Mr. Friendly the benefits of entering a rehab program.

Case 2

Jane Deaux is a 57-year-old woman with chronic bronchitis who is enrolled in your pulmonary rehab program. During walking exercises she reports dyspnea and will not continue with the walk.

43. What assessments would be useful in this situation?

44. Give several possible methods for modifying the exercise program to improve this patient's compliance.

► WHAT DOES THE NBRC SAY?

In the case of pulmonary rehabilitation, the examination matrix is very specific. Up to five questions may be asked. The matrix states:

"Initiate and conduct pulmonary rehabilitation . . . within the prescription," namely:

- Establish optimal therapeutic outcome
- Implement and monitor graded exercise program
- Explain and instruct planned therapeutic goals
- Conduct patient education and disease management programs
- Smoking cessation

In reality, however, you can expect fewer than five questions on the CRT exam because this area of the matrix also includes home care and assisting in special procedures. The Written Registry exam may ask more questions at a more difficult level. Chapter 48 goes into the subject in much greater depth than do the boards. The Clinical Simulation matrix includes identical items but also specifically mentions that you may encounter a case of a patient with COPD who needs pulmonary rehabilitation. This means that rehab is a small but very important part of the advanced practitioner testing.

Copyright © 2003, 1999 Mosby, Inc. All rights reserved.

45. A COPD patient has enrolled in a pulmonary rehabilitation program. The patient should be informed that the program will help provide all of the benefits *except*?
   A. Increased physical endurance
   B. Improved PFT results
   C. Increased activity levels
   D. Improved cardiovascular function

46. During an exercise test a patient is able to reach a maximum heart rate of 120 beats/min. His resting heart rate is 70 beats/min. What target heart rate would you recommend for this patient during aerobic conditioning?
   A. 70 beats/min
   B. 85 beats/min
   C. 100 beats/min
   D. 115 beats/min

47. Which of the following tests would be useful in assessing ventilatory reserve during exercise testing?
   A. Forced vital capacity
   B. Maximum voluntary ventilation
   C. Body plethysmography
   D. Single breath nitrogen washout

▶ FOOD FOR THOUGHT

Chapter 8 (and others) refers to the Borg scale (must be something to do with Star Trek!). This scale is a valuable tool that can be easily used at the bedside or in the rehab setting.

48. Describe the Borg scale.

49. What are the units of measurement on the scale?

50. What is the value of this instrument?

▶ INFORMATION AGE

A good place to start is the home page of the American Association of Cardiovascular and Pulmonary Rehabilitation:
www.aacvpr.org

Cheshire Medical has a nifty website devoted to their pulmonary rehab program:
www.cheshire-med.com/programs/ pulrehab/rehab.html

Postgraduate Medicine Online has a good overview:
www.postgradmed.com/issues/1998/ 04_98/celli.htm

There are lots more sites. The Internet is a very useful resource for the topic of pulmonary rehabilitation.

Copyright © 2003, 1999 Mosby, Inc. All rights reserved.

Respiratory Care in Alternative Settings

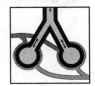

"Problems are only opportunities in work clothes."

Henry J. Kaiser

Egan's had to end with a beginning, and Chapter 49 introduces you to the fastest growing area of respiratory care. As healthcare is being redefined on many levels, the work setting for our profession is rapidly moving outside the boundaries of the traditional medical center. Alternative care settings provide special challenges for the RCP, particularly the new graduate.

► ACRONYMS

No matter what else you get out of this book, you're bound to have a brain full of odd letter combinations. Don't worry, be happy. This is the last of the acronyms. (I promise)

Write out the meanings, SVP.*

1. AHI

2. DME

3. HCFA

4. NPPV

5. SAHS

---

*S'il vous plait. ("If you please.")

Copyright © 2003, 1999 Mosby, Inc. All rights reserved.

6. SIDS

7. SNF

8. TTOT

▶ **RECENT TRENDS**

9. What is the most common alternative site for healthcare?

10. What is the overall effect of the prospective payment system?

11. What were the results of the Muse study?

▶ **DEFINITIONS AND GOALS**

12. Name the four areas of subacute or alternative care.
    A. _____
    B. _____
    C. _____
    D. _____

13. What is subacute care?

14. In what categories of subacute care are respiratory therapists usually involved?

15. Which age group most commonly receives subacute care?

Copyright © 2003, 1999 Mosby, Inc. All rights reserved.

16. State at least three of the benefits of respiratory home care.

A. _____

B. _____

C. _____

▶ STANDARDS

17. Why does government play a major role in setting standards for the regulation of postacute care?

18. What is the purpose of the Medicare Provider Certification Program?

19. Who is responsible for accreditation of companies that provide home care services?

20. What are the two types of accreditation for respiratory home care?

▶ TRADITIONAL ACUTE CARE

21. Why do many respiratory therapists prefer working in the postacute care setting?

22. Compare traditional and alternative settings in terms of the following areas (see Table 49-1):

Area	Traditional	Alternative
A. Diagnostic tests	_____	_____
B. Equipment	_____	_____
C. Supervision	_____	_____
D. Patient assessment	_____	_____
E. Work schedule	_____	_____
F. Time constraints	_____	_____

▶ DISCHARGE PLANNING

23. Explain the role of the following practitioners on the postacute care team (see Table 49-2):

A. Utilization and review

B. Social services

Copyright © 2003, 1999 Mosby, Inc. All rights reserved.

C. Physical therapy

▶ **OXYGEN THERAPY**

26. Why do so many people in the United States use home O_2?

D. Physiatrist

27. State two of the documented benefits of home O_2 therapy.
    A. _____
    B. _____

E. Durable medical equipment (DME) supplier

28. Describe the six elements that must be included in a home O_2 prescription.

    A.

24. How can you confirm that a nonprofessional caregiver is able to provide care?

    B.

25. Discuss the equipment requirements necessary in a home environment that must be assessed before discharge.

    C.

Copyright © 2003, 1999 Mosby, Inc. All rights reserved.

D.

E.

F.

29. What is the purpose of the Certificate of Medical Necessity (CME)?

30. What are the two primary uses of compressed O_2 cylinders in the alternative setting?
A. E cylinder

B. H cylinder

31. How do flowmeters used in alternative settings differ from those used in the hospital?

32. Let's compare the advantages and disadvantages of the O_2 supply systems available for use in alternative settings (see Table 49-3).

System	Advantage	Disadvantage
A. Cylinders		
1. _____	_____
2. _____	_____
B. Liquid		
1. _____	_____
2. _____	_____
C. Concentrator		
1. _____	_____
2. _____	_____

33. Liquid O_2 is weighed to determine the amount available. If a patient is using 3 L/min with a 100-lb system one-fourth full, how many hours would the gas last (see Table 49-4)?

Copyright © 2003, 1999 Mosby, Inc. All rights reserved.

34. Explain how an O_2 concentrator works.

35. What is the typical range of O_2 percentage a concentrator will supply at 2 L/min? 4L/min?
    A. 2 _____
    B. 4 _____

36. What effect will the concentrator have on a patient's electric bill?

37. Describe some of the methods for avoiding communication problems with patients receiving home O_2 therapy.

38. In addition to providing a backup supply, what other precautions should be taken in terms of concentrator power supply?

39. List at least four areas that should be evaluated when checking a home patient's O_2 concentrator.
    A. _____
    B. _____
    C. _____
    D. _____

40. When a patient is placed on an O_2 conserving device, how would you determine the correct liter flow to use?

41. What actions should a patient who is wearing transtracheal O_2 take if they believe the catheter isn't working properly?

42. In theory, how would a demand flow O_2-conserving system benefit the patient?

43. What are the two main drawbacks of demand flow systems?

Copyright © 2003, 1999 Mosby, Inc. All rights reserved.

44. In what situations should a patient or caregiver be instructed to alter the prescribed flow setting?

45. State the three main problems associated with insertion of a transtracheal catheter (see Box 49-4).
    A. _____
    B. _____
    C. _____

46. Describe the basic methods for avoiding complications of transtracheal catheters.

▶ VENTILATORY SUPPORT

47. Give examples for each of the three main groups of patients who are placed on ventilators in the alternative care setting (see Table 49-5).
    A. Nocturnal ventilation
       1. _____
       2. _____
       3. _____
    B. Continuous mechanical ventilation
       1. _____
       2. _____
       3. _____
    C. Terminally ill
       1. _____
       2. _____

48. Identify the three common settings in which ventilatory support is delivered outside the hospital.
    A. _____
    B. _____
    C. _____

49. Invasive long-term ventilation is always provided via what type of airway?

50. Describe the emergency situations a family must be able to deal with in caring for a home ventilator patient.

51. Identify at least three situations in which NPPV is partly contraindicated.
    A. _____
    B. _____
    C. _____

52. Identify at least three situations in which NPPV is absolutely contraindicated.
    A. _____
    B. _____
    C. _____

Copyright © 2003, 1999 Mosby, Inc. All rights reserved.

53. What options exist for patients who do not want invasive ventilation and cannot use NPPV?

54. What options are available on invasive PPV systems during power failures, or if a patient wishes to be mobile?

55. What is the biggest challenge associated with NPPV?

56. Identify the three basic types of negative pressure ventilators.
    A. _____
    B. _____
    C. _____

▶ OTHER MODES OF POSTACUTE RESPIRATORY CARE

57. What is the primary use of bland aerosols in the postacute setting?

58. What is the major problem with delivery of bland aerosols?

59. What are the two limits on Medicare reimbursement for compressor-driven SVNs in the alternative setting?
    A. _____
    B. _____

60. Identify the three requirements for approval of reimbursement for compressor-driven nebulizers?
    A. _____
    B. _____
    C. _____

61. How can you prevent bacterial growth on suction catheters that are used repeatedly?

62. State three common problems associated with sleep apnea hypopnea syndrome (SAHS).
    A. _____
    B. _____
    C. _____

63. What is the primary therapy for this condition?

Copyright © 2003, 1999 Mosby, Inc. All rights reserved.

64. When should nasal masks be replaced?

65. Discuss solutions to the common problem of nasal dryness.

66. What infant condition suggests the use of apnea monitoring?

▶ **PATIENT ASSESSMENT AND DOCUMENTATION**

67. Describe the main areas you would check during initial screening of a patient after admission to a postacute care facility.

68. What areas would be important to assess *besides* the usual vital signs and evaluation of the respiratory system?

69. Once the initial assessment is completed, a treatment plan is initiated. When is formal reassessment performed?

70. How often should a member of the home care team perform a follow-up evaluation for patients receiving respiratory care treatments? What factors should be considered in determining the frequency of visits?

▶ **EQUIPMENT DISINFECTION AND MAINTENANCE**

71. Describe the process for cleaning a home nebulizer (for example).
    A.

Copyright © 2003, 1999 Mosby, Inc. All rights reserved.

B.

C.

D.

72. Describe the American Respiratory Care Foundation (ARCF) guidelines for using water in humidifiers and nebulizers.

73. What is the most important principle of infection control in the home setting?

▶ PALLIATIVE CARE

74. According to WHO, palliative care involves control of what two debilitating symptoms?
    A. _____
    B. _____

75. What is hospice?

▶ CASE STUDIES

Case 1

Jim Billings is a 70-year-old man with COPD who is discharged with an order for home O_2. The patient's room air blood gas values before discharge are

pH	7.47
$PaCO_2$	33 mm Hg
PaO_2	62 mm Hg
SaO_2	92%

Medicare returns the CMN as disapproved because this patient does not meet the criteria for saturation of PO_2 for home O_2.

76. Make an argument for keeping the patient on O_2 based on your knowledge of respiratory physiology. (This is a real case and we did get reimbursement.)

Copyright © 2003, 1999 Mosby, Inc. All rights reserved.

Case 2

Steve Bete is a home care patient you are seeing who uses an O_2 concentrator. Mr. Bete calls you to say that he doesn't think he is getting an adequate amount of flow from his cannula.

77. What are some possible causes of this problem?

78. What would you suggest Steve should do at this time?

Case 3

Cathy Chow, an active 49-year-old with α_1-antitrypsin deficiency, is to be discharged with home O_2. The prescription is for 2 L/min of continuous O_2.

79. What system would you recommend for Ms. Chow to use at home?

80. What about a portable system?

► WHAT DOES THE NBRC SAY?

A small but important section of the examinations is devoted to home care. Because most respiratory therapists are working in acute or subacute care, it is easy to overlook this information. It is reasonable to expect that the newly revised tests will include some information on subacute care, but that hasn't happened yet. The matrix includes

- Monitor and maintain home care equipment
- Assure safety and infection control
- Modify procedures for use in the home
- Evaluate patient's progress
- Maintain apnea monitors
- Implement and monitor graded exercise programs
- Explain therapy in terms the patient can understand
- Counsel the patient concerning smoking cessation

The Clinical Simulation matrix adds that you may encounter a COPD patient in a home care setting.

Copyright © 2003, 1999 Mosby, Inc. All rights reserved.

81. A patient with a tracheostomy is to receive humidification via a nebulizer in his home. With regard to water for the nebulizer, which of the following would be the most appropriate choice for the home setting?
    A. Sterile distilled water should be obtained from the DME provider
    B. Tap water is sufficient for the home setting if the nebulizer is cleaned properly
    C. Bottled water can be used as long as it is distilled
    D. Tap water that is boiled may be used for up to 24 hours

82. Which of the following actions would an RCP perform during the monthly check of a home oxygen concentrator system?
    I. Replacement of the silica pellets in the sieve bed
    II. Analysis of the FIO_2 delivered by the concentrator
    III. Filter replacement
    IV. Evaluation of the concentrator's electrical system
    A. I, II only
    B. II, III only
    C. II, IV only
    D. II, III, IV only

83. A patient who is wearing a transtracheal oxygen catheter suddenly becomes dyspneic. The first action the patient should take would be to
    A. Call the physician
    B. Clean the catheter
    C. Increase the oxygen flow to the catheter
    D. Remove the catheter and proceed to the emergency department

84. A patient who is using oxygen at home occasionally needs to go out for healthcare appointments. What type of portable system would you recommend for this patient?
    A. E cylinder with standard flowmeter
    B. E cylinder with conserving device
    C. Small liquid oxygen reservoir
    D. Patients can go out for short periods without supplemental oxygen

85. A respiratory care practitioner determines that a cuirass-type negative pressure ventilator is now reading a pressure of -20 cm H_2O when it should be cycling at -35 cm H_2O. The patient is in no distress, but the measured tidal volume is 200 mL lower than the desired volume. The practitioner should
    A. Begin manual ventilation of the patient
    B. Check for leaks in the system
    C. Increase the vacuum setting
    D. Increase the amount of air in the cuff

▶ **FOOD FOR THOUGHT**

86. Where could you find the local regulations that apply to providers in your state?

Your textbook indicates that there is some controversy over the best way to disinfect reusable equipment and supplies in the home setting.

Copyright © 2003, 1999 Mosby, Inc. All rights reserved.

87. State three types of solutions that can be used.

A. _____

B. _____

C. _____

88. What are the advantages of using acetic acid (vinegar—white, not balsamic!) as a disinfectant?

89. What are the disadvantages?

▶ INFORMATION AGE

A wide variety of information is available to enhance your knowledge of respiratory home care, rehabilitation, and palliative care. You might want to look at the website of a national company such as Linde: **www.agalindehealthcare.com**

or Apria: **www.apria.com**

If you're looking for patient resources, Assist Guide is the most comprehensive national website. Here you can find resources for any home or senior need in almost any state: **www.assistguide.com**

Journals are useful as well. The May 2001 *Respiratory Care* has a good article at **www.rcjournal.com/ contents/12.00/12.00.1534.asp**

I think palliative care is pretty hot stuff for our profession. The November and December 2000 issues of *Respiratory Care* are devoted to palliative care. I highly recommend that you check them out.

Pulmonary rehabilitation is equally important. Check out the website of the American Association of Cardiovascular and Pulmonary Rehabilitation: **www.aacvpr.org**

or you might look to National Jewish at **www.nationaljewish.org/medfacts/ pulmonary.html**

Copyright © 2003, 1999 Mosby, Inc. All rights reserved.